THE VISUAL HISTORY OF COSTUME

THE VISUAL

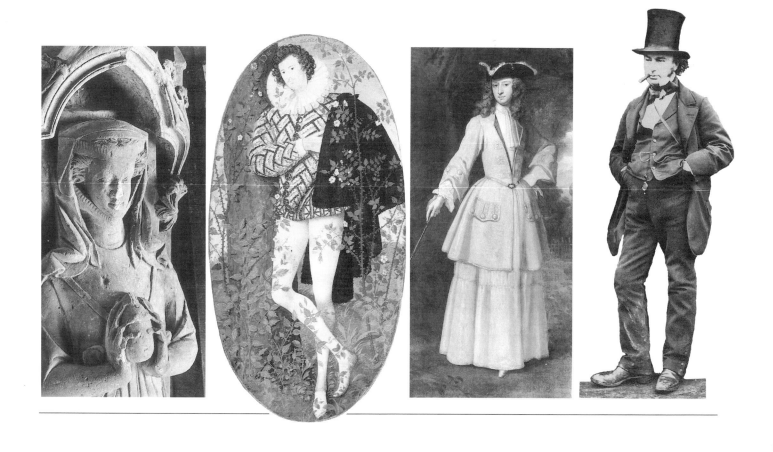

HISTORY OF COSTUME

Aileen Ribeiro and Valerie Cumming

original research and text for the
Visual History of Costume series

MARGARET SCOTT

JANE ASHELFORD

VALERIE CUMMING

AILEEN RIBEIRO

VANDA FOSTER

PENELOPE BYRDE

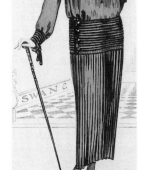

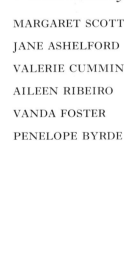

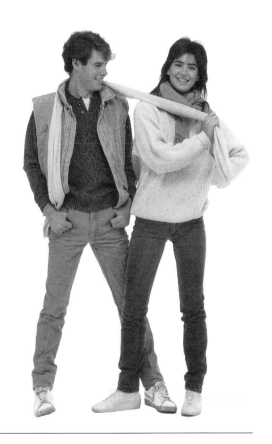

B.T. Batsford Ltd, London

Publisher's note
The visual material in this book has been selected from that appearing in the six-volume series *A Visual History of Costume*. The authors of that series are:

Fourteenth and Fifteenth Centuries	Margaret Scott
Sixteenth Century	Jane Ashelford
Seventeenth Century	Valerie Cumming
Eighteenth Century	Aileen Ribeiro
Nineteenth Century	Vanda Foster
Twentieth Century	Penelope Byrde

The Introduction in the present single volume owes a debt to those earlier books, but has been largely rewritten for present purposes, as has the Glossary. The commentaries to the illustrations remain substantially the same.

This edition © Aileen Ribeiro and Valerie Cumming 1989
First published 1989

ISBN 0-89676-113-4

Printed in Great Britain by
Courier International Ltd, Tiptree, Essex
for the publishers
Drama Book Publishers
260 Fifth Avenue
New York
New York 10001

CONTENTS

ACKNOWLEDGEMENTS

WE are grateful to our fellow authors in the *Visual History of Costume* series – Jane Ashelford, Penelope Byrde, Vanda Foster and Margaret Scott – for giving permission to use original material from each of their books.

We would like to thank all of the public and private collections which have assisted us in the compilation of this volume. Detailed acknowledgements relating to the use of illustrations are given in the *List of Illustrations*.

We are, as always, deeply appreciative of the support and resources afforded us by our respective employers, the Courtauld Institute of Art and the Museum of London.

We would like to acknowledge the help given us by the staff at Batsford, particularly Rachel Wright, Tim Auger, and Clare Sunderland.

The joint responsibilities of co-authorship and co-editorship tested our patience occasionally to the limits, but ultimately our professional association and personal friendship allowed us to find the task both amusing and rewarding.

PREFACE

THE *Visual History of Costume* is a series devised for those who need reliable, easy-to-use reference material on the history of dress. Each of the six published volumes deals with a specific period in a fair amount of detail, but it was thought that a single work bringing together a selection of key images from 1300 to the present day would provide a valuable visual survey of dress in Britain.

This book follows the successful pattern of the series, by providing contemporary illustrations – including sculpture, brasses, manuscripts, oil paintings, line drawings, engravings and original photographs – selected from each individual volume in the *Visual History of Costume*. Each picture is captioned in a consistent way, under the headings, where appropriate, of 'Head', 'Body' and 'Accessories'; the clothes are not just described but their significance explained in a prefatory 'Note' where relevant. The illustrations are arranged in date order, and the colour plates are cross-referenced with the black-and-white, so that the processes of change can be clearly followed.

The *Introduction* is, like Gaul, divided into three parts. The first provides background information on the inspiration for fashion through the ages, how styles were communicated, and the ways in which clothing was bought and sold; the second provides an outline survey of dress; and the third part discusses the sources, especially the visual, with some of the problems involved. Much of this introductory section relies on the work of the individual authors in the *Visual History of Costume* series; as far as possible we have retained each author's opinions and the thrust of our/their arguments. However, in order to avoid repetition and in the interests of a coherent theme, we have had to re-arrange this material, and make some additions of our own, in the hope of creating a reasonably seamless robe. A detailed *Glossary* has been provided which is designed also to act as an *Index*. The reader will find a *Select Bibliography* at the end of the book.

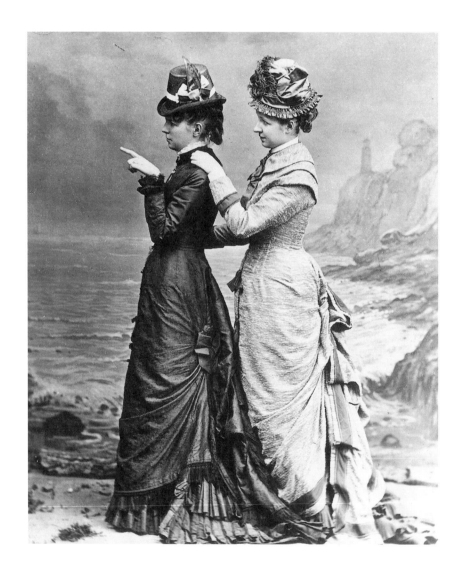

LIST OF ILLUSTRATIONS AND PICTURE ACKNOWLEDGEMENTS

The subject is followed by the artist, where known (attr. = attributed) then the medium or nature of the artefact and then the collection or location.

RCHME = Royal Commission on Historical Monuments (England)

Colour Illustrations (between pages 128 and 129)

I Chaucer reciting before an elegant audience
English School
Manuscript illumination from Chaucer's *Troilus and Criseyde*, MS 61 f.lv.

II Lady Donne and her daughter
(detail from the Donne Triptych)
Hans Memlinc
Oil on panel
National Gallery, London

III Unknown girl
Master of the Countess of Warwick (attr.)
Oil on panel
Tate Gallery, London

IV Sir Jerome Bowes
Anon.
Oil on canvas
Ranger's House, Blackheath (English Heritage)

V Queen Henrietta Maria
Anon.
Oil on canvas
National Portrait Gallery, London

VI 'Homme de qualité garny de rubans . . .'
J.D. de St. Jean
Coloured engraving, fashion plate 1689
Private Collection

VII Prince James Stuart with his sister
Nicholas de Largillierre
Oil on canvas
National Portrait Gallery, London

VIII John Conyers
Francis Hayman
Oil on canvas
Marble Hill House (English Heritage)

X 'Miss Eleanor Dixie'
Henry Pickering (attr.)
Oil on canvas
Nottingham Museums and Art Galleries

X The Morning Walk
Thomas Gainsborough
Oil on canvas
National Gallery, London

XI The Cloakroom, Clifton Assembly Rooms
Rolinda Sharples
Oil on canvas
City of Bristol Museum and Art Gallery

XII The Dancing Platform at Cremorne Gardens
(detail)
Phoebus Levin
Oil on canvas
Museum of London

19. **William Welley, merchant and his wife Alicia**
English School
Brass rubbing, Church of St James, Chipping
Campden, Glos.
Photograph: RCHME

20. **Margaret of Anjou, Queen of Henry VI, receives a book from John Talbot, 1st Earl of Shrewsbury**
English School
Manuscript illumination, Royal MS 15 E VI, f. 2b
British Library, London

21. **Edward Grimston**
Petrus Christus
Oil on panel
National Gallery, London, on loan from the Earl of Verulam

22. **Two female weepers from the tomb of Richard Beauchamp, Earl of Warwick**
John Massingham (?)
Gilded bronze figurines, church of St Mary, Warwick
Photograph: B.T. Batsford Ltd

23. **Flemish street scene, with presentation of a book to Duke Philip the Good**
Jean le Tavernier
Manuscript illumination, *Conquestes de Charlemagne*, MS 9066, f. 11
Bibliothèque Royale, Brussels

24. **William Gybbys and his wives Alice, Margaret and Marion**
English School
Brass rubbing, church of St James, Chipping
Campden, Glos.
Photograph: RCHME

25. **Sir John Curzon and his wife Joan**
English School
Brass rubbing, church of St Mary, Bylaugh, Norfolk
Photograph: B.T. Batsford Ltd.

26. **Henry Stathum and his wives Anne Bothe, Elizabeth Seyntlow, and his widow Margaret Stanhop**
English School
Brass rubbing, church of St Matthew, Morley,
Derbys.
Photograph: Victoria and Albert Museum, London

27. **Sir Thomas Peyton and his two wives, both called Margaret**
English School
Brass rubbing, church of St Andrew, Isleham, Cambs.
Photograph: Victoria and Albert Museum, London

28. **The Lover greets the God of Love**
Flemish School
Manuscript illumination, *Le Roman de la Rose*, Harley
MS 4425, f. 24
British Library, London

29. **Jean and Jeanne, Comte and Comtesse de la Tour d'Auvergne, with St John the Baptist and St John the Evangelist**
The Master of the de la Tour d'Auvergne Triptych
Mixed technique(?) on panel
North Carolina Museum of Art, Raleigh, North Carolina, Gift of the Samuel H. Kress Foundation

30. **Robert Serche and his wife Anne**
English School
Brass rubbing, church of St Peter and St Paul,
Northleach, Glos.
Photograph: RCHME

31. **Henry VII**
Pietro Torrigiano
Terracotta
Victoria and Albert Museum, London

32. **J. Wyddowsoun**
English School
Brass rubbing
Victoria and Albert Museum, London

33. **J. Marsham and wife**
English School
Brass rubbing
Victoria and Albert Museum, London

34. **Thomas More and his family**
Hans Holbein
Drawing
Kupferstichkabinett, Kunstmuseum, Basel

35. **An unknown English lady**
Hans Holbein
Drawing
British Museum, London

36. **Henry VIII**
After Hans Holbein
Oil on panel
Walker Art Gallery, Liverpool

37. **An English lady walking**
Hans Holbein
Drawing
Ashmolean Museum, Oxford

38. **Lady of the Bodenham family (?)**
John Bettes (attr.)
Oil on panel
Thos Agnew & Sons Ltd, London, 1987

39. **Lady Jane Grey**
Master John (attr.)
Oil on panel
National Portrait Gallery, London

40. Unknown man
Anon.
Oil on panel
Reproduced by gracious permission of Her Majesty the Queen

41. The Earl of Surrey
William Scrots
Oil on canvas
National Portrait Gallery, London

42. Mary I
Hans Eworth
Oil on panel
Fitzwilliam Museum, Cambridge

43. Mary, Queen of Scots
School of Clouet
Oil on panel
Victoria and Albert Museum, London

44. Sir Nicholas Throckmorton
Anon.
Oil on panel
National Portrait Gallery, London

45. Sir Henry Lee
Antonio Mor
Oil on panel
National Portrait Gallery, London

46. Four English women
Lucas de Heere
Watercolour; Add. MS 28330, f. 33
British Museum, London

47. Queen Elizabeth I
Anon.
Oil on panel
National Portrait Gallery, London

48. Robert Dudley, 1st Earl of Leicester
Anon.
Oil on panel
National Portrait Gallery, London

49. The Falconer
The Book of Falconrie, George Turbervile
Engraving
British Museum, London

50. Sir Philip Sidney
Anon.
Oil on canvas
National Portrait Gallery, London

51. Jane Bradbuirye
English School
Brass rubbing
Victoria and Albert Museum, London

52. Sir Christopher Hatton
After Cornelius Ketel
Oil on panel
National Portrait Gallery, London

53. Thomas Inwood, his three wives and children
English School
Brass rubbing
Victoria and Albert Museum, London

54. Unknown girl
John Bettes
Oil on panel
Governors and Headmaster of St Olave's and St Saviour's Grammar School, Orpington

55. Unknown man
Nicholas Hilliard
Miniature
Victoria and Albert Museum, London

56. Mary Huddye
English School
Brass rubbing
Victoria and Albert Museum, London

57. A courtier and a countryman
Frontispiece to *A quip for an upstart courtier*, 1592
Woodcut
British Museum, London

58. Thomas Kennedy of Culzean
Anon.
Oil on panel
National Trust for Scotland

59. Elizabeth Vernon, Countess of Southampton
Anon.
Oil on panel
The Duke of Buccleuch and Queensberry

60. Lady Elizabeth Southwell
Marcus Gheeraerts the Younger (attr.)
Oil on canvas
The Viscount Cowdray

61. Sir Walter Raleigh and his son
Anon.
Oil on panel
National Portrait Gallery, London

62. Anne Vavasour
Marcus Gheeraerts the Younger
Oil on canvas
Private Collection

63. Mary, Lady Scudamore
Marcus Gheeraerts the Younger
Oil on panel
National Portrait Gallery, London

134. Lord Byron
Count Alfred D'Orsay
Pencil and wash
Victoria and Albert Museum, London

135. Portrait of a woman
'Mansion' (André Léon Larue)
Oil miniature on ivory
The Trustees of the Wallace Collection, London

136. Mrs Ellen Sharples
Rolinda Sharples
Oil on canvas
Royal West of England Academy, Bristol

137. Benjamin Disraeli
After Daniel Maclise
Drawing
National Portrait Gallery, London

138. Florence and Parthenope Nightingale
William White
Watercolour
National Portrait Gallery, London

139. Lady Elizabeth Villiers
After Alfred Edward Chalon
Engraving
Witt Library, Courtauld Institute of Art, London

140. Unknown gentleman
William Huggins
Oil on canvas
Walker Art Gallery, Liverpool

141. Two Dandies
'Crowquill' (Alfred Henry Forrester)
Engraving, *Punch* magazine, 1843
Museum of London

142. Mrs Bell
David Octavius Hill and Robert Adamson
Original photograph
National Portrait Gallery, London

143. Angela Georgina, Baroness Burdett-Coutts
Sir William Charles Ross
Watercolour on ivory
National Portrait Gallery, London

144. Queen Victoria and Prince Albert
Roger Fenton
Original photograph
Victoria and Albert Museum, London

145. 'Derby Day' (detail)
William Powell Frith
Oil on canvas
Tate Gallery, London

146. Isambard Kingdom Brunel
Robert Howlett
Original photograph
National Portrait Gallery, London

147. Unknown woman
Anon.
Original photograph
Gallery of English Costume, Manchester City Art Galleries

148. 'The Travelling Companions'
Augustus Egg
Oil on canvas
Birmingham City Art Gallery

149. 'Woman's Mission: Companion of Manhood'
George Elgar Hicks
Oil on canvas
Tate Gallery, London

150. 'On the Beach' (detail)
Charles Wynne Nicholls
Oil on canvas
Crescent Art Gallery, Scarborough Borough Council

151. An August Picnic
Anon.
Engraving, *The Girl of the Period* magazine, 1869
Museum of London

152. The Marchioness of Huntley
Sir John Everett Millais
Oil on canvas
Royal Academy of Arts, London

153. Travelling scene
William Ralston
Engraving, *Punch* magazine, 1874
Museum of London

154. Woman in day dress
James Tissot
Oil on canvas
Tate Gallery, London

155. Two women in day dress
Elliot and Fry
Original photograph
Victoria and Albert Museum, London

156. Scarborough Spa at Night
Francis Sydney Muschamp
Oil on canvas
Crescent Art Gallery, Scarborough Borough Council

157. Couple in aesthetic dress
George du Maurier
Engraving, *Punch* magazine, 1880
Witt Library, Courtauld Institute of Art, London

158. Marion Hood
Elliot and Fry
Original photograph
Victoria and Albert Museum, London

159. 'The First Cloud'
Sir William Quiller Orchardson
Oil on canvas
Tate Gallery, London

160. Sir Arthur Sullivan
Sir John Everett Millais
Oil on canvas
National Portrait Gallery, London

161. City Scene
'P. Naumann'
Engraving, *The Family Friend* magazine, 1890
Victoria and Albert Museum, London

162. Middle-class couple, holidaying in the country
Anon.
Engraving, *The English Illustrated Magazine*, 1894
Victoria and Albert Museum, London

163. 'The Bayswater Omnibus'
Thomas Matthew Joy
Oil on canvas
Museum of London

164. 'In the Holidays'
'HAAR'
Engraving from *The Windsor Magazine*, 1897
Victoria and Albert Museum, London

165. Fashionable walking dress
Alfred Chantrey Corbould
Engraving from *Punch* magazine, 1900
Witt Library, Courtauld Institute of Art, London

166. The family of George Campbell Swinton at Pont Street, London
William Orpen
Oil on canvas
Collection: Brigadier Swinton, Kimmerghame House, Duns
Photograph: National Galleries of Scotland

167. Seaside wear
George Lorraine Stampa
Engraving, *Punch* magazine, 1902
Museum of London

168. Sir Max Beerbohm
William Nicholson
Oil on canvas
National Portrait Gallery, London

169. Three gowns by Paul Poiret
Paul Iribe
Les Robes de Paul Poiret, Paris, 1908
Hand-coloured print
Courtauld Institute of Art, London

170. Day dresses
Anon.
Illustration from Harrods catalogue, 1909
Fashion Research Centre, Bath
Photograph: B.T. Batsford, Ltd

171. Horace Annesley Vachell
Gaston Linden
Oil on canvas
Victoria Art Gallery, Bath

172. Bank Holiday
William Strang
Oil on canvas
Tate Gallery, London

173. Costume by Liberty
Anon.
Engraving, Liberty's *Novelties for the Season*, 1916
Fashion Research Centre, Bath

174. Edward, Prince of Wales
William Orpen
Oil on canvas
Collection: The Royal and Ancient Golf Club, St Andrew's Fife; photograph: National Galleries of Scotland

175. Fashions by Swan & Edgar
Anon.
Illustration, 1924
Fashion Research Centre, Bath

176. Grafton Fashions for Gentlemen
Autumn and winter catalogue 1924/5
Lithograph
Fashion Research Centre, Bath

177. The Ranee of Pudukota in a Chanel suit
Anon.
Original photograph
Fashion Research Centre, Bath

178. Alfred Duff Cooper, 1st Viscount Norwich with his wife Diana
David Low
Chalk on paper
National Portrait Gallery, London

179. 'The Botanists'
Joseph Southall
Tempera on silk
Hereford City Museums

180. Evening dress by Paquin
Anon.
Pencil and watercolour on paper
Fashion Research Centre, Bath

INTRODUCTION

The Background

DRESS is one of the obvious ways in which we communicate to each other, for it defines Man and his place in society. The history of dress, however, requires us to understand the problems and possibilities of the past, and we have to abandon our preconceptions about our ancestors if we are to begin to understand why and how they dressed the way that they did. This becomes harder the further back in time we go. It is difficult, for example, to feel much sympathy with people whose values are so different from our own. In the case of the Middle Ages, so much of the visual information about people comes down to us in the guise of things the late twentieth century prefers not to think about – unquestioning expressions of faith and acceptance of mortality. Even their aesthetic values find few echoes in ours, for, though we may be overwhelmed by the beauty of the great Gothic cathedrals, few of us would care to wear the dress of their builders, so alien is it to our images of ourselves. Therefore, perhaps the initial steps to appreciating late medieval dress should lie in wonder at the ingenuity of its designers who sometimes cared little for practicality but much for splendour.

By the sixteenth century more emphasis was placed on the senses, and clothes were intended to please those of the wearer and the viewer – the sense of sight by colour and pattern, the sense of touch by embellishment of the surface and the combination of different fabrics, and the sense of smell by perfumed ornaments and accessories. Dress could also act as a visual statement of an idea or mood, as is apparent in the clown's comment to Orsino in Shakespeare's *Twelfth Night*: 'Now the melancholy god protect thee: and the tailor make thy doublet of changeable taffeta, for thy mind is a very opal.'

Fashions changed relatively slowly until the end of the seventeenth century, despite the fact that both the sixteenth and seventeenth centuries were characterized by a restless exuberance, partly explained by political upheavals, but prompted also by increased travel and communication between countries. The English in particular seem to have been fascinated by novelties, often adopting a foreign style or a new accessory simply because it was available, although this eagerness for change frequently militated against elegance. If contemporary commentators are to be believed, this period saw one absurd fashion after another, exciting derision and ridicule from the more balanced and sober-minded 'average' Englishman. However, this is not a phenomenon of these centuries alone, but a concomitant of all fashions throughout history. Those who believe that there are more important considerations than the minute details of personal appearance will always mock exquisitely dressed contemporaries.

By the eighteenth century a sense of ingrained 'Englishness' in dress was an established feature of fashionable society. The English might acquire foreign clothes, adopt Continental fashions – usually French – and they might even export their own styles for informal dress, but it was with a sense of being set apart from the rest of Europe, both in terms of political and social institutions and, to a certain extent, in appearance. It is, of course, but a short step from feeling apart to feeling superior, and throughout the nineteenth century the British effortlessly – or so it seemed – demonstrated a political, moral and social superiority which both amused and irritated their European and North American neighbours. In dress this superiority was translated into fine but sombre tailoring for men and women, backed up by the technical achievements in textile production which flowed from the Industrial Revolution. It was a century in which the distinction between purposeful and businesslike men's clothing, and constrictive but exquisitely decorative women's costume was at its apogee. Dress reform and female emancipation movements met, on the whole, with derision, but they presaged a future in which sharply drawn definitions of the male and female roles would be challenged and overthrown.

Fashion, of course, does not regulate itself according to the calendar and respond to the opening of a new year or a new century with a different style or change in direction. The early twentieth century parallels in many respects the early nineteenth century, showing a similar experimentation in styles of dress – particularly women's – against a background of political unease and sabre-rattling in Europe; but the similarities ended in 1914. The First World War and the ensuing period have demonstrated that freedom, for both sexes, and all classes in society, married to the English delight in novelty and an international restlessness of purpose, translates itself into a dizzy search for new fashions from every imaginable source. Change and individuality have grown in importance, and continuity and coherence are valued less, producing a confused but exciting situation for future dress historians to analyse.

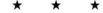

In all periods before our own century, it is true to say that fashions were mostly set by the top ranks of society. This could be the royal family itself, or a fashionable aristocratic group at court. In the fourteenth and fifteenth centuries, when there was a comparatively small court circle (and a restricted middle class of limited importance), this was even more the case. Obviously some kings were more interested in fashion than others; in the late fourteenth century, for example, Richard II was particularly fond of lavishly trimmed luxury in dress, and almost a century later Edward IV laid stress on a brilliant court. Generally, medieval kings had to tread a careful path between an over-indulgence in personal display (this was held by contemporaries to be a contributory factor in the downfall of Richard II) and the desire to show the rest of the world a civilized and visually appealing face through the elegance, taste and wealth of a glittering court. The propaganda benefits of dress at royal and princely courts were never underestimated by the wise ruler.

Unlike later periods, when we can discern fashion signals as deriving from identified countries, the situation in the late Middle Ages is less clear. There was no one country which seemed to have a monopoly of taste or fashion, although claims were made by some of the Italian states, by France and by the Netherlands. Although it is often impossible to identify the source of particular styles in the fourteenth and fifteenth centuries, what sense of 'fashion' that can be said to exist, was spread via travel to foreign lands or by noting what visitors wore. As in later periods, there was a fascination with the sartorial peculiarities of foreigners who were often blamed for anything which their contemporaries did not like.

The mobility of all ranks of men – as diplomats, merchants, soldiers of fortune etc, helped by repeated English invasions of France during the Hundred Years War – meant that within the triangle of Britain, Flanders and France there was almost complete uniformity in men's fashions. Women had far less opportunity for travel; their lives and what they wore were more closely defined within a narrower world, more subject to regional variations. Dynastic marriages may have created short-lived interest in the fashions of other countries, but as women were expected to be absorbed entirely into their husbands' families, so a queen had to forget her old loyalties and acquire those of her husband, the most obvious symbol of which was to dress like the women of her adopted country.

However the expansionist ambitions of Edward III *did* offer the ladies of his court a chance to see some of the world, and the English court was occasionally established across the Channel; in this way information on foreign fashions percolated through, although the impact on dress back in England is hard to assess. In the following century, there is no indication that English ladies travelled as much; for much of the time England was involved with internal strife, and less international in outlook. Although the court was still a centre of fashion, it was less so than in the fourteenth century, because there were, in a sense, a number of rival courts throughout the kingdom; this state of affairs continued until peace was restored at the end of the fifteenth century.

One of the effects of a stratified society in the England of the late medieval and early modern period was a recurring belief that clothing had to be regulated according to class. From the beginning of the period covered by this book, high fashion was frequently defined by law as being only for the upper classes, with a sliding scale of diminishing privileges from the Royal Family downwards. Occasional concessions were made to the merchant classes who were, after all, largely responsible for the trade which created the wealth of the country. Although the aim of this sumptuary legislation (from the fourteenth century until the end of the sixteenth century) was ostensibly protective of native textile industries, there is no doubt that it was basically intended to reinforce the class system, to keep the luxurious materials – imported gold and silver tissues, fine woven silks and rich furs – as the prerogative of the higher, wealthier reaches of society; there were penalties for the misuse of such luxuries by the lower classes. Such legislation divided the population into distinct categories, with detailed descriptions of what should, or should not, be worn (usually the latter). It was constantly being repealed, and then reissued in an updated form, which suggests that it was a virtually useless exercise. It is worth looking at, however, as a documentary source of interest to the dress historian, for it provides a considerable amount of information on what *were* the desirable styles and luxurious fabrics, which had to be limited in this way.

In the early seventeenth century the remaining sumptuary legislation was finally repealed. Although in the later seventeenth century, and during the eighteenth century, various measures were passed to prohibit silks and laces from abroad, they do not seem to have had much impact, for it became increasingly fashionable to acquire luxury foreign goods and exotic novelties. It is perhaps no accident that France and England were leaders of fashion from the late seventeenth century onwards, because they were largely untrammelled by sumptuary concerns, and a relatively wide choice of both native and imported goods was available to most sections of society. Once dress was totally open to market forces, the momentum of fashion – defined as an increasingly rapid series of changes in style – became unstoppable.

By the sixteenth century, the most splendidly dressed person in England, safeguarded in this grandeur by sumptuary legislation, was the monarch. The Tudors were aware of the political advantages that could be gained from wearing magnificent clothes and jewels. The dazzling outfits worn by Henry VIII on the Field of the Cloth of Gold (1520), and by Elizabeth I when she received foreign dignitaries, were not chosen solely for reasons of personal vanity; they also impressed foreigners with the wealth and hence the strength of England. Naturally the monarch expected his or her courtiers to reinforce this appearance of substance and power by dressing richly. Queen Elizabeth chastized anyone who appeared at court in unfashionable or unflattering clothes; this engendered an atmosphere of sartorial rivalry as courtiers vied with each other to wear the latest fashions.

Court fashions would happily incorporate attractive foreign styles; various European fashions entered the English wardrobe during Henry VIII's reign and Spanish dress, for example, became popular with the visit of Philip II and his entourage in 1554. By Elizabeth's reign, the dress of Englishmen was an eclectic mixture of foreign influences, such as, for example, a French doublet, a Spanish hat, German or Dutch hose, and Italian neckwear. To a certain extent, such internationality was inevitable as silks were imported from Italy, fine leathers from Spain, linen from Germany and Holland, and lace from Italy. In addition, the dress of foreigners could be observed at first hand, for travel abroad became more usual during this period. Interest in the modes and manners of every country in the known world was also reflected in the spate of illustrated costume books published from the second half of the sixteenth century onwards.

Increased expenditure on dress was not limited solely to courtiers and wealthy members of country society; a higher standard of living and an influx of imported goods meant that all classes in society wanted to purchase more clothes (and clothes more in the mainstream of fashion) than their forefathers. Fashions spread from the court into London society, and then filtered slowly out to country districts. Naturally the humbler members of the social order had neither means nor interest in more than modifying, in the simplest manner, their style of dress. Such innocence, in the minds of social commentators, was preferable (especially when married to industry) to the expensive and indiscriminately chosen fashions of the aristocratic courtiers. However, in pursuit of the contrived fantasy of court life which, by the late Elizabethan period 'aym'd wholly at singularitie', courtiers were immune to carping criticism.

Throughout the seventeenth century, the monarch, his immediate family and his courtiers provided the circle within which new fashions were generated or adopted. Not all kings were interested in fashion; James I, his grandson James II, and William III were not noted for their sartorial elegance, but they understood the propaganda use of splendid dress, and encouraged lavish display when appropriate. A round of public ceremonies and private parties dictated fine clothes and magnificent jewellery, and courtiers spent a great deal of money on the newest materials and the latest styles of dress. The hiatus provided by the Commonwealth, with its tendency towards sobriety in dress, its dislike of merrymaking, and a Puritan emphasis on spiritual values, ensured that the Restoration court was, much like an antidote, extravagant, frivolous and luxurious.

Imported materials and styles in dress were essential ingredients in the costume worn at the Stuart courts. Charles I, when Prince of Wales, visited France and Spain, and was impressed by the dignified fashions worn in both countries. He and his French wife Henrietta Maria epitomized the understated grandeur which characterized English dress from the mid-1620s to the late 1640s. The future Charles II, exiled in France and Holland, developed a keen sense of how kings could and should influence fashion. His court was less formal than that of his cousin Louis XIV, but its styles were primarily French in inspiration. Even under William and Mary, when England was in political and military opposition to France, the flow of ideas and goods from that country was barely affected.

During the eighteenth century it was the nobility rather than the king and his family, which initiated fashions; the court of the Hanoverian monarchs – described by one visitor as 'the residence of dullness' – was not a centre of style until the 1780s under the aegis of the Prince of Wales. On the whole, France was the dominant influence on high fashion in English society, particularly with regard to women's styles. The rules of good taste both in dress and etiquette had been well established by the French court at Versailles during the later seventeenth century, and the English upper classes, especially in the first half of the eighteenth century, looked towards France as the fount of wisdom regarding elegance in dress and refinement of manners. Although Italy continued to produce high-quality silks throughout the eighteenth century, France captured the initiative in the design of patterned dress silks and also inaugurated the concept of seasonal changes in silk designs, the latter being an important factor in the speeding up of fashion changes as the century progressed.

The fact that the court was not the sole focus of power – the lives of the aristocracy and the gentry encompassed in many cases the practical care of landed property and a parliamentary career – ensured the existence of more 'democratic' English fashions, particularly for men. Many men made a virtue out of the relative simplicity of English country clothing which they claimed reflected the relative freedoms enjoyed by English political and legal institutions, compared to the absolutism which they saw on the Continent, and particularly in France.

By the early nineteenth century two main influences can be seen in fashionable dress: the continued pre-eminence of France with regard to women, and further confirmation that England was the new guiding star for men. The paradigm was no longer the male peacock, but a soberly dressed worker, a merchant, a banker, a professional man, whose calling was expressed in his understated, impeccably cut clothing. English tailoring, the *ne plus ultra* of the art, relied on the plastic, draping qualities of fine woollen cloth; it has retained its dominance for almost two hundred years. The allegiance of the fashionable woman, on the other hand, was given to France; it was admitted that Paris alone possessed the secrets of style and elegance with regard to women's dress. The prevailing taste of the English court under Queen Victoria was towards expensive frumpishness, although some members of the Royal Family such as the Prince of Wales (the future Edward VII) and his wife Alexandra, took an informed interest in fashion. By the middle of the nineteenth century the roads of high fashion led towards Paris, and in particular to the court of the Emperor Napoleon III and his wife Eugénie. The presiding sartorial genius of this court was the designer Charles Frederick Worth who elevated the dressmaker to the status of *couturier* and became the virtual dictator of the fashionable woman. Provided she could pay, such a woman could be of any class; she could be an aristocrat (Worth's clientèle was international) or a member of the somewhat raffish *demi-monde* who starred in the flashy court of the Second Empire. In political terms, in spite of the continuation of the monarchical system (some stable like the British, some rather more fragile like the French), the nineteenth century saw the triumph of the bourgeoisie. The prevailing image was one of wealth, opulence, and a lifestyle of comfort and ease.

The twentieth century differs from previous centuries in several important respects. Firstly there has been a gradual but distinct erosion of the idea that royals, aristocrats and the wealthy should provide a model for fashionable existence. This is perhaps inevitable in a century which has placed increasing emphasis on people's talents and achievements rather than on the place in society in which they were born. Certain royal persons and members of the aristocracy have been admired for their stylishness of dress but, generally speaking, as a group in society they have become gradually more conservative in the fashions that they adopt – sons going to the tailor patronized by their father and grandfather, daughters preferring to look agreeably turned-out rather than eye-catchingly fashionable. In the latter part of the century the most elegantly dressed men and women are often newly rich, able to buy from exclusive shops and order clothes from fashionable designers; they view their appearance as extension and confirmation worldly success.

As the century has progressed the couturier or designer has become much more influential, drawing upon artistic movements such as *Art Deco* and *Surrealism* for inspiration, and travelling the world in search of new materials and ideas. The new fashions they create, their favourite models and notable clients, attract the kind of attention and emulation which has little to do with 'old money' or breeding. Chanel, for example, was her own best advertisement, admired and copied for her relaxed elegance as well as for the innovative stylishness of her designs and accessories.

Better communications and increased opportunities to observe foreign ideas have influenced fashion. Films have popularized new fashions and styles of beauty to a growing international audience, and television has had an equally important impact, as have pop stars and media celebrities. Fashion has become, to all intents and purposes, classless, instant and disposable, with new fashions reproduced in versions which range from the wildly expensive to the incredibly cheap, allowing everyone, irrespective of income, to be as fashionable as they choose.

While mass-production has given us greater amounts of clothing than our forebears would have possessed, there has been a steady diminution in the actual garments worn. Simpler, lighter undergarments and lightweight materials have replaced the rigid, structural layers worn earlier in the century. This has been partly prompted by the improved heating and ventilation in houses, offices and transport, but is also due to a changing way of life which has encompassed a gradual decrease in sartorial formality. Women's clothes, in particular, have changed radically, allowing them freedom to work and to play sports untrammelled by cumbrous garments. Although retaining certain distinctively feminine features, these have become more practical, borrowing elements from the male wardrobe such as tailored suits and trousers. In the 1980s many casual garments for both sexes are virtually interchangeable. However, there are still occasions which require a degree of formality; professional men are still expected to wear suits to work, and, if mourning has largely disappeared, weddings are still elaborate affairs.

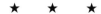

In the Middle Ages and the early modern period, both sexes were equally interested in their clothing, as can be inferred from a survey of the gorgeous textiles worn by the aristocracy. These included luxurious furs from the far north of Europe, silks of all kinds from Italy, and high-quality woollen cloths from Flanders and East Anglia. Clothing was expensive, and must be regarded as representing a far greater capital investment than it does today; except at the very top of society, even the well-to-do would have a fairly limited wardrobe, containing only a few garments of expensive, imported materials, and relying to a considerable extent on locally produced stuffs. Contemporary inventories and letters reveal that much alteration and refurbishment of clothes took place; clothing was often 'recycled', the silks being made into vestments, and the poorer fabrics turned into children's and servants' costume.

Ordering clothing was often difficult, complicated and time-consuming. The fabrics and accessories had to be bought from the relevant merchants, and then put in the hands of the tailor. In the days before ready-to-wear clothing, the tailor played a vital part in the chain from fabric to finished garment. Royal and aristocratic households had their own tailors; those lower down the social scale relied on tailors resident in the nearest large town, or on the services of itinerant journeyman tailors. To a large extent women also used tailors in the making of their costume; in addition, being more confined to the home than men, they relied also on the skills of seamstresses within their own households especially in the provision of linen, children's clothing etc.

At this distance, it is impossible to know how fashions were disseminated, and what processes went into the choice of certain styles. Maybe a customer took along an existing garment to the tailor, who then suggested slight modifications in style or trimming; maybe there were rough and ready patterns in tailors' workshops, although there are no surviving tailoring manuals until the sixteenth century. Imitation – of those who were perceived to be stylish people at court and among the aristocracy – must have played a major part in the momentum of fashion, but due to lack of adequate communications, there was often a considerable time-lag between styles in London and those in remote rural areas.

London, where the court was increasingly based, was the centre of fashion, as well as of government and trade. It was one of the international market places for the luxury textile trades, and home to an increasing number of specialist merchants and shopkeepers who could cater for every fashionable requirement. By the sixteenth century London was well supplied with drapers, silk and linen mercers, milliners, etc; the most exclusive mercers and jewellers were located in Cheapside. Fashionable accessories could be ordered and purchased from the hatter, glover, shoemaker, and so forth. After its opening in 1571 the Royal Exchange quickly became known as a treasure house of desirable goods. In this one building there were wig shops, feather shops, milliners – with their expensive imported accessories and some ready-made items such as falling bands and cuffs, embroidered nightcaps, ruffs etc. – sempstresses who made linen garments, 'starchers' to stiffen linen, and 'drawers' who devised and drew embroidery patterns for customers.

Unlike the formal garments which used the rich, expensive imported silk fabrics from Italy or Spain and consequently could not be trusted to the unskilled, informal linen garments were often made at home. These were embroidered by female members of a family or, in great households, by sempstresses and maids trained to fine sewing and to the charming embroidery which is such a pronounced feature of English costume during the second half of the sixteenth century, and the early seventeenth century. The poor (a term that of necessity encompasses, for example, the upper servants in a wealthy household, down to the beggar in the streets) wore what they could get, and – depending on their occupation – with varying pretensions to fashion. In the country, locally woven stuffs were the basic source of apparel, sometimes decked out with accessories obtained from pedlars and from visits to fairs. Those who could not afford new clothes, or who preferred the aura of the fashionable even at one remove or more, could buy second-hand clothes from the dealers whose stalls existed in most of the major cities.

During the seventeenth century, certain provincial cities (for example, Bristol and Newcastle) prospered and grew. Increasingly they offered a wide range of goods in specialist shops of the sort to be seen in London. London, however, acted as a kind of magnet, attracting the fashionable through the quality (and novelty) of its luxury goods and its sense of style in all matters pertaining to dress. Many families outside the capital commissioned visitors to London, or relatives who lived there, to buy them the latest materials and accessories and to send news of the latest fashions.

With regard to dress and textiles, some important developments took place in the later seventeenth century. There was, for example, a new division between the making of male and female clothing. In the 1670s seamstresses evolved into mantua-makers, taking over responsibility from tailors for the making of women's formal dresses. Tailors, however, continued to make the more structured female garments such as riding habits.

An increased range of fabrics was available to the tailor and mantua-maker. With the growing fashion for Indian printed cottons in the late seventeenth century, William Sherwin, an engraver of West Ham, took out a patent for 'printing and stayning such kind of goods' in 1676. The first English calico printing factory was established at West Sheen near London, and by 1700 calico printing was flourishing in many parts of south-east England. By the middle of the eighteenth century printed cottons (of home manufacture or imported from India) and linens (from Ireland and Scotland) printed in their place of origin or in England, were popular for informal fashionable wear.

With the influx of French Protestant refugees in the 1680s came the skills required for silk-weaving. The main centre for this new industry was Spitalfields in London, which produced silks rivalling those from Lyons for design and quality, especially during the first half of the eighteenth century. Foreign silks, particularly figured silks from France, and fine velvets from Italy, continued to be the staples of the fashionable wardrobe; on the whole the quality of tailoring and dressmaking was poor and it relied on the beauty of the fabrics and the luxury of the trimmings rather than on excellence of cut. Increasingly, however, while silk remained *de rigueur* for formal dress, woollen fabrics of high quality were adopted by Englishmen of the upper and middle classes for simpler styles – a development which aided more expert tailoring by the end of the century.

For most of the century, however, Paris was the Mecca for fashionable men and women. Easier travel enabled the wealthy to visit the French capital and to order their clothes there. Those remaining in London could have their clothes made by French tailors and *modistes*; every capital city of Europe had numbers of these people making the most of the general perception that France had a monopoly of taste with regard to high fashion. Information on French female fashions also came via dressed dolls which were sent from Paris to the capital cities of Europe, including London. Such dolls, having been used by the court dressmakers and those catering to a wealthy upper- and middle-class clientèle, would then be sent to the provinces so that within a comparatively short period of time (on improved roads) the country lady could copy metropolitan modes. Such dolls were largely replaced, in the last quarter of the eighteenth century, by the first regularly produced fashion plates which depicted and described every month's new fashions and accessories in minute detail. Such magazines included as many

English fashions as French, for by this time London was being considered as an international centre of style, particularly with regard to men's wear, and women's informal costume. From the late seventeenth century the fashionable shopping area had moved from the City westwards to the Strand and Covent Garden; a hundred years later Oxford Street and Bond Street had assumed the importance they still have today.

In an age of better communications and with an increasingly mobile population, fashion, by the late eighteenth century, was a concept familiar to all but the very poorest members of society. Fashions could be seen, not just in London, but in other big cities such as Bath and Birmingham; styles in dress could be copied with relative ease, and this factor, plus the existence of a fairly homogeneous society, ensured that there was little in the way of distinctive regional costume – though there might be local interpretations of current fashions. Unbridgeable sartorial gulfs did not separate the upper classes from the middle classes, nor the middle classes from the respectable artisan class. This state of affairs was particularly true in the second half of the century as everyday clothing generally became simpler and less adorned in style.

The poorer classes wore, at different levels, scaled-down versions of fashionable dress. Throughout the eighteenth century some ready-made garments were available to all classes including the poor who could also, like their wealthier compatriots, have clothing made up, albeit of far cheaper, usually locally produced stuffs. Such clothes were, however, quite expensive when compared to the other costs of living, as were the cast-off garments which formed the basis of many a poor person's wardrobe. It was technological change in the textile industries, initiated in the eighteenth century, which made possible the large-scale production of fabrics such as cotton and enabled a much wider section of the population to buy cheaper clothes first-hand. A series of inventions in both spinning and weaving were first applied to the cotton industry in the north-west of England (and further encouraged by expanding colonial markets) and then adapted for the woollen industry of Yorkshire. Until well into the nineteenth century Britain had the only effectively industrialized economy in the world; it had a headstart in mechanized textile production, enabling people of fairly humble means to buy more than just the most basic clothing. However, profit not philanthropy guided the entrepreneurial spirit of the Industrial Revolution. The production of wealth and the immense technical achievements of the nineteenth century were not accomplished without massive social problems and insensitive urbanization, exacerbated by

a vast population increase from the mid-century.

It was a period of great ingenuity and dynamic change, a century characterized by a delight in progress, and a vast expansion of commerce. More people than ever before had greater buying power, some of which was inevitably directed towards the conspicuous consumption of clothing. This is particularly true with regard to women's dress; while the masculine ideal in appearance was deliberately low-key (though expensively so), a man's wealth was demonstrated in the costume worn by his wife and daughters. Female dress was complicated, elaborate and subject to rigid etiquette – a fashionable woman needed a whole series of costumes for various times of day and the different functions she took part in. Her sartorial needs were catered for by an army of couturiers and dress-makers in London and Paris.

It is a paradox, given the English obeisance to the fashion dictates of Paris, that it should have been an Englishman, Charles Frederick Worth, who almost single-handedly established the *haute couture* system in mid-nineteenth-century Paris. The dress designer, hitherto a shadowy figure of uncertain status was – particularly in the person of the imperious M. Worth – the arbiter of taste to royalty, aristocracy and *nouveaux riches* in the moneyed world of the second half of the nineteenth century. Worth only dealt with those who by their vast wealth or exalted social position merited his expensive attentions. Those of less exalted status, who could not have their dresses made in Paris, had them made by London or provincial dress-makers; riding habits continued to be made by tailors.

Both the professional and the home dressmaker were aided by sewing manuals, and by the expansion of fashion magazines. From the early nineteenth century these magazines had published occasional embroidery patterns, or instructions for the making of such accessories as knitted purses; by the middle of the century patterns for such items as bodices, mantles and underwear were commonplace. From the 1860s there was a rapid increase in the use of paper patterns, covering all but the most complicated or tailored garments, and this was given a further boost when the American firm of Buttericks opened an English branch in 1873. Also from America came the sewing machine, an invention of the mid-1840s, a version of which was soon widely sold in Britain, marketed by the American firm of Singer. During the last quarter of the nineteenth century traditional hand sewing was increasingly limited to lingerie and some couture garments; machine work revolutionized both the dressmaking techniques of the individual at home and the production in clothing factories.

The greater mechanization of clothing helped the ready-to-wear industry. During the second half of the century there were department stores in the major cities (the earliest in London, Whiteley's shop in Westbourne Grove, was opened in 1863), which provided dressmaking services and a selection of ready-made and partly made garments – the latter could be altered by the customer herself or her personal maid. By the late nineteenth century, except at the top of society, it was gradually becoming more acceptable to be dressed in ready-made clothes. However, with the sartorial conservatism which was so much a part of men's dress in the nineteenth century, traditional ways were more entrenched; upper-class men continued to have their clothes made to measure, as they do – although to a much more limited extent – today.

Improved travel (the railways) and the mass-production of fashion periodicals ensured a far more informed interest in fashion than had hitherto been the case, although of course there were regional variations and interpretations of certain styles depending on income, status, peer acceptability, and personal preference.

In addition, a number of technical developments have to be noted. These included, for example, the introduction in the 1830s of the Jacquard loom which revolutionized the production of woven silks. In 1856 the first aniline dyes were discovered (these were fast dyes for printing all types of material), and in 1892 the first synthetic silk was created from chemically treated wood pulp, the forerunner of twentieth-century man-made fibres.

Thus, many of the technical developments associated with twentieth-century dress had their roots in the nineteenth century. The sewing machine, chemical dyes, paper patterns, and the first man-made fibre had all been invented before 1900. It is the last that has made the most notable contribution to the production of practical, inexpensive clothing for both men and women. The first such fibre had imitated silk, and was known as rayon after 1924; it was followed by nylon in 1938. These generated a number of other synthetic fibres – acrylics, viscoses and polyesters – called by various brand names; they have been used on their own to produce new fabrics, or blended with natural fibres. Modern clothes also incorporate new types of fastenings such as the press stud and the zip, and also use elastic to a considerable extent; consequently, clothes have become easier to put on. This fact, combined with the use of 'easy care' fabrics, and the invention of the washing machine, synthetic detergents, coin-operated dry-cleaning machines and the electric iron, has made clothing easier to look after and more hygienic.

At the beginning of the twentieth century it was still more usual for clothes to be individually made, although a range of ready-to-wear garments was available. The most affluent and fashionable had their clothes made to measure, by a tailor (for men's clothes) and by a couture house or Court dressmaker (for women's). Middle-class ladies could have a similar but less expensive service at the larger shops and department stores (which ran their own dressmaking departments) or by going to an individual dressmaker; and many women made their clothes at home. Britain tended to look to France for the lead in female fashion, and in Paris the *haute couture* houses set the style. Their clothes were imported to England, or made under licence for rich customers, or simply plagiarized by shops and dressmakers who could skilfully interpret fashion illustrations. During the twentieth century the couturier became an important figure, regarded more as an artist than as a craftsman, and such figures (both men and women) held sway in most of the European capitals. However, since the 1950s, fashion has become much more international, with designers in London, New York, Italy and Japan being recognized on an equal footing with those in Paris. Furthermore, those in the ready-to-wear market are now as influential, if not more so, than those in traditional *haute couture*. Since the end of the Second World War there has also been the phenomenon of fashion emerging from amongst groups of young people who have evolved original styles of dress which owe little or nothing to the fashion establishment, but which have made a vital contribution in terms of ideas and direction.

The increasing importance of ready-made clothing has been one of the more striking features in the history of twentieth century costume, and this led to a new standardization of dress. The mass-production of clothing followed the invention of the sewing machine, but during the first half of the twentieth century off-the-peg garments (particularly for men) were sometimes regarded as inferior to those made to measure. However technical advances and improvements in sizing resulted in the eventual manufacture of well-made and well-fitting garments at reasonable prices, and these have been worn by the majority of people since the end of the Second World War.

The ways in which clothes are bought and sold have also changed. The Edwardian period saw the expansion of the department store and the establishment of new clothes shops. Later there followed the multiple or chain stores, of which perhaps the most popular is Marks & Spencer; this firm started life as the Penny Bazaars established by Michael Marks in the 1890s, offering cheap goods made so by self-selection and a fast turnover. From the late 1950s there appeared boutiques, small specialist shops with a sympathetic environment. Today good shopping facilities have become accessible to almost everyone, with virtually the same range of goods available almost simultaneously in London and the provinces. This fact, and new methods of marketing and promoting fashion, have ensured that information on changing styles is rapidly transmitted. The fashion show, the professional fashion model, and even the mannequins in shop windows are twentieth-century developments which have made it possible to package and present new ideas and images very effectively to the widest of audiences.

The Dress

IN the fourteenth and fifteenth centuries dress should be seen firstly as a struggle to develop the mastery over cloth implied by the word 'tailoring', and then as an expression of delight in that mastery in some of the most fantastic fashions ever devised. At the start of the fourteenth century the dress of both sexes was based on the simple T-shaped garments of the previous century (the tunic and super-tunic), with cloaks on top. Women's clothes always covered their ankles and, sometimes, trailed on the ground, but men's clothes could be shortened to the knee if violent activity was to be undertaken. Men's hair was much easier to manage, worn in soft waves with a small fringe and curls over the ears, whereas married women had to swathe their heads and necks in a series of veils. Unmarried girls, however, were allowed to display their hair in increasingly elaborate plaits.

By *c* 1320 there were attempts to make the clothing of both sexes fit more tightly round the chest and arms. This was achieved by buttoning the sleeve of the under-tunic and, by the 1340s, through an increasing use of buttons on the torso of gown or tunic. In addition, men shortened their garments to just above knee level, provoking a charge of indecency from older and more conservative citizens, an accusation levelled also at women for their wide, increasingly revealing necklines. The surface of dress became more broken with, in the 1320s, the addition of peaks and then pendant strips on the sleeves; hoods also developed these strips at the back. As a counterbalance to the tightness of the bodice, the skirts of tunic and super-tunic flared out, and clothing generally became more interesting with the use of *mi-parti*, embroidery and 'dagging'. Hairstyles for women became more elaborate, and were frequently revealed; men grew their hair longer, in soft waves, and some sported beards.

The late 1350s saw the start of a movement away from extreme tightness and shortness in men's dress, with the introduction of a full-length garment known as a 'goun'/*houppelande*, buttoned down the front and loose in the body. The sleeves, originally tight, gradually grew wider, towards the end of the century, into great open or closed funnel shapes, often edged with decorative 'dagging', as was the hem of the 'goun'. Underneath, men wore short, tight, often padded, tunics to which were tied *mi-parti* hose.

Until *c* 1380 women continued to wear tightly fitting super-tunics, laced at the front; then they adopted the goun/*houppelande* with a V-shaped front opening and high collar and vast sleeves which often, like the train, trailed on the ground. By *c* 1360 women had begun to cover their hair again, and many were depicted in head-dresses which consisted of a number of veils with fluted edges framing the face from shoulder to shoulder, with or without a box-shaped understructure. By the late 1380s, as the gown collar rose higher, the veils grew smaller and, by the mid-1390s, small 'horns' of hair appeared at women's temples. By *c* 1420 these horned headdresses were at their widest. This period of the late fourteenth and early fifteenth centuries, which was dominated by the goun/*houppelande*, marked a return to very similar outer garments for both sexes, although, for men the waistline was set at natural height, whereas for women it was immediately below the bust. Men, too, had high-collared gowns, which led to their hair being cropped very short; and they wore hoods which were fantastically twisted, dagged and trimmed.

The frivolity of dress began to diminish after *c* 1420 when 'dagging' slipped from fashion, being replaced by padded rolls in men's hoods, and by fur linings in gown sleeves. The skirts and sleeves of the goun/*houppelande* also shrank into the narrower lines of the straight-sleeved gown worn by both sexes by 1440; in the case of women's dress it retained a V-shaped neckline into the 1480s. By the 1460s the female gown had become so tight that it must have been almost impossible for a fashionable woman to breathe deeply or move her arms. In men's dress, however, the impulse to impose tight control affected the clothing rather than the body, with excess material left from the shortened goun/ *houppelande* drawn into carefully set folds down the back and the front, with sleeves built up at the top of the arm. By *c* 1450 fashionable men were very wide-shouldered, narrow-waisted creatures, walking around on long, slim legs which ended in the tapering toes of pointed shoes or boots. By this time padded hoods were being replaced by modest, acorn-shaped caps. For women, however, the urge to increase the size of the headdress seemed to have become irresistible. They began to wear horned or steeple-shaped caps over which veils were draped or suspended from wires in a manner resembling huge butterflies. By the 1470s the most popular style in England was a butterfly veil worn over a small pillbox hat.

In the 1470s men's dress altered radically. By the middle of the decade the most fashionable men had discarded bulkiness in the upper body, replacing it with a skimpy look; the sleeves were not joined to the body at the top of the armholes, and the doublet and gown were left unfastened. This slimness of line was enhanced by the reappearance of full-length gowns and shoulder-length hair. In the 1480s gowns were cut more generously, developing lapels often made of exotic furs; by the 1490s gowns were so bulky and loose that they seemed to be in danger of slipping off at any moment. So, by the end of the century, the male silhouette was solid and wide; the hair was cut in a long, square 'page-boy' style and, at the other end of the body, the feet were shod in square-toed shoes.

While men moved right away from Gothic spideri-ness, women clung to their tightly-fitting, flat-chested gowns, but with the introduction of a square neckline in the mid-1480s. One way, however, in which they imitated the male gown was by adopting loose sleeves, with the cuff gradually widening into a bell-shape by the mid-1490s and the whole sleeve developed into an ever-lengthening funnel shape by *c* 1500. The accep-tance of the square neckline in the 1480s probably marked the beginning of the end of Gothic forms, and, in the next decade, this was followed by a more sober headdress consisting of a box-shaped under-cap covered with a veil of black satin or velvet slit up the sides.

People looked more solid in their square, bulky clothes by the end of the century, and colours were less frivolous. The bright reds, greens and blues, which had formed the basis of most wardrobes in the fourteenth and fifteenth centuries, gave way to more sombre hues. Black, which has always been worn, but selectively, now became *the* colour which all classes could wear and feel fashionable.

In the sixteenth century male dress consisted of five basic items – shirt, doublet, jerkin, hose and gown. The shirt, made of linen, was usually visible above the doublet collar, and, at first, was gathered into a low-necked band. By 1525 it was cut higher and given a band round the neck; by 1530 this had evolved into a standing collar edged with a frill. This frill gradually developed into a ruff, and became a separate article, gaining in size and complexity of construction after the 1560s.

The doublet was a close-fitting garment, shaped to the waist. Until *c* 1540 the waistline was fairly high, then worn at the natural line until it extended lower, into an exaggerated point, during the last quarter of the century. The style of doublet favoured by Henry VIII and his courtiers fitted round the neck, fastened down the front with hooks and eyes or ties, and extended into skirts which were knee-length or longer. After *c* 1540, the doublet had a standing collar which increased in height until the end of the 1560s. Sleeves varied in shape; they could have puffed-out fullness at the shoulder, or be full and 'paned' (strips of material caught into a band, or held with a few stitches) from shoulder to wrist, or be so wide that they were shaped into a close fit around the wrist. Detachable sleeves were joined to the doublet armhole by 'points' (laces with metal ends), and, from the late 1540s, it was fashionable to disguise the join with a curved section of material called a 'wing' which quickly developed into an ornamental feature. In addition, hanging sleeves of a different colour or material could be worn over the actual sleeves. The doublet and hose were held together by points tied between corresponding sets of eyelet holes around the waistline of the two items of clothing.

Until the mid-seventeenth century the term hose applied to all masculine outer garments worn below the waist, not just to stockings. The hose was constructed in two sections, 'trunkhose' or breeches and the closer-fitting stockings (also called 'nether-hose'). Until *c* 1570 the two garments were often sewn together, but after that date they tended to be worn as separate items held together with points or garters. By the late 1550s the most popular form of the upper hose were trunk-hose; these were padded and stiffened to achieve a fashionably swollen shape. The central front opening of the hose, over the crotch, was both disguised and emphasised by a 'codpiece', a padded, ornamental pouch; initially a controversial fashion, this style was soon accepted as an integral feature of men's dress in the sixteenth century.

Over the doublet a jerkin might be worn; sleeved or sleeveless, its shape was dictated by the style of doublet underneath. During the reign of Henry VIII, the jerkin had a wide U-shaped opening to the waist so that the doublet could be seen. By c 1540 this style had been replaced by a close-fronted jerkin with a low standing collar. A broad-fronted and open loose gown, falling in ample folds from a fitted yoke to the ankle, and then to mid-knee, was worn over the doublet and jerkin. The sleeves of this garment were cut in a variety of ways, but, invariably, revealed all or part of the sleeves of the garments worn beneath. The European fashion for cloaks, introduced into England in the mid-1540s, soon ousted the gown from fashionable dress, although it retained its popularity amongst the professional classes, and as a warm, informal garment for wear in the home.

The most notable feature of fashionable male dress in the first half of the century was its swaggering bravado. This was personified by Henry VIII in the many portraits which display a burly virility, achieved by the use of massive padding across the shoulders and chest, and a defiantly emphatic codpiece. Rich materials were slashed, 'pinked', embroidered and trimmed with lace and braid to create a wide range of decorative effects. Amongst male accessories the most distinctive were bonnets with soft crowns and turned-back brims which acted as foils for aglets, jewels and ostrich feathers. Shoes were flat, with broad spatulate toes, often slashed in the same manner as the garment they complemented.

The contrast between male and female dress in the first half of the century was that between dominant, self-assured and active masculinity, and subservient, static femininity. This was expressed in that unique English contribution to fashion, the rather cumbersome gable or pediment headdress. It was worn over a coif which completely hid the hair; the latter was not seen until the advent of the French hood in the 1530s.

Until the middle of the century the basic elements of female dress, worn over the ubiquitous linen shift, were a united bodice and skirt, called a 'kirtle', covered by a voluminous gown. The side-fastening bodice of the kirtle encased the upper half of the body in a rigid shape with, until c 1540, a rounded waistline. The square, slightly curved neckline was cut very narrow and tight on the shoulders, and the arms were weighed down by massive oversleeves with turned-back cuffs and stiff undersleeves. This type of bodice was worn with a gored skirt that expanded from the waistline in a smooth, unbroken surface which might have an inverted V-shaped opening to display a decorative underskirt. From the mid-1540s the skirt was given a pronounced bell-shape by means of a Spanish device called a 'farthingale'; this was an understructure, similar to a petticoat, but stiffened with a series of hoops that increased in circumference from waist to ankle.

In the first 40 years of the sixteenth century the kirtle was masked by the gown worn over it; this had a square neckline, was fitted to the waist, and fell to the ground in voluminous folds. By the mid-1540s the bodice and skirt were made as separate items, with the term 'kirtle' applying to the skirt only. The gown changed in style, and two types, loose and fitted, appear in portraits of the 1550s. The loose or open gown fell in folds from the shoulders. The fitted gown, ankle-length like the loose gown, fastened at the front and was worn both semi-formally and informally. The majority of these items of fashionable women's dress relied, like men's, upon rich, imported materials and decorative ornamentation for their impressive grandeur.

If sixteenth century dress is personified by individuals, Henry VIII (1509–1547) and Elizabeth I (1558–1603) would be the most readily identifiable personalities. In effect the century can be divided into masculine domination (1500–1553: Henry VII, Henry VIII and Edward VI) and feminine ascendancy (1553–1603: Mary I and Elizabeth I). Clothing, to a certain extent, followed this unnatural (to contemporary minds) reversal of the natural order. Men's dress retained the basic garments, discussed earlier, undergoing little in the way of change in the reign of Edward VI, but assimilating various features of Spanish dress under Mary I. In the course of Elizabeth's reign men's dress lost the assertive outline of the earlier part of the century, becoming more dandified and romantic, evolving, finally, into the self-conscious elegance epitomized by the young man in Hilliard's miniature of 1588 (Fig. 55).

In the late 1550s men's dress was generally restrained and dignified: rich, dark-coloured doublet, hose and cloak set off by white ruffles at neck and wrist, and enlivened by gold and blackwork embroidery, slashing and a profusion of aglets. The garments followed the lines of the body fairly closely and, apart from the shape of the trunk hose, there was little exaggeration of any one feature. However, in the 1560s and 1570s the doublet absorbed more and more padding until its belly, often called a 'peascod belly', could be extended into an artificially curved point. Sleeves were padded and trunkhose shrank in size until, in the 1580s, they were a narrow pad around the hips with 'canions' (a type of fitted thigh-warmer) enclosing the area from thigh to knee. The head was either encircled by a ruff or framed by a collar known as a 'falling band', and, for the first time since early in the century, hair was worn long. This new silhouette was both top-heavy and somewhat effeminate but, in the 1590s, the line relaxed as the fit of the doublet loosened, and it began to be worn undone. Large-brimmed hats, soft boots or round-toed shoes complemented the smooth line of long hair and unwrinkled stocking. The style was predominantly French, but the materials were still imported from Spain and Italy.

As in men's dress, so in women's. The closely pleated and decorated layers of the frilled neck ruffle of the female shift of the late 1590s soon developed into a separate accessory, wide enough by the 1580s to accommodate flowers and jewels in the pleats. In Elizabeth's reign the rigid and emphatic style of female dress moved quickly from the dignified sobriety of the 1550s into the livelier style of the 1560s. The surfaces of gown, bodice and skirt were broken up by applied decoration and jewellery, puffs and slashes exposed materials of differing colour, and the contrast between plain colours and black-and-white embroidered patterns on sleeves, cuffs and ruffs became more marked. The brighter colours of the 1560s can be seen in the portrait of An Unknown Girl of 1569, now in the Tate Gallery (Colour Plate III).

During the latter half of the 1570s the female silhouette became fuller and stiffer, and in the 1580s the shape that is thought of as typically Elizabethan had evolved. A stiff, heavily boned bodice compressed the bust, and a 'stomacher' (a triangular piece of decorated or embroidered material, worn at the front of the bodice) provided an extended point which rested on the skirt. Sleeves were an important feature, their swollen, padded surface embellished with substantial embroidery. The steep lines of the farthingale and narrow, elongated bodice emphasized a waist rendered narrower by the enormous width of skirt and broad shoulder-line. A slightly tilted ruff projected outwards from the neck, completely separating the head from the body. In the 1590s the stomacher became longer and narrower, extending well into the farthingale skirt. The shorter skirt length and higher hairstyle, decorated by wired ornaments, unbalanced the natural symmetry of the body. The evolution of fussy, decorative surface effects reached its apogee in the 1590s; the sharp, spiky shapes and encrusted, irregular decoration suggested a carefully contrived fantasy of appearance which reflected a social context in which female dress was of paramount importance, a visual stimulus to awe and admiration. This virtuosity drew upon a new 'phantasical' range of colours, and a widening range of luxury materials, ornaments and embroidery designs.

At the beginning of the seventeenth century the exaggerated fashions of the late Elizabethan period were still worn. Menswear still favoured padded doublets with distended peascod bellies combined with wide trunkhose and canions, or with breeches. Women continued to wear the elongated, tightly-boned bodices and tilted wheel-farthingales which encased the lower half of their bodies like enormous cages. Distortion of the natural shape of the body was admired and, throughout the century, these distortions increased and decreased in turn; the emphasis shifted but always drew attention to one area of the body at the expense of the others. As the exaggerated bulk around the hips of both sexes disappeared from high fashion in the mid- to late teens of the century the waistline rose, creating an elongated line which, when married to the lustrous plain satins and simple accessories recorded by van Dyck in the 1630s, produced the Caroline restraint which was the hallmark of the most elegant period of English dress in the seventeenth century.

The almost total disappearance of ruffs from fashionable dress in the mid-1620s allowed the head to appear, once again, as a coherent whole with the style of dress. Men's hair lengthened into loose curls, often with one 'love-lock' worn longer over the shoulder, and women's hair was smoothed back into a high chignon with soft curls around the face. Falling bands widened into full, wide collars for both sexes, often lavishly edged with fine Italian or Flemish lace, the men's collars falling over the neckband of their buttoned doublets, those of women edging their square-cut décolletage.

By the end of the 1630s menswear was looser and less formal, as depicted in the van Dyck portrait of Prince Rupert, c 1637 (Fig. 72). Buttons were left undone, the ample shirt linen billowed over fuller breeches, and boots were worn even by those without pretensions to country or martial pursuits. This evolution continued throughout the 1640s and 1650s, producing a tubular silhouette, with short doublets no longer attached to the wide breeches that stood away from the body – the style that became the voluminous 'petticoat' breeches of the 1660s. This chunkiness of line was broken only by the busy surface decoration of braids and ribbons which proliferated in all but the strictest Puritan circles. Women's dress, however, became increasingly rigid around the upper torso, and this dichotomy in style between the sexes prevailed until the mid-1680s.

The easier, more relaxed style of menswear developed into the 'vest', tunic and breeches of the mid-1660s, settling down, after an experimental phase, into the happy combination of coat, waistcoat and breeches. The unstructured, almost smock-like looseness of the early coat was replaced by a more fitted line in the late 1680s, with the coat-skirts stiffened by inter-lining, and the fullness arranged into pleats at sides and centre-back. These coats were worn with vests (early waistcoats, often with sleeves which turned back over the coat cuff) and narrow breeches. The falling band was replaced in the late 1660s with a cravat, a long rectangular band of linen, sometimes edged with lace, which was knotted at the neck in a variety of formal and casual ways. Throughout the century men's and women's wear had kept pace in the use of colours, materials and decorative accessories, if not in stylistic emphasis. England's excellent wool cloth remained a relatively unfashionable material except for riding-habits and travelling cloaks, and the majority of fashionable materials were still imported. Silks came from Italy and, later in the century, from France; lace from Italy and the Low Countries; linen from the Netherlands and Germany, and braids, fringes, buttons and ribbons from a wide range of sources.

Women, constricted by the tightly boned bodices and stiff sleeves of their formal gowns, signalled a change of style in the late 1670s. The bodice, skirt and petticoat, all separate garments worn over a shift, were replaced gradually by the mantua. This was a one-piece gown which evolved from the popular but informal 'nightgown'; it was belted at the waist and fitted smoothly, but relatively easily and comfortably over stays and petticoat. In the 1680s this new style widened to complement the increasing width of men's coat skirts, with a bustle or shallow hoop worn to support the looped-up fullness of the mantua skirts. So, by the end of the century, a restrained rigidity of style was apparent once more in the dress of both sexes.

The basic lines of men's clothing had been laid down during the later seventeenth century, and consisted of the three-piece suit – coat, waistcoat and breeches; with little alteration this lasted for most of the eighteenth century. The main changes to be seen involved a progress from a heavy fullness of cut with large cuffs, wide side pleats and baggy breeches, to a slimmer line with short waistcoat and coat curving away from the chest, and a change, also, from a baroque richness of fabric (silk velvets, ornate brocades and damasks) to plain, untrimmed light silks and woollen cloths.

The first 30 years of the period were a time of ponderous solidity in male dress, with long waistcoat reaching almost to the hem of the stiffly padded coat and both virtually hiding the amply cut breeches. Adding to the bulkiness of the silhouette was a large powdered wig, the most popular styles being the short 'full-bottomed' wig, and the 'campaign' wig, the latter a way of tying-up the flowing locks for greater comfort and ease of movement. In the 1730s the front edges of the coat began to curve slightly towards the back, the waistcoat to shorten slightly, the breeches to buckle over the knee, and small, neat wigs with the back hair tied with a ribbon or in a black silk bag were adopted. It was in this decade also that the 'frock' coat was taken

from the wardrobe of the working man into fashionable country and later, town wear, and by the 1780s the frock was worn everywhere except at court. It was characterized by functional simplicity of style, demonstrated by the absence of stiffened side pleats, by its plain or slit cuff and its small, turned-down collar.

Female dress in the eighteenth century was subject to greater change and greater variety. France continued to be the most important arbiter of taste and fashion, especially with regard to formal dress. The most notable example of this was the *grand habit* with its heavily boned bodice and separate lavishly trimmed skirt and train, a style based on French fashions of the 1670s which was worn at courts all over Europe, although its use in England was limited to royal weddings and occasions of similar high formality. More usual at court, particularly in the first half of the eighteenth century, was the mantua, an open robe with increasingly stylized back drapery, worn over a trimmed skirt, known as a 'petticoat'. Formal occasions in fact demanded the wearing of an open robe worn with a separate 'stomacher' piece, which was either laced across, embroidered, or covered in ribbons (*échelles*), and a 'petticoat' which usually matched the robe. The robe was either fitted into the waist at the back, a style to which the English were particularly attached, and which was known in the last quarter of the century as a *robe à l'anglaise*, or it fell in folds from the shoulders at the back, a type of dress known as a *sacque* (sack to the English) or *robe à la française*. This latter style, perhaps the most characteristic and graceful dress of the first half of the eighteenth century, was, in origin, a loose informal gown, becoming more formal from the 1730s, with regulated back pleats and tighter-fitting at the sides; at about this time it entered the wardrobe of the fashionable English lady. It reached its apogee in the middle years of the century under the influence of the rococo styles popularized by Madame de Pompadour, when the surface of the dress was broken-up with frills, ruffles and three-dimensional 'robings', and the air of frivolity and playfulness enhanced by tiny headdresses made of lace, flowers and feathers. Fabrics for formal dress included lustrous silk satins (often lavishly embroidered), velvet, brocade and damask; the ever popular floral designs of the eighteenth century ranged from heavy foliage and flower patterns to delicate botanical designs, most notably Spitalfields silks.

On less formal occasions women in England had, from the earliest years of the century, shown a fondness for being portrayed in simpler styles, such as 'wrapping gowns', nightgowns (a term encompassing a multitude of meanings, including a dressing-gown, a loosely fitted closed robe, and a more fitted open gown worn with a contrasting petticoat), and a jacket and skirt style. However informal, they were usually worn over hoops, an English contribution to fashion first seen *c* 1710. The early hoops were full-length, made of rings of cane or whalebone, and fastened from waist to hem with tapes, forming a conical shape; they became large and circular in the 1730s and, with the introduction of side hoops, became wide and square in the 1740s. By the 1760s hoops, if worn at all, were small and extended at the sides, but the large hoops persisted at court until 1820.

The second half of the eighteenth century saw a growing simplicity in male dress; in spite of the 'macaronis' of the 1770s, whose brightly coloured, exaggerated costume was a last flicker of luxury, the trend was towards sobriety in colour and cut. A constant theme in men's dress in the eighteenth century is the contrast between the imported silks and lace worn formally, and the plain, high-quality woollen cloths worn for informal, country or sporting dress, along with natural hair, simply styled. In addition, by the last quarter of the eighteenth century, England set the trend both in dark, cloth suits for urban wear, and in country costume which consisted of a simple frock coat (shades of brown and blue were popular), buff waistcoat and breeches, and boots. Male clothing was distinguished by excellence of cut, with tailoring triumphing over luxury of fabric and trimming.

Women, too, were increasingly seduced by notions of 'natural' simplicity in their informal clothing, characterized by a growing distinction between formal and informal costume. The *sacque*, by the 1770s, was increasingly limited to formal occasions, and the dress that was most often worn as everyday wear was the *robe à l'anglaise* or fitted English gown. Fullness and bounce at the hips and the back – the newly fashionable line – was achieved by lifting the overskirt and draping it at the back, or by wearing small pads. The rounded, ample appearance of women was further achieved by starched muslin 'kerchiefs' called *buffons* at the bosom, towering coiffures, and vast hats. The increasing popularity of a healthy outdoors existence was reflected in the fashion for tailored walking costumes, such as the riding habit and the greatcoat, both of which derived originally from masculine wear.

Typical of the growing informality in dress in the late eighteenth century was the popularity of newly fashionable fabrics such as printed cotton and fine muslin. In the 1780s, *the* fashionable dress was the 'chemise dress', revolutionary in its simplicity, for, in its early form, it was merely a tube of white muslin with a drawstring at the neck and a sash at the waist.

Originating from the French West Indies, it was popularized by Queen Marie Antoinette at the French court, and then spread all over Europe, developing into the neo-classical gown of the French Revolution, and heralding the temporary relaxation in women's dress which characterized the early years of the nineteenth century.

To the eighteenth century the supposed simplicities of the countryside as expressed in the natural, informal costume of the Englishman, and the simple cotton and linen dresses worn by many fashionable women, were tantamount to a belief in democracy, and were enthusiastically adopted on the eve of the French Revolution. To contemporaries who lived through the startling social and political changes brought about by the French Revolution, the links between the informality of dress seen in the immediate pre-revolutionary years and the subsequent advance of democracy (however short-lived) were clearly apparent.

It was in the nineteenth century that fashion, in terms of an interest in dress and its changing styles, became a predominantly female concern. From the early years of the century, the sexes began to adopt diverging roles in society. The masculine ideal became one of solid integrity and economic reliability which was expressed in safe, conservative styles of clothing, and in discreet and sombre colours. On the other hand, the female was seen as a mere dependant, a decorative accessory who could display the family wealth and social status in fashionable dress. While men's clothing became increasingly standardized over the century, women's dress demonstrated a wide variety of styles, which changed more rapidly than in any previous period.

Women's dress, in the first two decades of the century, was distinguished by a high-waisted and narrow appearance, owing much to the general wave of neo-classicism. Hair was arranged in styles popularly thought to be 'antique', either short and tousled *à la Titus*, or long and bunched in ringlets on the crown, and soft cotton muslins were almost universal for day and evening wear. In imitation of the clinging draperies of antiquity, the fashionable style was graceful and softly rounded, with a low neckline, short sleeves and a high waistline over a closely gathered skirt. After *c* 1805, long sleeves and a narrower skirt created a more rigid vertical line. Outerwear either followed the line of the dress, with fitted 'spencers' and 'pelisses', or added draperies in the form of loose mantles, cloaks and shawls.

From 1815, the year of the long-awaited peace with France, 'Romantic' influences (always popular in England) began to prevail; Elizabethan ruffs, 'vandyke' trimmings, and ostrich-plumed bonnets were fashionable revivalist touches. The softly draped white muslins were gradually replaced by stiffer printed cottons and silks; the skirts were now gored, producing an 'A-line' shape, further emphasized by being stiffened at the hem by flounces or padded ribbons.

After 1820 the waistline began to drop, reaching its natural level by 1827; this produced a longer fitted bodice which usually fastened at the back, worn over increasingly wide skirts. By the late 1820s, female fashions were exuberant, with highly elaborate curled hairstyles, vast hats, huge 'gigot' sleeves and wide, gored skirts supported by stiff, cotton petticoats; wide capes and 'pelerines' gave additional emphasis to the shoulders. From 1830 steadily inflating sleeves and skirts began to billow and sag like overblown roses, and the centre of gravity began its descent towards the hemline. The bodice became more pointed, the sleeves, set low on the arm, gradually collapsed in size, and the main focus of interest was the increasingly wide skirt; from 1841 straight widths of fabric were gauged to the waistline, producing a distinctive dome-shape. By this time the Gothic arch influenced the fashionable appearance, its narrow apex a sleek, smooth hairstyle and a face-framing bonnet; the look was one of modesty and reticence.

By the 1850s the waistline had risen slightly and the skirt had increased in size, so that the prevailing shape was a wide-based triangle; an increasingly horizontal effect was created by wide-brimmed bonnets and hats, and flared sleeves. Lightly patterned fabrics, such as printed muslins, warp-printed silks, and draped bodices, flounces, pinked edges, and fringe decoration all added to the softer silhouette. By the mid-1850s it was usual to wear as many as five stiffened petticoats, including one of horsehair, in order to create the fashionable full skirt. In 1856, however, this intolerable weight was lightened by the introduction of a hooped petticoat, not unlike that of the eighteenth century. Called a crinoline (from the French crin, horsehair), it had an immediate impact on female fashions and, although widely criticized for its impracticalities, was adopted at almost every level of society, and dominated fashion up to 1868. During the 1860s the crinoline was modified in shape. From 1860 it began to flatten at the front, and skirts were gored to follow this line; by 1865 tunic-dresses or double skirts gave added emphasis at the back, with the lower skirt extending as a train. By 1868 many women had discarded crinolines, adopting the narrower skirt with a train. The newly fashionable back emphasis required support in the form of a bustle, initially a kind of half crinoline, but soon reduced to a large flounced pad of horsehair tied around the waist.

A vertical look dominated the 1870s, emphasized by a rising hairstyle, with the hair dressed high on the head, usually with a chignon or heavy ringlets at the back, the whole topped with a small hat or bonnet. Skirts were flat and narrow at the front, curving in a soft undulating line at the back; overskirts, either separate or attached to the bodice in the 'polonaise' form, were draped to give an additional puffed 'pannier' at the back. The whole ensemble was encrusted with layers of pleated frills and lace flounces. By the middle of the decade an even narrower look was being created by the long, 'cuirass' bodice which fitted snugly over the waist and hips. This was worn with a skirt which, according to The Ladies' Treasury (1876), was 'so tight that our sitting and walking are seriously inconvenienced'. Indeed, it was found necessary to reduce the volume of underwear by replacing the separate chemise and drawers with fitted combinations.

This narrow style continued into the 1880s, with variations created by the draping of the skirt and overskirt, and by the range of bodices, many of which were cut en Princesse, with an attached polonaise overskirt almost as long as the underskirt. After 1880 the skirt was a straight tube, but this was soon replaced by a new form of bustle, a narrow angular construction, forming a shelf-like profile at the back, which reached its maximum size in 1887, but which had disappeared by the end of the decade. After 1884, although formal and evening wear demanded complicated skirt draperies and trains, the general trend was towards a simpler style in everyday dress. This was inspired by the increasing popularity of travel and sport, for which many women wore a woollen tailor-made dress, or a jersey (a simple bodice of knitted wool or silk) with a plain skirt.

The elaborate costume of the 1870s, with its bright colours and complex draperies, was, in artistic circles, compared unfavourably with the supposedly plainer forms of medieval dress. Aesthetes and dress reformers, eschewing tight-lacing, developed a distinctive style of their own – loose-fitting dresses in the soft muted oriental silks being popularized by Liberty's of London. Some dress reformers also recommended simpler, functional styles, and although relatively few women were brave enough to adopt masculine bifurcated garments such as knickerbockers, in the 1890s many women wore tailor-made outfits based on the male suit. Some women even wore straw sailor hats and neckties with the blouse and skirt which were worn on all but the most formal occasions.

Appearances were deceptive, however. As the informal blouse became more fashionable, it was shaped to the figure by a heavily boned lining and high stiffened collar. From *c* 1890 the top of the sleeve began to grow, producing by the middle of the decade a revival of the huge, impractical gigot sleeve of the 1830s; and as in the 1830s, a wide hat and a tiny waist were *de rigueur*. At the end of the 1890s a more fluid silhouette was apparent; bodices were pouched at the front and skirts were cut to fit tightly over the hips, flaring into a train at the back, helping to form the art nouveau curves of the Edwardian age.

In contrast to the constant changes in female fashions, men's dress was very conservative. Post-revolutionary Europe continued in reaction against the brightly coloured silks and lavish trimmings so identified with the *ancien régime*, but which were on the wane from the 1780s onwards. In the early years of the nineteenth century dark cloths and plain styles were the order of the day, and following the tenets of Beau Brummell, the fashionable emphasis was on fit rather than on novelties in cut and design.

During the first two decades of the century, the neo-classical ideal was expressed in hair *à la Titus*, and in a narrow, high-waisted silhouette, produced by short-bodied coats and waistcoats, and almost skin-tight pantaloons. By the late eighteenth century, knee-breeches were being replaced by tight-fitting calf- or ankle-length pantaloons which were then replaced by looser-fitting trousers during the second decade of the nineteenth century. Knee breeches were retained for full court dress and pantaloons for evening wear.

At the beginning of the period, the main coats worn were the dress tailcoat with its straight front waist, and the less formal morning or riding coat with sloping fronts. From 1816 the nineteenth century version of the 'frock coat', with its distinctive straight front edges, made its first appearance, becoming the usual garment for formal day wear in the second half of the century. In the 1820s men's coats, like women's dresses, featured full, gathered shoulders and low, narrow waists, and men's baggy trousers complemented widening skirts. By the 1840s the masculine waistcoat (the only garment in which a sense of colour and pattern could be given free rein) shared not only the same fabrics, colours and patterns as women's dress, but also their waistline.

A number of new, informal garments were introduced into the male wardrobe during the nineteenth century. A short, loose-fitting 'pilot coat', or *paletot*, began life as an overcoat in the 1830s, but soon evolved into a variety of short, informal jackets. Of these, the lounging jacket was soon given the addition of matching waistcoat and trousers, producing, in the 1860s, the early form of the lounge suit. The Norfolk jacket was fashionable country wear in the second half of the

century. In line with all of these changes, the 1880s saw the dinner jacket competing with the tail-coat for evening wear; and in the 1890s the reefer and blazer jackets evolved from sporting garments as popular leisure clothing.

With the prevailing sobriety in male dress, fine white linen was a status symbol; collars, cuffs and shirt fronts were often heavily starched to keep them clean as well as smooth. Initially, collars were attached and swathed in fine linen cravats but, during the 1840s, detachable collars appeared, and the cravat narrowed around the neck to be fastened as a loose scarf or large bow at the front. Turn-down collars and shaped neckties finally appeared in the 1860s.

The top hat was worn throughout the century, but from the 1850s a range of less formal styles appeared, including the hard felt 'bowler' and the straw sailor hat. The soft felt hat with a dented crown, known as a 'trilby', emerged in the 1870s, and by the 1890s there was also the harder 'Homburg', together with a range of caps, helmets and boaters. Light shoes or pumps were worn with evening dress, but in the daytime boots were usual. With the advent of trousers, 'hessians' and top-boots were replaced by half-boots.

Changes in male fashion during the nineteenth century were slower and more limited than those adopted by women; variations in style were subtle and often difficult to distinguish even in the exaggerations of fashion plates and caricatures. By the end of the century, however, it is possible to be able to identify, in their early form, all the items of men's clothing which can be found in the twentieth century.

At the turn of the century, women's clothes were still constructed on the principle of a very firm foundation: a tightly laced and rigidly boned corset, which produced as slim a waist and as elegantly rounded a figure as possible. A new type of corset, which appeared *c* 1900, with a straight centre-front busk, induced a characteristic S-shaped stance, and this threw the bust forwards and the hips backwards. Dress bodices and blouses were softly draped over the bust; skirts were fluted in shape to skim the hips and sweep outwards at the hem, with a short train at the back. Tailored suits and skirts were worn with elaborately trimmed high-necked blouses in the daytime; in contrast evening wear consisted of low-cut dresses of light, airy textures in pastel colours, trimmed with froths of lace, net, chiffon, beads, ribbons and artificial flowers. Hair was dressed in soft, undulating styles, and hats were large with curved brims.

After 1905 this line gradually eased out and straightened up, inspired by neo-classical models of the late eighteenth and early nineteenth centuries. The waistline rose above its natural level, the skirt narrowed, and a new, longer and straighter-fitting corset was introduced in 1908. This new line was refined and promoted by Paul Poiret, the French designer, and, despite its apparent simplicity, was a particularly restricting form of dress. Aptly called the 'hobble' skirt, this fashion reached its extreme form in 1911/12, but the severity of line was blurred as overtunics were added and bodices lengthened into jackets. By 1914 the skirt began to shorten, and was several inches above the ankle, and had a wider hemline by 1915. A more traditionally feminine shape, with a bell-shaped skirt, often flounced, was evident in 1915/16, but towards the end of the War the earlier cylindrical line was re-adopted, but retained the shorter hemline.

The tubular line of the 1920s allowed women complete freedom of movement, as the position of the waistline dropped to the hips in c 1920–22, eliminating any shaping over the natural female contours. An even greater contrast, which had appeared towards the end of the War, was that between daytime wear of practical, sober, tailor-made suits and evening dresses made from vibrant and luxurious fabrics. Such clothes required little expertise in cut and construction, and evening dresses, in particular, were virtual tubes reliant upon surface decoration for interest, the most spectacular being the all-over bead embroideries.

Towards the end of 1924 hemlines began to rise, reaching knee-level in 1926; the silhouette began to be pared down so that by 1927 women seemed increasingly streamlined. This provides the most familiar image of the 1920s – the knee-length waistless dress worn with a helmet-like cloche hat pulled down to the eyebrows. The neat effect was enhanced by cutting the hair short and dressing it close to the head in flat waves. Startling jewellery and flamboyant cosmetics mitigated this uncompromisingly functional line.

By 1929 the Paris collections were showing a gentler line, which hinted at the natural contours of bust, waist and hips. The new silhouette was smooth and uncluttered as before, but, after 1930, it encompassed a soft, supple, diagonal line. This new fluidity was achieved by cutting the dress material on the bias or cross-grain, and this style of dress design, particularly associated with the French designer Madeleine Vionnet, dominated fashion during the first half of the 1930s. By day women's clothes looked neat and disciplined, with crisply smart accessories; in the evening they were softly draped.

From 1933 the shoulder-line was widened and accentuated; towards the end of the 1930s the waistline tightened and the hemline rose, producing by 1938 a trim, tailored suit for women, cut on rather masculine lines. Dress design of the later 1930s was also characterized by elements of eccentricity and fantasy, influenced by Surrealism, by nostalgia for late Victorian and Edwardian fashions, and by the glamour of the American film industry.

During the Second World War the need in Britain to economize on cloth and other materials essential for the war effort resulted in clothes rationing in 1941, quickly followed in 1942 by the Utility Scheme which strictly governed the design and production of cloth and clothing for both sexes. Although rationing continued until 1949, as early as 1946 French, British and American collections were attempting changes in women's dress. These were expressed in a coherent form in Christian Dior's 'New Look' collection of spring 1947. This style, a nostalgic revival of the fashion for slim waists and wide, ankle-length skirts, dominated fashion until the mid-1950s, developing an alternative long, slim skirt; both versions had fitted bodices, natural shoulder-lines and slender waists. Shorter hairstyles and a wider range of cosmetics combined with this look to create an appearance of well-tailored, well-groomed femininity. In the late 1950s there were experiments with new shapes, and variations in waistline, producing a more structured outline, which, at its best, depended upon skilful cutting and construction, at which practitioners of Parisian *haute couture* excelled.

However, such styles were formal, expensive and designed for the mature woman; they were challenged by a group of talented, young, British designers, who, in the 1960s, produced lively and provocative ranges for their own age group. By 1965 mini-skirts were several inches above knee-level, and their brevity was enhanced with stark simplicity of line, colour, minimal pattern, geometrical hair-cuts and stylized make-up featuring dark eyes and pale lips. The young appeared innovative and classless in these fashions, as they did in their blue denim jeans, and their inventiveness inspired a new generation of young French designers, like Courrèges and Yves St Laurent.

The late 1960s saw experiments with softer, more tentative styles – new 'midi' and 'maxi' hemlines, and a diffusely romantic, quasi-exotic style which drew upon earlier fashions, Antique Market finds, and eastern garments. In the mid-to-late 1970s, Japanese dress designers posed a challenge to western clothing by introducing features of the wrapped, layered and unstructured styles of oriental dress. At much the same time, the street fashions of the 'Punk' movement, with their bizarrely dyed, sculpted and spiky hair, black tattered clothes and chains, studs and safety-pins, startled observers until certain modified elements were incorporated into fashionable dress. This seeming anarchy was at variance with the casual but essentially health-conscious vogue for sportswear, which passed across into fashionable dress certain key features for longer, looser, unstructured clothing. Throughout the late 1970s and early 1980s daytime fashion has helped to blur the distinctions between male and female dress, but evening wear continued to enhance and emphasize the differences.

Men's dress, when the century began, was generally formal, and regulated according to a man's occupation and the time of day. Frock coats and morning suits, with appropriate accessories, were correct for day wear, with three-piece lounge suits as alternatives for less formal occasions in town, and for country wear. In the evening, dress suits with tail-coat, white waistcoats and white bow-ties were usual for formal functions, while dinner suits (evening versions of lounge suits, worn with black bow-ties and waistcoats) were worn at other times. The cut of all of these suits was fairly narrow.

A new informality appeared in the 1920s and 1930s. Shirt collars were lowered, and gradually the starched, winged style was replaced by soft, turned-down collars; frock coats disappeared, and morning suits were relegated to more formal wear. Single- or double-breasted three-piece lounge suits were worn during the day. For informal occasions, tweed sports jackets (adapted from riding or hacking jackets) or blazers (originally worn for yachting) were worn with flannel trousers in the country and at weekends; golfing clothes – a rough tweed knickerbocker suit and knitted pullover – also became acceptable casual wear.

By the mid-1920s the shape of the male suit had changed quite considerably. Trousers had widened, and the jacket had widened at the shoulder and loosened at the waist, becoming much squarer in outline. This slacker fit and more geometrical line echoed developments in the female silhouette, and in the 1930s there was a parallel emphasis on the slimness and flatness of the hips, accentuated by the width of the shoulders. Men's jackets became increasingly boxy in shape, assisted by shoulder-padding, wide lapels and double-breasted fastenings. Trouser legs were wide with turn-ups at the ankle. Knitted informal wear included sweaters, sleeveless pullovers and waistcoats.

After the rationing, Utility wear and uniforms of the War, menswear in the late 1940s retained the square, loose cut of coat and trousers which had appeared in the late 1930s, and which is so familiar through the styles seen in the American films of the period. In the 1950s, however, men's suits began to narrow, and an elegant minority of neo-Edwardians pursued a new ideal of stylishness which was compared with the line and exquisite tailoring of the early years of the century. These ideas were adapted and popularized by 'Teddy Boys', with their long jackets, 'drainpipe' trousers, 'bootlace' ties and heavy crêpe-soled shoes. This was the first of many youthful/teenage cult styles of dressing; followed in the early 1960s by 'Mods' ('sharp' Italian suits) and 'Rockers' (studded leather). Later in the 1960s and in the early 1970s 'Hippies' (Indian cottons, beads and long hair) and 'skinheads' ('crew-cuts', collarless shirts, braces, shortened trousers and 'Bovver' boots) appeared, closely followed by Punks and 'New Romantics' (longer hair, make-up, Byronic frills and silks).

In the mainstream of menswear the 1950s and early 1960s saw a progressive paring-down of the male silhouette. Slimmer trousers, more fitted jackets with natural shoulder-lines, smaller lapels and single-breasted fastening owed much to the influence of Italian designers. Crease-resistant suitings and drip-dry shirts added to the neat, well-pressed look of clothes. Footwear was lighter, but with pointed toes. As the 1960s progressed the new boutiques specializing in inexpensive and vibrant clothes for men, often influenced by the dress of pop groups, added vitality to menswear. Men's clothes, albeit briefly affected by patterns and colours popularized by innovators, retained their traditional format of the two-piece suit and sports jacket and trousers. Details changed – flared trouser hems appeared in the late 1960s, shirts became skin-tight with long collars, and broad 'kipper' ties were popular. Teenagers and younger men wore denim jeans, T-shirts, sweaters and running shoes for cheapness and practicality.

Inevitably, as casual clothing became more important, it was seized upon and refined by international couture designers. 'Blouson' jackets, ribbed polo-necked sweaters and styled trousers with pleated fronts and wider legs were introduced. Like women, men were offered an increasingly wide range of sportwear, and the informality of loose, unstructured garments offered an alternative to the classic styles for suits and casual wear.

The Sources

HISTORIANS of dress have, with regard to the late medieval period onwards, a wealth of documentary, literary, and visual sources to help them in their recovery and depiction of the past. As the title of this book indicates, and because dress is basically about perceived images, we have concentrated on the visual sources, their range, usefulness and their problems, especially when considered beside other evidence such as surviving costume.

The almost total lack of garments surviving, relatively unrestored, from the Middle Ages, means that anyone studying the late medieval period has to rely on other sources. These include the documentary evidence which encompasses the day-to-day business of recording the expenditure on dress of the wealthy and powerful, and the literary evidence which embraces drama, verse, and the works, often moralistic in tone, of chroniclers and poets.

To the general reader, however, many of the documentary sources are rather inaccessible, such as the still largely unpublished English royal wardrobe accounts, written in rudimentary Latin or French. The chroniclers, being mainly monastic, tended to write in Latin, and translations – where they exist – do not adequately cope with the semantic problems of dress terms. In addition, such chroniclers are often selective in the choice of fashions singled out for censure, choosing to discuss such styles which (according to these authors) resulted in natural disasters as a sign of God's punishment for sartorial offences.

Even works in medieval English can be difficult to read, because they look so strange, although they are less so when read aloud. Some individual poems may, like the chronicles, decry certain fashions, but others offer useful and appreciative references to dress, such as *Sir Gawain and the Green Knight* of the late fourteenth century; few, however, can be dated at all precisely. Chaucer's works have often been plundered for references to dress, but the standard literary practice of his day – that of re-working or translating the works of other writers – makes this occasionally a dangerous exercise. The pilgrims of the *The Canterbury Tales* are presumably wearing the dress of the author's time, but when the narrator of *The Romaunt of the Rose* describes, for example, in the process of getting dressed the sewing shut of his sleeves, we have a reference not to the customs of Chaucer's day, but to that of the date of the original French poem, over 150 years before.

The surviving visual sources in continental Europe in the late medieval period are almost entirely pictorial (i.e. paintings and illustrated manuscripts) while those in the British Isles are predominantly funerary (i.e. effigies, brasses and incised slabs). However, especially towards the end of the fifteenth century, there are high quality English illustrated books, as well as a number of wall paintings; the latter, however, present many problems, for not only have they suffered the ravages of time (and the attentions of nineteenth-century 'restorers') but they are often an indecipherable amalgam of English and foreign (mainly Flemish) costume.

One of the realities of the late Middle Ages is the fact that England was not particularly important in the development of fashionable dress; in north-western Europe, France in the fourteenth century, and its north-eastern neighbour Flanders in the fifteenth century, were arbiters of late Gothic taste and magnificence. Some of the late medieval painted portraits and illustrated manuscripts in this book are, therefore, by foreign artists, but they have been included because in some cases they are of British sitters, and in other cases they may depict native dress, as well as French or Flemish costume. With regard to men's dress, due to their greater mobility, a spirit of internationalism largely prevailed; thus, dated portraits in particular can provide useful information as to the details of upper-class masculine costume. Illustrated books are included, for they contain scenes of everyday life, and people of different classes, allowing one to build up a series of 'coat-hangers', as it were, of dated or datable material on which to hang the stages of the development of a fashion, as well as an understanding of its appearance from different angles; they can also show how fashions are interpreted by various classes according to the demands of practicality and finance.

Sculpture alone can reproduce the three-dimensional effect of clothing on a body, but tombs have distinct problems as sources of information, for they were sometimes commissioned within the lifetimes of those they were to commemorate, and sometimes long after. Consequently, any dates of death which they may bear can be quite misleading if taken to represent the date of commission. They cannot always be relied upon to give an accurate likeness of the deceased, or any real indication of age or even of social status. One of the most curious features of tomb effigies is that they seem to depict people who are still alive, and who have been carved as though standing upright before being laid flat on their backs; when the bright paints in which the effigies were originally covered were undamaged, the sensation of the figures being alive must have been profound. Because of the conventions of the sculptors, and because the effigies are being examined as sources of information on dress and not as pieces of sculpture, they are mostly reproduced here as upright figures.

The merchant classes seem to have preferred brasses or incised slabs as memorials, possibly because they were cheaper. These are often so standardized in their representations that it looks as though the pattern books for them remained unchanged over a period of many years, or that they were often ordered well in advance of being needed: therefore they have to be treated with caution as a source of information on dress. In addition, there is a tendency for monuments of all types to be concentrated in the wealthier south of England, so that it is difficult to establish the extent to which dress was regionalized within the British Isles.

In life, men had open to them a far wider range of occupations, and hence outfits, than women had, and yet – paradoxically – they are on the whole depicted in memorial works of art either in their official dress, or – due to the prevailing cult of chivalry – in armour. Men tend to appear in fashionable dress usually only if they are in the subsidiary role of weepers (small figures of the family of the deceased, set along the front and sides of the tomb). Women, on the other hand, are mainly shown in the fashions they had loved in life.

The visual sources for British dress gradually increase in number and diversity during the sixteenth century, but they do not begin to match the richness of visual material found in many other European countries. Inevitably, there are brasses, funerary sculpture, and some manuscript illustrations, as in the earlier centuries, but the iconoclastic depredations of the Reformation, and, in the seventeenth century, the Puritan excesses of the Civil War and the Commonwealth, have robbed us of much stained glass and religious wall painting which would have provided some additional evidence for different styles and changes in dress.

There was no established British school of painting in the sixteenth century which can provide us with drawings and easel works comparable to those found in other European countries. During the reign of Henry VII, his son and grandchildren, major artists such as Torrigiano, Holbein and Mor were occasionally commissioned (some even visited England) to undertake sculpture and paintings on behalf of royal and aristocratic patrons. These works were supplemented by the portraits (after the Reformation, portraiture was the preferred form of secular art in England) produced by humbler artists, often French or Flemish in origin and Protestant in religion. Such artists made a respectable

living portraying the nobility and gentry who, as the century progressed, were busily rebuilding their houses, and incorporating a long gallery in which portraits (of themselves and their ancestors) were a prominent feature.

However, portraiture in Britain, after the brief glories of Holbein's sojourn at Henry VIII's court, was on the whole a pedestrian affair, enlivened only – later in the century – by the exquisite miniatures of Hilliard and Oliver. Artists were not well treated at the English court; they were considered artisans and paid accordingly. Neither Henry VIII nor Elizabeth I, despite their pretensions to Renaissance scholarship and culture, seem wholly to have sympathized with, or understood, the important propaganda role that a great artist might fulfil at a European court. This, however, is not of paramount importance for the student of costume history, as the many surviving portraits, although not major works of art, provide accurate and detailed depictions of the fashions worn in England throughout the century.

Apart from portraits, there are illustrated broadsheets and books in which some evidence of dress can be found. There are also, during the second half of the sixteenth century, a number of costume books (published mainly in France, Italy, the Netherlands and Germany) which include the dress of the British Isles; this was sometimes misunderstood, or cribbed from a variety of European sources, and the information that is provided must be treated with circumspection. A minor but attractive source of visual detail is to be found in the books of embroidery designs, often taken from contemporary herbals, upon which both professional and domestic embroiderers relied for inspiration; many of the delicate embroideries found on the dress of sitters in sixteenth-century portraits can be traced back to these books. Such embroidery skills formed an essential part of the education of young women, and it is perhaps not surprising that of the small number of sixteenth-century garments that survive unaltered, the majority should be of embroidered linen – coifs, nightcaps, shirts, shifts and gloves. Embroidery and miniature painting – not dissimilar in effect – are two of the main artistic English contributions to European civilization in the sixteenth century.

The major cultural contribution, however, was literature. The English language was an expressive tool, forged during the Renaissance of the sixteenth century, and was used by both poet and polemicist with equal vigour. Throughout the country, in plays, poetry, pamphlets, wardrobe accounts, inventories and sermons, there are vivid descriptions and allusions – both complimentary and disparaging – about dress.

Foreign visitors also reported on what they saw in England, and there are many accounts, some in translation, of what such travellers thought about English costume. That they were both impressed and amazed tends to confirm the view of native commentators, to whom the dress worn by their contemporaries was often – by the end of the century – an awkward and bizarre mingling of French, Spanish, German, Dutch and Italian styles.

In the seventeenth century, the written evidence regarding dress extends well beyond the sources available to students of sixteenth-century costume. In addition to the type of evidence mentioned above, there are also diaries, many more letters (as literacy increased), larger numbers of printed (and illustrated) books, and the introduction of the newspaper alongside the broadsheet.

Visual evidence also increases in both range and subject matter. Painting in England during the seventeenth century continued to be mainly concerned with portraiture; with few exceptions, portraits were the principal stock-in-trade of all artists working in England, whether native or foreign. The patronage of art became a growing royal enthusiasm from the accession of James I onwards; foreign artists of international stature, like Rubens and van Dyck were welcomed and lavishly rewarded. Inevitably, portraiture became fashionable amongst the wealthier classes, from great nobles to rich City merchants, and individual portraits, family groups and delicate miniatures were executed in profusion to meet the seemingly insatiable demand for personal images. By the middle of the century, artists of stature had evolved from craftsmen into men of influence and social consequence. Fortunately for the costume historian there are many artists – from influential court painters to provincial journeymen – who provide images of fashionable dress as worn by the social categories of those who could afford to have themselves portrayed.

However, this rich and diverse range of seventeenth-century portraiture poses certain problems, as does the growing importance of the portrait painter. For example, let us take a group of figures painted at a known date, say 1665, and ask the following questions. Are the figures depicted fashionable city dwellers or provincial conservatives? Are they elderly, wearing a style of dress once fashionable to which they cling for reasons of habit or sentiment, or have they adapted a current fashion to fit this 'fly in amber' image of themselves? Are they young, rich, experimental? Are they from the lower orders in society, or do they practice a profession which dictates a certain style of dress and distorts contemporary fashion? Or do they subscribe to an artistic and social admiration for a form of stylized dress, perhaps pseudo-classical or pastoral, which they and/or their chosen artist wished to translate into a timeless costume, thus conveying to posterity their ability to transcend the ephemeral modes of a particular year, decade or era? These are the kind of questions that – with slight variations – have to be asked about dress in portraiture from this time onwards; sometimes the answers are clear, at other times less so.

Fashions changed relatively slowly in the seventeenth century; new styles were assimilated at different rates depending on age and status. This social digestion of fashion is easier to understand than the admiration for the classical and pastoral worlds as translated into a stylized 'romantic' dress. Van Dyck introduced this theme in the 1630s via a process of reducing the minutiae of fashionable detail in his portraits; by concentrating on the lyrical, shimmering folds of material and adding vaguely 'antique' touches (billowing white chemise sleeves, asymmetrical draperies etc.) the artist virtually invented a fashionable 'uniform' for his upper-class sitters. This kind of artistic convention was continued and accelerated by Lely, Kneller and other major (and minor) artists working in England from the 1640s onwards, well into the eighteenth century. Within our chronological survey, there are certain portraits which contain elements of this stylization. Yet, however much the artist wished to omit the ephemeral elements of fashionable dress, the sitter never whole-heartedly co-operated; hairstyles, jewellery, the fit of a sleeve, these and other small details place each individual firmly into a particular period. Ironically, children, whose costume has often been described as that of miniature adults, were subjected less frequently than their parents to stylized portraiture. For this reason children are included in this book, providing accurate evidence, on a small scale, of fashions that their elders wore but sometimes preferred to discard when being recorded for posterity.

At certain times in the seventeenth and early eighteenth centuries, even the selective use of children as miniature models for adult fashion is not enough to provide a comprehensive survey of fashionable dress. The 1650s, the 1690s and the first two decades of the eighteenth century are particularly bare of useful portraits, but, by the late seventeenth century it is possible to refer to French fashion plates to fill some of the gaps. Examples of such plates, which began to appear in the 1670s, are included because the post-Restoration English court looked to France for supplies of luxury fabrics, styles in dress and accessories.

Other important illustrative sources in the seventeenth century include woodcuts and engravings taken from books and broadsheets about topical events; although crudely executed, they capture the overall look of the participants and the line of their clothes. However, such engravings of major public events may have been executed by someone who was not a witness, working with inaccurate descriptions of the occasion and its personalities. Caution must also be used when looking at engraved portraits of distinguished people; these were often copied from earlier portraits but given the later publication date. Sophisticated engravings, often published in a series, provide more detailed information; the work of painstaking and accurate artists working in England, like Hollar (in the 1640s and 1650s) and Marcellus Laroon II (in the late 1680s) are particularly useful. These artists, however, were more interested in recording a range of existing styles and types than suggesting new fashions. Although fashion plates were circulating in England before the end of the century and were, perhaps, influencing fashionable taste with regard to new colours, materials and styles of dress, it was not until the last quarter of the eighteenth century that a regular series of English fashion plates appeared to challenge the supremacy of the French.

The eighteenth century has been described as the 'coming of age' of British painting; for the first time in our history native artists of first-class talent (and some with international reputations) appeared. The work of such great portraitists as Gainsborough and Reynolds comes immediately to mind, and perhaps our view of the period is coloured – some might say distorted – by an image which they help to perpetuate, of civilized felicity enjoyed in fact only by a small section of society. Yet, as well as portraiture – both formal and informal – commissioned by an aristocratic clientèle, there is also the kind of portraiture ordered by an increasingly important middle class; this includes portraits of individuals, and conversation pieces, often by lesser artists, but sometimes by artists of originality and vigour such as Hogarth. In addition, we are fortunate in the wide range of genre scenes which exist, serving to balance our knowledge of upper- and middle-class costume by giving information on dress and manners through the whole social spectrum. With this veritable outpouring of works of art, however, a word of caution should be sounded. Dates and attributions often change in what can seem sometimes to be a game of art-historical musical chairs; even when a painting appears to be firmly dated on the canvas, or by exhibition, the actual work may have taken several years to complete, or it may have been altered by later additions. This is true of all periods, but it ought perhaps to be stressed in the eighteenth century, when not only is there a vast increase in the number of works of art produced, but there are also problems with regard to the composition of a painting especially when it involved the services of a drapery painter.

The drapery painter made his living by painting the costume only, a custom introduced by van Dyck, and carried on by Lely and Kneller. In *The Spectator* (1712) Addison explains the practice: 'Great Masters in Painting never care for drawing People in the Fashion, as very well knowing that the Head-dress or Periwig that now prevails and gives a Grace to their Portraiture at present, will make a very odd Figure and perhaps look monstrous in the eyes of Posterity'. The low ebb of painting during the reign of George I, which Horace Walpole later recalled, he attributed to the stranglehold on portraiture by Kneller, an artist whose widespread use of drapery painters and stock poses contributes to the dreary uniformity of much of his work.

The use of drapery painters and conventional, somewhat hackneyed poses, persisted well into the second half of the eighteenth century, and can be seen even in the work of a great artist like Reynolds when his sympathies were not engaged, especially in his portraits of society ladies. One of Reynolds's beliefs, as expounded in his famous *Discourses*, was that dress in portraiture should be timeless and above fashion; this partly explains his use of 'classical' draperies in many portraits, particularly of the 1760s and 1770s. Given the propensity of his sitters to keep to their fashionable hairstyles, corsetry and the indefinable 'lines' of the contemporary mode, it proved impossible to achieve a kind of costume above the fleeting whims of high fashion. Another way of escaping from contemporary dress in painting was to return to the costume of the historic past (the late sixteenth and early seventeenth centuries were particularly popular periods) and the exotic present, especially that of the orient, mainly Turkey. The historian of dress must therefore be aware that when looking at eighteenth-century portraiture, there will be a considerable amount of fancy dress, sometimes real (due to the immense popularity of the masquerade), sometimes part of the current artistic vocabulary, and sometimes mingled with fashionable costume.

In the first two decades of the eighteenth century there are relatively few dated or datable pictorial sources for dress. Apart from the sometimes almost 'Identikit' portraits by Kneller and his contemporaries (only a few of these are firmly dated), there are a few rather stiff family groups, some portrait drawings and the occasional genre scene and landscape with figures. In the 1720s and 1730s, with the introduction of the conversation piece – groups of identified people, sometimes indoors and sometimes outside – it is possible to see a more lively and detailed depiction of the costume of the upper and middle classes. Favourite themes include somewhat self-conscious tea-parties, (a fashionable occupation which also served to show off the latest styles in interior decoration) and groups of families and friends out of doors surveying their estates with proprietorial satisfaction. Such scenes which depict a range of fashionable activities serve as a particularly useful source of information on both formal and informal costume. Conversation pieces, however, show society on its best behaviour, and if we want to see *la comédie humaine* in all its aspects both high and low, there is the incomparable Hogarth; no other artist has such a satirical and yet sympathetic view of mankind, or so uses dress to define status and personality, to point a moral and adorn a tale.

By the middle of the century there were large numbers of artists working in the British Isles to supply the growing demand for portraits. The dress historian should take note not just of the works of the fashionable metropolitan society painter, but also look at portraits painted by artists resident in the provinces; in the latter case, with a predominantly middle-class clientèle, the costume depicted is often more likely to reflect reality, less prone to follow the sort of artistic fads which romanticized the sitter.

During the first half of the century, Britain continued to depend on visiting foreign artists, who brought with them not just their international experience, but new ways of looking at British dress and manners; their practice and teaching helped to inspire a native school of art, particularly from the mid-century onwards. By the late eighteenth century there were a number of British artists resident abroad, particularly in Italy, who found it profitable to paint groups of their countrymen on the Grand Tour, following in the footsteps of such Italian artists as Batoni who had a lucrative practice of this sort.

As well as portraits, both of individuals and groups, in a range of media – oils, pastels, watercolour, line drawing etc. – the dress historian will find a useful source of information in the work of the caricaturists. Caricature, although a form of art invented by the Italians, became a virtual English monopoly from the 1760s onwards. The comparative freedom of English government and society allowed caricaturists licence to make fun of politics and manners, including the foibles of fashion. While it is true that caricatures are often grossly exaggerated, the artists were perceptive enough to fasten on to the essentials of 'extreme' forms of high fashion, such as the macaroni styles of the 1770s.

At about the same time, the first regularly produced fashion plates were beginning to be published in England. While subject to a certain amount of stylization, these somewhat stilted fashion images add considerably to our knowledge of the bewildering array of female costume, as the pace of sartorial change quickened during the last quarter of the eighteenth century. Fashion plates of a higher quality from France were also available either in their original form or copied by the English fashion magazines. The French *magasins des modes* ceased to appear in 1793 after the demise of the monarchy, and were only restored in the late 1790s by which time the English fashion plate, under the aegis of *émigrés* like Heideloff, had immensely improved.

The work of the artist is one of the most important primary sources for the historian of dress, for it reveals not just the details of costume and its visual impact, but *how* and *when* certain styles were worn; it makes intellectual and artistic statements which tell us much about the century's image of itself. Visual sources, however, supply only a part – if an important one – of the story of dress in the eighteenth century. In addition to the kind of documentary and literary sources that existed in previous centuries – published and unpublished inventories and accounts, letters, diaries, plays and poetry – we have, for the first time, the novel. This new literary form, described by Jane Austen as a 'work in which the most thorough knowledge of human nature, the happiest delineation of its varieties, the liveliest effusions of wit and humour are conveyed to the world in the best chosen language', was as much about manners as emotions, revealing society to itself in a kind of mirror image. In eighteenth-century novels dress plays an important part; it is described as interesting in its own right (see Richardson in particular), it furthers plot and character (see Fielding and Smollett) and it is used to pinpoint social distinctions and the comedy of manners, as in the novels of Fanny Burney, and, later, Jane Austen.

We also have, throughout the century – but rather more in the latter half – a sequence of surviving garments. These are mainly of upper-class provenance, but there is also – increasingly as the century progresses – some middle-class costume, and a few items of working-class dress. Although much eighteenth-century dress has been altered, there is much to be gained by looking at what survives; not only does it help in furthering our knowledge of the actual styles worn, their fabrics, colours, cut and construction, but it puts flesh on the visual and written evidence of the history of costume.

It is when we turn to the nineteenth century that we are almost overwhelmed by the amount of material available to the dress historian; it may be true that we know more about dress during the last century than about any other period, even, perhaps, our own, as we cannot, as yet, stand back and view our own time dispassionately, picking out the themes which will prove important only with the passage of time. For the nineteenth century there is a wealth of documentary material, both published and unpublished, about the costume of all sections of society. The Industrial Revolution, brutal in much of its impact on the lives of the poor, can be said to have inspired the work of crusading journalists and parliamentary commissions in documenting the existence of the poorest members of society, including their clothing. Further information on working and occupational dress – evidence of the period's interest in the wider community – can be gained from such early nineteenth-century illustrated costume books as Pyne's *Costume of Great Britain* (1808), and Walker's *Costume of Yorkshire* (1814). There are vast numbers of published accounts, letters and diaries which give factual information (and personal experience) of the dress of all classes. In addition there are works by philosophers such as Carlyle (*Sartor Resartus* 1838) and economists such as Veblen (*The Theory of the Leisure Class* 1899) which analyse the significance of dress in society. Among the many literary sources of the nineteenth century, the foremost is the novel, a flexible and powerful instrument in the dissection of an often rapidly changing social order. Novelists of the stature of Dickens, Trollope, Mrs Gaskell, George Eliot and Arnold Bennett etc. illuminate the part played by dress in metropolitan and provincial societies.

As we would expect, the visual sources are overwhelming in their variety. They include the garments themselves, for a large number survive in museums and private collections. These are particularly useful when studied in conjunction with patterns found in tailoring guides, and – after the mid-century – in fashion magazines. Yet for an understanding of the *total* look – dress, accessories, hairstyle, appropriate underwear and correct posture – one must turn to painted, printed and photographed images.

For the upper and middle classes, an obvious visual source is to be found in portraiture. Although some artists and sculptors preferred to give their sitters a 'classical'/'historical' guise to set them above the mediocrity of everyday life, most painters, even when critical of contemporary costume, were content to depict it in their portraits, reserving their grand style for other types of painting. In the hands of a master like Ingres, even a simple pencil sketch can communicate much information on cut, construction and drape,

while an oil painting can convey even more about colour, pattern and texture. From the most detailed work, it is possible to distinguish a satin from a plain-weave silk, or a blonde lace from one made of linen. Where the artist *does* attempt to idealize his sitter, however, the result is often a simplification of dress, draperies, fabric patterns and hairstyles; the historian of costume should be aware of this occasional tendency, but there are far fewer examples of it than in the eighteenth century.

In some ways a more accurate rendering of dress is to be found in narrative paintings of contemporary life, a tradition dating back to Hogarth, and given new impetus by the work of artists such as Frith and Hicks. The subjects were deliberately chosen to demonstrate a wide range of characters in typical dress, and they are a most valuable source of information. It must be stated, however, that there was a limit to what was socially acceptable, and there is not all that much of the seamier side of life unless it is depicted with a sentimental varnish. Only in the 1870s and 1880s did a school of social realism enjoy a brief popularity with artists like Herkomer and Fildes who tried to depict the real poverty and misery of contemporary life; even they, however, succumbed to sentiment and melodrama, and their dramatic use of light and shade tends to blur details of dress. By the 1890s painstaking detail and social realism were almost superseded by the painterly, atmospheric designs of artists influenced by the Impressionists, and inspired by the concept of 'art for art's sake'. Even an artist like Sargent, while brilliantly conveying the character, pose and silhouette of his fashionable sitters, often presents their dress in a shimmering haze of brushstrokes, expressing general effect rather than specific detail.

Fashion plates are another source of information. They vary enormously in quality, from the fine, often hand-coloured plates of the early nineteenth century, to the commercialized steel engravings, colour lithographs and prints issued by mass-produced fashion publications from the mid-century onwards; in the latter case, the colours depicted can often be misleading, since the range was limited by the print-maker's palette. The usefulness of fashion plates lies in their visual information concerning costume and accessories complete with descriptions in contemporary terminology. However, although they depict actual garments, the illustrations are highly stylized, for they aimed to show the fashionable ideal rather than the reality.

A complementary viewpoint is provided by the caricaturists, many of whom depicted fashion and the fashionable. Through the wit of artists like Gillray, Cruikshank and du Maurier, we are shown not just the fashion plate ideal, but clothing as it was being worn, albeit in a highly exaggerated form. Some changes in fashion – like, for example, a temporary shortening of the hemline – seem imperceptible to the modern eye, but through the intensified vision of the caricaturist we are able to recognize that a change has taken place, something that must have been glaringly obvious to contemporaries.

In the first half of the nineteenth century caricatures were usually published and sold individually, but the removal of the paper tax in 1861 produced a flood of illustrated newspapers and journals, providing new outlets for writers, caricaturists and illustrators alike. These publications are a mine of information, not just for fashion but for dress generally; in illustrations to such subjects as popular fiction and advertisements, ordinary people of all classes are shown in a variety of situations and portrayed without the distorting bias of the fashion plate. Outside such magazine illustrations, this combination of social range and various formal/informal situations can only be found in the later developments of photography, the other major visual source for the study of Victorian dress.

It was in 1837 that Louis Daguerre first produced a clear, permanent photographic image, and within a few years his 'daguerrotype' technique was widely used to create small mirror-image portraits. Although unsophisticated by later standards (poses were stiff and wooden due to the fact that exposures lasted up to a minute) these photographs from the 1840s can provide surprisingly clear details of contemporary costume. Photography became cheaper in the following decade and thus available to more people, but the real impetus came with the craze for *cartes de visite* in the 1860s; portrait photographs of relatives, friends and celebrities were printed the size of visiting cards and sold in thousands. Later, new technical advances led to the development of the snapshot, and – via the new continuous film – to photographs of crowd scenes, outdoor groups and portraits, often taken without the knowledge of the subjects, and therefore more relaxed and less self-conscious. Such photographs are unique sources for the study of informal, occupational and working-class dress, although they lack the fine detail of the studio portrait. By the end of the century, photography had changed from being just a curiosity to perhaps the most important source for the appearance of all classes in society; major developments in the twentieth century were to confirm this status.

When we reach the twentieth century we have a bewilderingly wide range of closely dated visual evidence to draw upon: paintings, portraits, drawings, engravings, cartoons, book illustrations, posters, sculpture, fashion plates, advertisements and trade catalogues, and an additional dimension is offered by ciné film, the cinema and television. These sources provide details of fashionable silhouettes and the styles of beauty favoured in each decade, and give us an impression of that elusive and indescribable element, the 'atmosphere' of a period. Fortunately for the student of costume history, many original garments from the twentieth century have survived in near-perfect condition, and can be viewed in museum displays and exhibitions. This opportunity allows the look of garments, their shapes, proportions, materials, colours and decoration to be seen in three dimensions. However, a static figure, usually behind glass, can only *suggest* how the outfit might have looked when it was worn. To appreciate what the wearer looked like in such clothes, how they behaved and how they affected the wearers' posture and gestures, and how well they expressed the fashionable ideal, it is necessary to look at contemporary illustrations.

Photography only began to be widely used to illustrate fashion from around 1900. Since then, fashion photography has developed as a distinct branch of this form of art, and provides a continuous and invaluable source of visual information on high fashion during this century. Most of these photographs have become available in the form of published illustrations in newspapers and magazines, but some archives of the original photographs are now housed in museums. Photography has gradually replaced the traditional methods of fashion illustration, although drawings and sketches are still used to some extent today. The engraved plate, lithograph or print, often coloured by hand, had little life beyond the 1920s, but, during the first three decades of the century it was still used to illustrate the more expensive fashion periodicals such as the *Gazette du Bon Ton*. Fashion plates, drawings, and, on occasion, fashion photographs have the disadvantage, as a source of information, in stressing the ideal image often to the point of distortion at the expense of reality. Consequently they need to be used with care, balanced by more straightforward images, such as firmly dated professional studio and press photographs, amateur snapshots and family groups.

The widespread use of photography contributed to, though was not wholly responsible for, the decline of painted, drawn or sculpted portraits in the twentieth century. In addition, the move away from representational painting and sculpture towards more abstract and conceptual art forms has meant that costume historians have fewer works of art to which they can go for realistic depictions of appearance and clothing. Portrait painting, of the traditional kind, continued, but generally depicted the wealthy strata of society, and such works are not easily accessible to students. Sculpture is equally problematic (being, on the whole, less representational than painting), but one minor but significant branch of the art should be considered: the shop-window display mannequin, a twentieth-century phenomenon. Like fashion illustrations, these figures reveal the aspirations of a period – facial features, shapes of body, and styles of posture.

New techniques of printing and reproduction have made a wider range of visual material available during this century, and the many magazines, books, shop catalogues and advertisements represent additional areas which can be explored. These also provide useful written evidence to supplement the visual statements that they make. There is a superabundance of written commentary on fashion in the twentieth century, ranging from the hyperbole of trade advertisements to the often waspish comments by published diarists and authors of memoirs. The seemingly insatiable demand for the 'inside story' has led everyone, from royalty to fashion models to commit their reminiscences to paper. These reveal, often inadvertently, the importance of fashion and changing styles of dress in the lives of their authors. Placed alongside novels, magazine and news-paper articles, they help to fill the gap in twentieth-century archives which has developed as wills and inventories concentrate upon money and property rather than clothes, bills are discarded as meaningless wastepaper, and telephone calls replace letters as the most regular means of communicating information.

Given the wealth of visual information available to the dress historian for the period of almost 700 years which this book covers, the authors are only too aware of the restrictions imposed on them by having to choose a limited selection of images from the six volumes of the *Visual History of Costume* series. The illustrations have been chosen to reflect the main developments in costume, to make statements about personal appearance and the desired image, to indicate social customs and manners relating to dress, and to reveal some of the problems which the historian of dress will come across when studying the visual sources of any period. As well as describing the main fashion changes from the late medieval period to the present day, the chief purpose behind this book, as of the original series, is to show how visual evidence may be read and assessed, with a view to recognizing, understanding and dating the costume portrayed.

THE HISTORY OF COSTUME

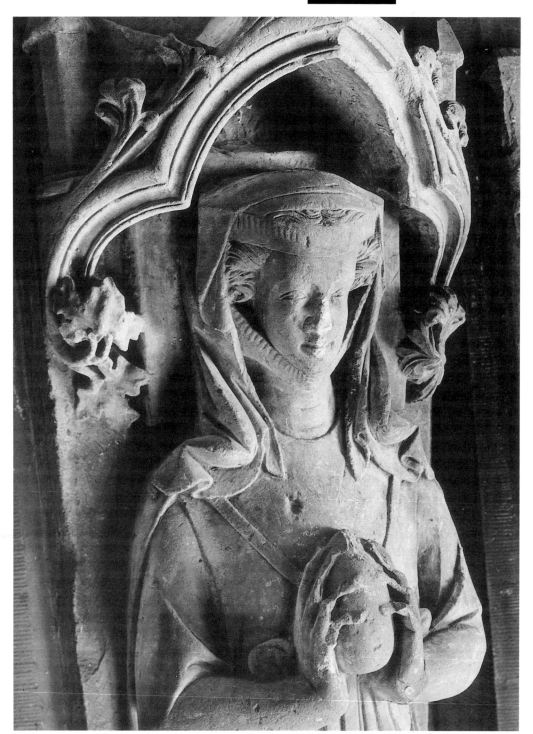

1. A lady of the Heriz (?) family, c. 1300–10

English School, effigy

Note At this date it is impossible to draw hard-and-fast divisions between the fashions of the thirteenth and fourteenth centuries. The structure of the headdress recalls that of the earlier century, while its revealing of so much hair looks forward into the later century.

Head The headdress is the most elaborate part of a woman's outfit at this time. Here it is composed of a series of (probably) linen bands with fluted edges wound round the head and under the chin, while allowing the waved and curled hair to show at the top and sides of the head. A shoulder-length veil is worn on top.

Body The outermost layer, which is not much in evidence at this time, is a cloak worn at the points of the shoulders and prevented from slipping back and choking its wearer by the looping of the thumbs through its cord at chest level; this is a relic of the behaviour of the previous century, as is bunching up the cloak in folds and holding it against the body with the forearms. Beneath is a sleeveless supertunic which fits well around the chest and round the base of the neck, but falls loosely below the bust. The arms are covered by the sleeves of a tunic worn as the final visible layer of women's clothing; as yet its sleeves fit only on the forearms, and the bunching of the upper parts will be developed into a shorter oversleeve by 1320. The combination of cloak, supertunic and tunic forms the basis for the fourteenth-century idea of a suit, known as a '*robe*'. The underwear would consist of a linen smock, and stockings worn with flat shoes.

2. Lady Joan Cobham, *c.* 1320–5
English School, effigy

Note This figure shows an early attempt at making dress fit more tightly.

Head The hair appears as curls at the temples and is dressed somewhat unconvincingly into sharp points about the ears; these points have no effect on the angle of the outer edges of the wimple, which is presumably meant to be attached to them under the shoulder-length veil.

Body The supertunic is developing new features: a more clearly scooped neckline; three-quarter-length sleeves with a slight peak at the cuffs; and a tendency to 'bind' across the chest as an attempt is made to make it fit more closely. As yet, however, only the sleeves of the tunic fit well, because they are so precisely buttoned.

Accessories Shoes with pointed toes appear from among the folds at the hem.

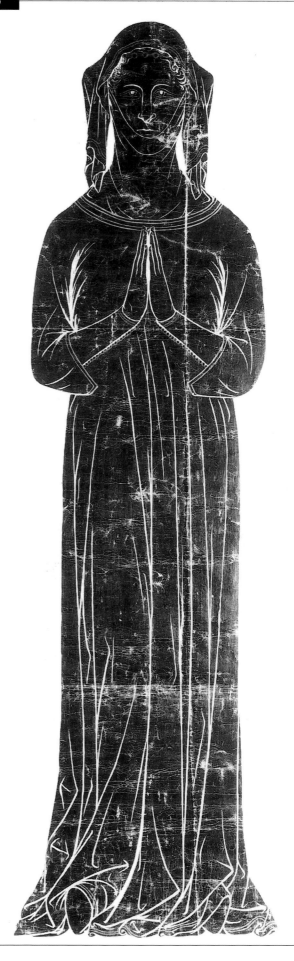

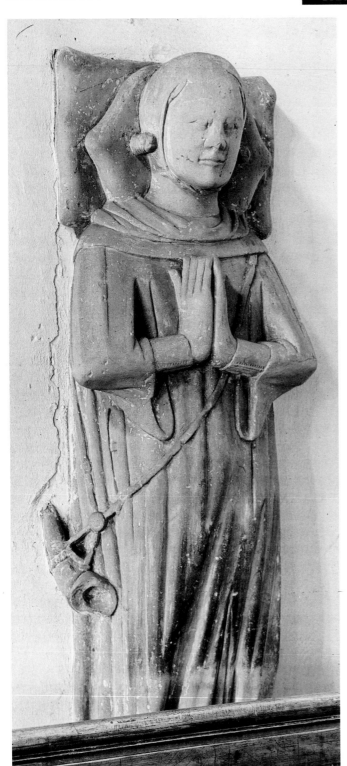

3. An unknown official of Sherwood Forest, *c.* 1325–30
English School, effigy

Note This figure combines fashionable dress with symbols of office, and it shows that the tunic and supertunic were basically the same for both sexes.

Head The man's hair, except for two sausage-shaped curls at the sides, is confined within a coif which has a narrow edging and is tied beneath his chin. This coif is probably part of his 'uniform'.

Body Around the shoulders is the hood with shoulder cape which remained in fashion until the end of the century. When the hood was worn pulled up on to the head, it looked like a loose Balaclava helmet with a small cape. Beneath is a rather loose supertunic with three-quarter-length sleeves which now have a more pronounced bell-shape at the ends. The original supertunic would probably have been in *mi-parti*.

Unseen but present beneath the forester's clothing would be a linen shirt, linen drawers, stockings of woollen cloth, and boots or shoes with pointed toes.

Accessories On a belt slung over the left shoulder is a hunting horn, another part of the 'uniform'.

4. A girl having her hair dressed, *c.* 1335–40
English School, manuscript illumination

Note The thick comb used in the Middle Ages lies at the girl's knee.

Head The girl's hair is parted in the centre before being plaited with ribbons and bunched up at the side of the head. The maid's lower status is shown by her having no such elaborate arrangement to disturb her veil.

Body Both the girl and her maid are in their tunics, which still fit well only on the lower arms. The girl, however, has a lower and hence more fashionable neckline. The tunics are belted at natural waist level.

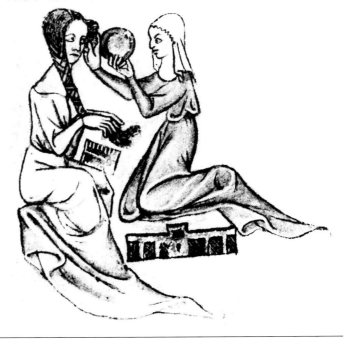

5. Male figure from the Percy Tomb, *c.* 1340

English School, effigy

Head The hair is worn in a short fringe and corkscrew curls in front of the ears. The hood is worn on top and its point is now long enough to be brought forward and to reach almost to the wearer's left elbow.

Body The man wears a tunic which seems a bit too long and a bit too tight in the body as it crinkles and binds at the same time. The buttons and buttonholes on the lower sleeve are quite clearly carved. The skirt of the tunic must be open at the centre front, as was usual at this date, because it manages to reveal most of his right leg while concealing most of his left.

Accessories A purse with a dagger thrust through it is worn at the front in exactly the way Henry Knighton said dissolute women wore them when they appeared at tournaments in 1348, dressed in men's clothes. This figure also has short boots, laced across the top of the foot.

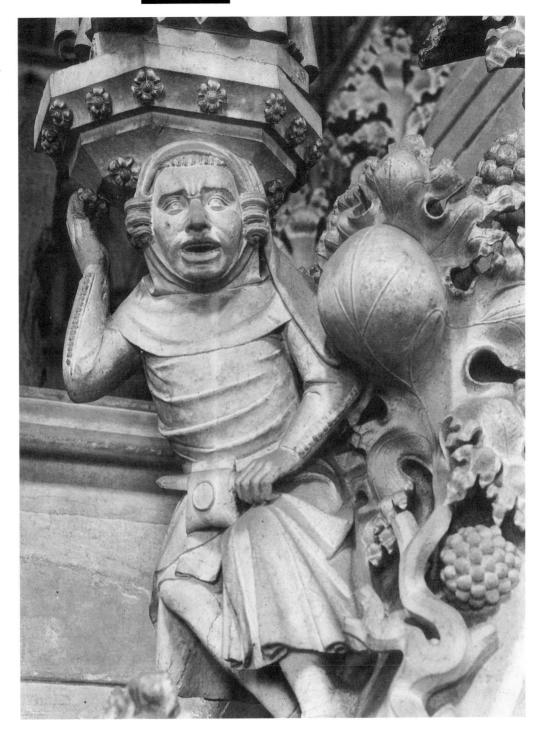

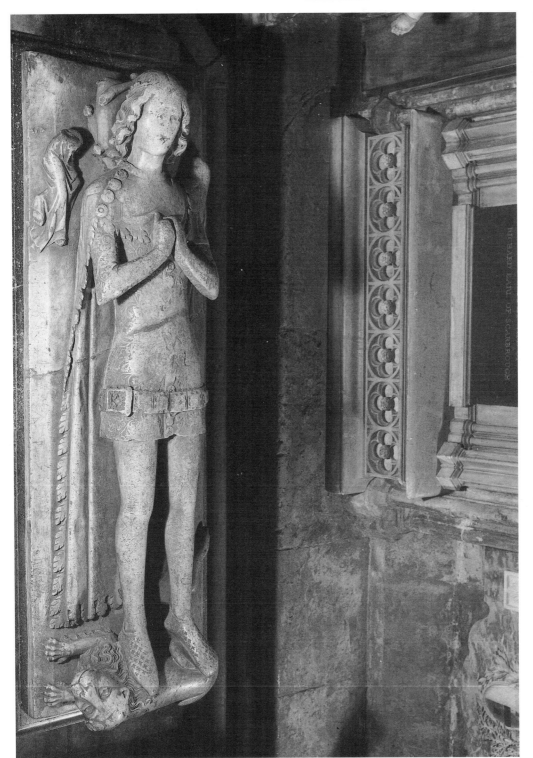

6. Called Prince William of Hatfield, *c.* 1344
English School, effigy

Note William, the second son of Edward III and Philippa of Hainault, died in 1344 at the age of eight. The dress of this figure, which offers us a rare glimpse of the elaborate textiles used, accords well with the traditional identification.

Head The hair is parted in the centre and waved almost to the shoulders. There is a small circlet on top.

Body The prince wears a cloak with leaf-shaped dagging, fastened with four large flower-shaped buttons on the right shoulder, and flung back over the left shoulder. Dagging was one of the follies of 1344, according to John of Reading; he also disapproved of short, tight garments such as the supertunic we see here. Although the surface of the stone is worn, it is still possible to make out the scrolling plant pattern of the textile; such a pattern could be woven or embroidered.

Accessories A belt with large studs and a large square buckle, decorated with a stylized flower, is worn at the top of the thighs. The legs must now be covered in tights rather than stockings. The ankle-length boots are elaborately punched with small cruciform holes.

7. Robert Braunche and his wives Letice and Margaret
c. 1350–5
Flemish School, brass rubbing

Note Robert Braunche was a merchant of King's Lynn, trading with the Low Countries from where this brass must have been imported. Although he died in 1364, the small figures in the feast scene at the bottom below have the whiplash stance and short tunics of the early 1350s.

Head Braunche's hair is worn in large curls over his ears. His wives' hair is worn in two vertical columns at the side of the face, under a fine veil, and another veil is worn as a wimple.

Body Braunche wears his hood down over his shoulders, on top of a waisted ankle-length supertunic, slit up the front to the thighs. The tippets of the supertunic sleeves are almost lost against the background; they reach his knees.

His wives wear much longer supertunics which they have gathered up to one side to reveal their lavishly patterned tunics. The pattern can be seen on the tunic sleeves to be a scrolling plant (*compare* Fig. 6). Their tippets stop short of the knee.

Accessories The pointed tips of the women's toes can be seen; Braunche has longer toes on his short boots.

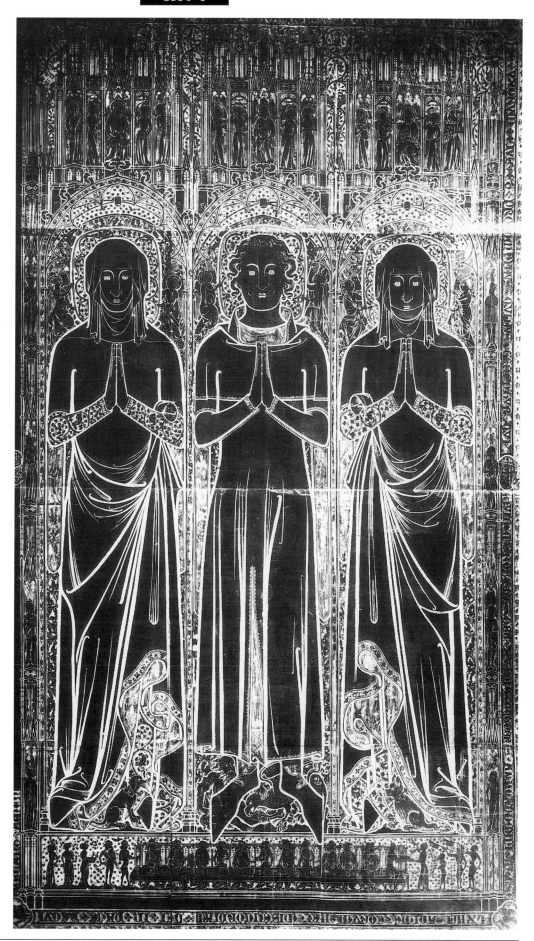

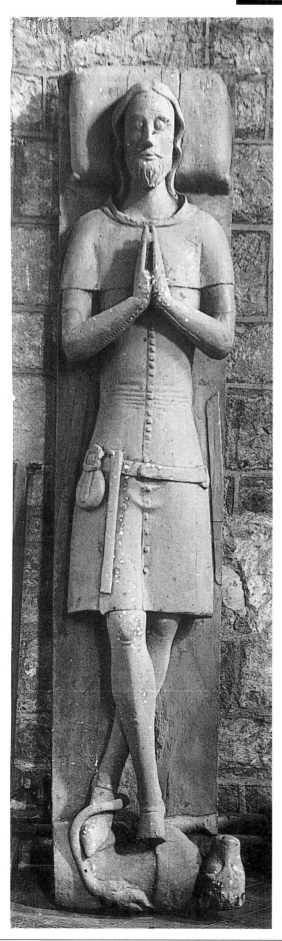

8. Walter Helyon, franklin of Marcle, *c.* 1355–60
English School, effigy

Note Walter Helyon was alive in 1357 and this effigy probably dates from about that time. A franklin was not a particularly important person in rural society (he was freeborn but a non-noble landowner on a fairly small scale), and his clothing can therefore be expected to be a bit old-fashioned.

Head The hair reaches to the shoulders and there is a pointed beard.

Body The hood is worn around the shoulders. Beneath is a supertunic so tight at the waist that it wrinkles there; the skirt section is more generously cut from the hips to the knees. This particular garment is interesting because of the relationship which it displays between the circumference of the area to be clothed, the tightness of the clothing, and the size and spacing of the buttons: the sleeves are the smallest area and have the smallest and most closely set buttons; the 'bodice' and the skirt use buttons of the same size, but they are much more closely set when required to take the strain of the tight fit of the bodice.

9. Queen Philippa of Hainault, wife of Edward III, *c.* 1365–7
Hennequin of Liège

Note This effigy was made just before the queen died in 1367 in her mid-fifties. It makes no attempt to flatter her, or to disguise the fact that skin-tight bodices suited only the young and slender.

Head Although damaged, the headdress can be seen to have consisted of two 'columns' of plaited hair framing the face, with a band running between them. The whole structure was probably extremely rigid, and has more in common with the headdresses of contemporary France and Flanders than with the headdresses of her English subjects.

Body A cloak is worn out at the points of the shoulders, giving a clear view of the supertunic (or tunic?), with its wide neckline and centre front lacing.

Accessories A narrow belt is worn round the hips, and dips down under the stomach.

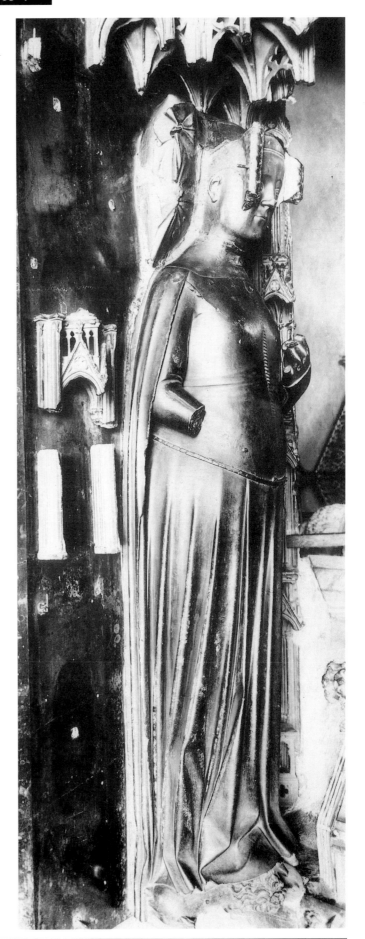

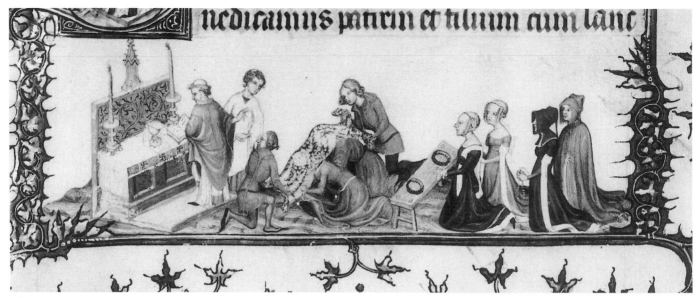

ncdicanius partan et filuun cum lauc

10. A wedding, *c.* 1380
The Parement Master

Note This scene shows French fashions.

Head The men are clean-shaven and have their hair curled round the back of their necks. Two of the women wear *chaperons* with front flaps pointed at the chin; the pointed effect is repeated in the stiff plaits worn in front of the ears of the other women.

Body The men wear mid-thigh-length *surcotes* with tight waists and padded chests. The *chaperons* are too small to be pulled on to the head; one is worn folded and draped around the shoulders. The women wear the tightly fitting dresses with wide necklines which were called *cotes hardies*, and white *cornettes* hanging from above the elbow. One woman wears a cloak, which was a fairly common thing for middle- and working-class women to do when they went to church.

Accessories The men have belts at the hips, and tights or stockings with leather soles.

11. Male and female weepers from the tomb of Edward III, 1377–86
John Orchard (?)

Note Although the king died in 1377, his tomb was not completed until 1386.

Head The man's hair is worn in a centre parting and drawn out in small curls above the ears. The woman's hair is dressed in two stiff plaits with a jewelled band, perhaps a link between their supports, crossing the top of the forehead.

Body There appears to be no distinction made in the overlap-and-button arrangement in the dress of men and women. The woman wears the usual long-sleeved dress with tippets, but extra interest is created by the pocket-like slits below the buttons. The man's supertunic follows the usual pattern in its buttoning, but the chest is less aggressively padded than it would have been in the 1370s. The rather tight-kneed look of the male figure suggests the problems encountered by the 'heroes' of a satirical poem written in 1388: their hose were so tightly laced to their doublets, and their toes were so long that they could not kneel in church without great care for fear of 'hortyng of here hose' (hurting their hose).

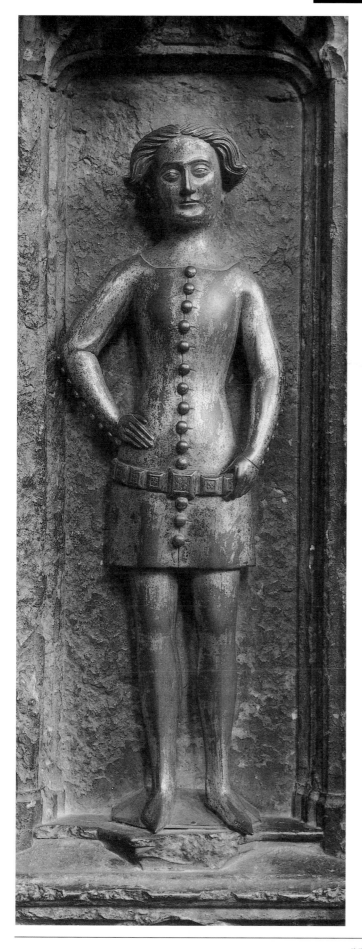
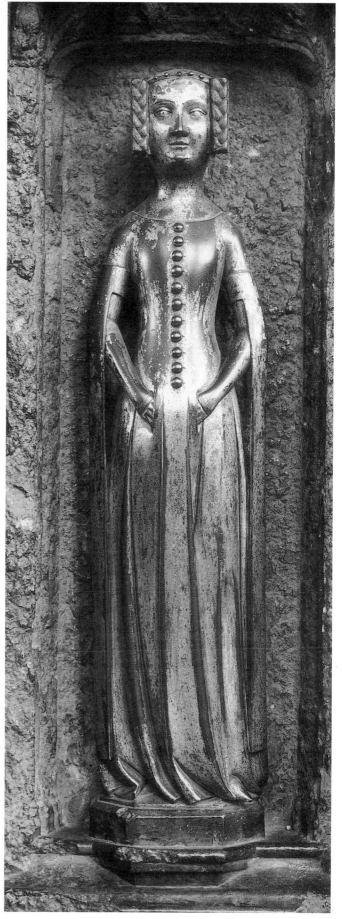

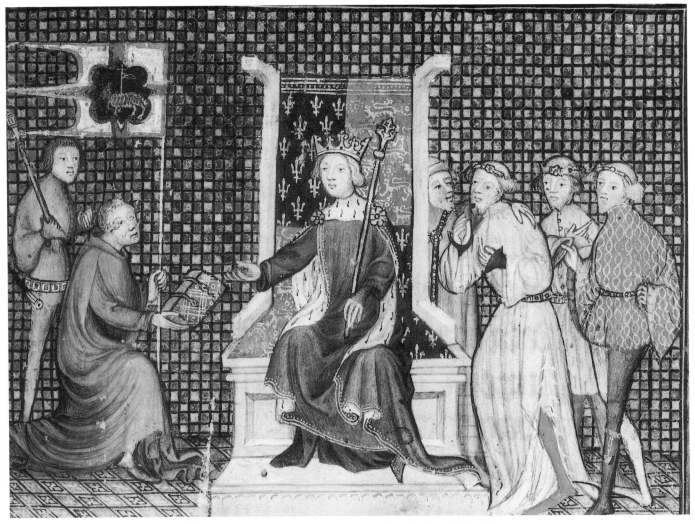

12. **The monk Philippe de Maizieres presenting a book to Richard II, 1395–6**

French School, manuscript illumination

Head The hair is almost shoulder-length but the dandies of the court have fluffed theirs around their ears, and wear jewelled circlets on top. Forked beards are becoming increasingly common.

Body The padded doublet of the mace-bearer on the left explains the shape of the chests of gowns of the courtiers on the right. Collars are beginning to choke their wearers and the cuffs of the tunic sleeves are widening into nuisances. The sleeves of the gowns are also widening. Dagging has been re-introduced up the side of the longest gown.

Accessories With the doublet the belt is worn at hip level; with the gown, at natural waist level. Hose can be in *mi-parti* or plain. The very long toes of these hose are rarely depicted but often denounced as having to be chained up to the knee before their wearer can walk; perhaps the chain worn by the man on the right is for that purpose. Richard II bought whalebone for the points of his shoes in 1393–4.

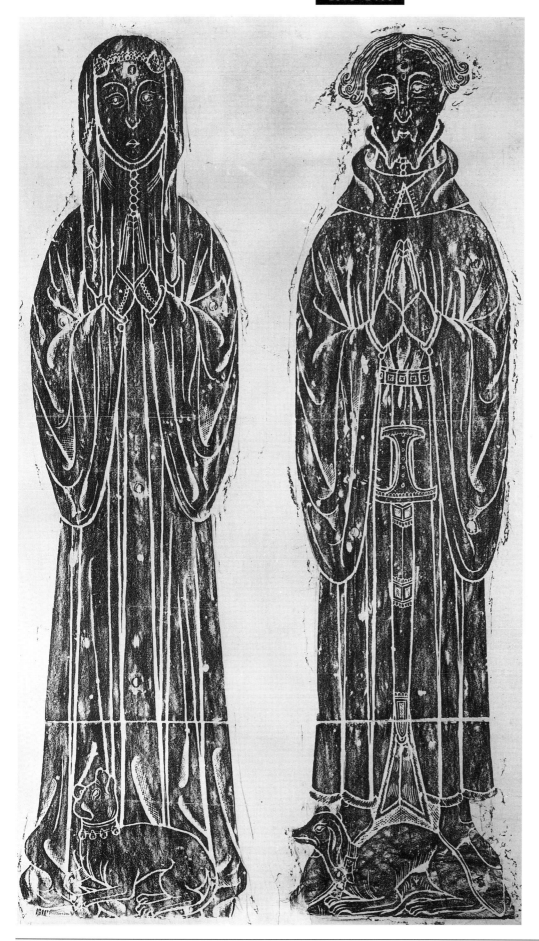

13. Unknown man and his wife, *c.* 1395–1400
English School, brass rubbing

Note These figures show very clearly how the dress of men and women followed the same aesthetic principles at this time.

Head The man's hair, beard and moustache are all quite fashionable. The woman's headdress, a single veil with fluted front edge worn over two small horns of hair on the forehead, shows that some women had tired of the more elaborate arrangements of several veils.

Body Both wear gowns with collars buttoned up the neck and bag-shaped sleeves buttoned at the wrists. They also have mitten-like undersleeves. The differences lie in the vestigial buttoned hood on the man's shoulders, the length of his gown, its being open at the calves and its being belted.

Accessories The fashionably studded belt supports the short sword carried by civilians. The shoes are cut away at the top and have clearly defined soles.

Chaucer reciting before an elegant audience, *c.* 1400
Colour illustration, between pages 128 and 129.

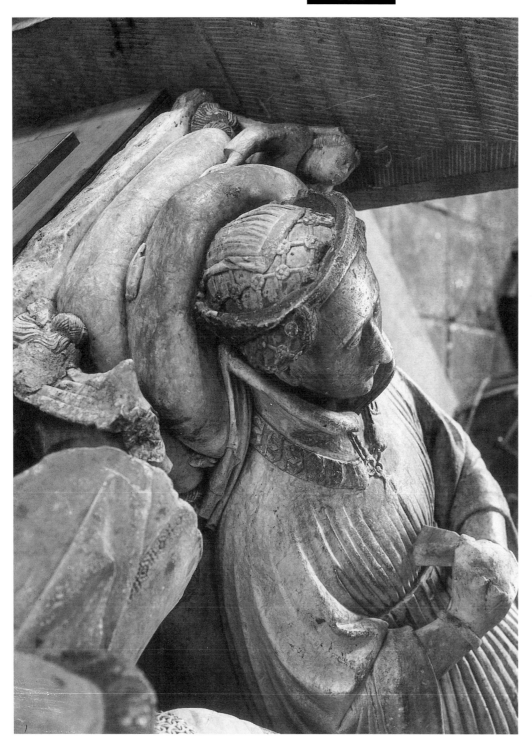

14. Lady Mainwaring, *c.* 1410
English School, effigy

Note There is some confusion over the Christian name of the lady's husband, but general agreement that he died in 1410.

Head Lady Mainwaring wears an elaborately decorated caul which forms two large 'bumps' over the ears, and is topped by a circlet. A shoulder-length veil is pleated into a narrow strip and attached to the caul at the top of the head.

Body She wears the upper half of her collar unbuttoned and has undersleeves which stop at the wrist in a small cuff.

Accessories Lady Mainwaring wears a collar of SS. This livery collar was established by John of Gaunt and may mean 'Souvente me souvene' ('remember me often'); it was associated with the Lancastrian cause.

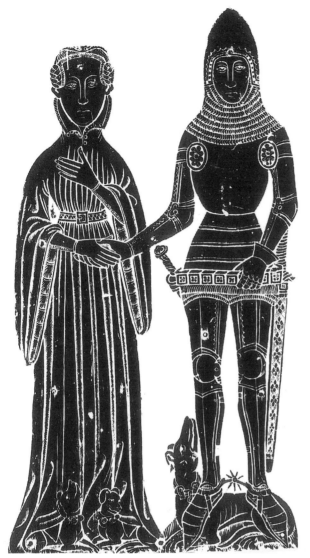

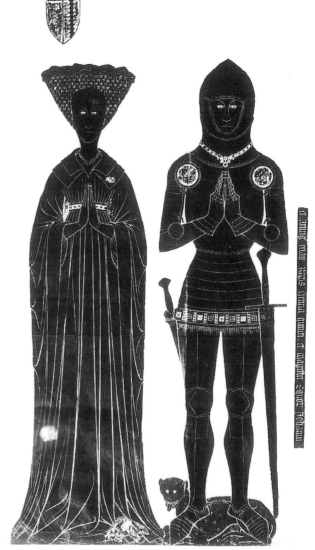

15. Clarice, wife of Robert de Frevile, c. 1410
English School, brass rubbing

16. Joan Risain, wife of John Peryent, c. 1415
English School, brass rubbing

Head The fashionable small horns are achieved here by plaiting the hair.

Body The fur lining of the gown sleeves shows as a series of stripes, each stripe marking the division between the skins used. The undersleeves lack the falling cuffs of very high fashion.

Note Joan Risain and her husband were Bretons, naturalized English in 1412 and 1411 respectively. She was chief lady-in-waiting to Henry IV's queen, the former Duchess of Brittany; and her husband was esquire of the body and pennon-bearer to Richard II, and esquire to Henry IV and Henry V. The uncertain position of Bretons in England at this time, as well as a record of service to Richard II, may have made it advisable to make prominent display of loyalty to the king through the devices worn. Joan died in 1415.

Head This headdress is unique among brasses with its triangular structure and scrap of veil thrown on top. Women's headdresses do, however, increase in size very rapidly in the second decade of the fifteenth century.

Body With the increasing size of the headdress it becomes impossible to wear the gown collar up; here it is spread over the shoulders, and the smock collar appears over it. The undersleeves are tight for a few inches above the wrist and then bell out.

Accessories A very high-set belt, a collar of SS and a swan badge on the collar. Like the collar of SS, the swan was a Lancastrian device.

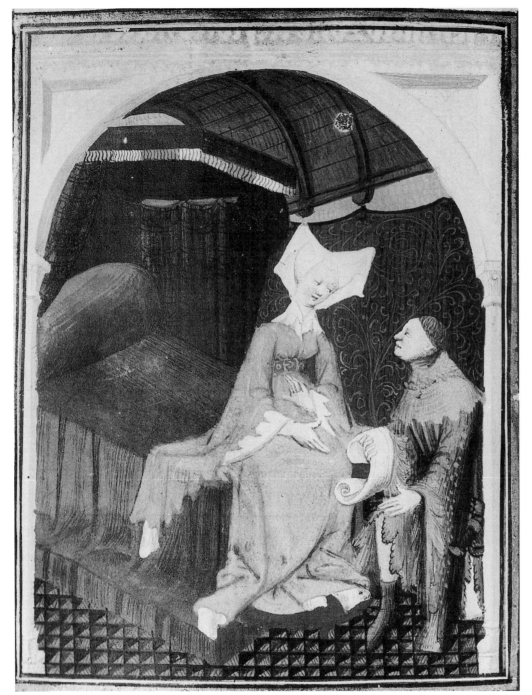

17. A lady receives a suitor, *c.* 1415–20

French School, manuscript illumination

Head The man's hair is cropped very short. The horned arrangement of the lady's veils is typically French, and they would be held out on strips of whalebone or dried plant stalks.

Body The man wears his dagged *chaperon* pushed down on his shoulders, over a *houppelande* with dagged sleeves and hem; the dagging is continued up the side seam of the 'skirt' where it has been left open. The sleeves are covered in what are probably embroidered teardrops, designed to soften the heart of his lady. Her *houppelande* has dagged sleeves and a turned-down collar which sits more closely round the neck than its English counterparts, although it is partly covered with the *chemise* collar.

18. Duke John IV of Brabant, early 1420s

Flemish School, drawing

Head The start of the *bourrelet* on the *chaperon* can be seen quite clearly; the dagging seems half-hearted.

Body The *houppelande* is as sumptuous as before but it seems less frivolous because of the way the dagging on the sleeves is now edged with the thick fur which also lines the garment.

Accessories A belt at natural waist level, and boots with long pointed toes.

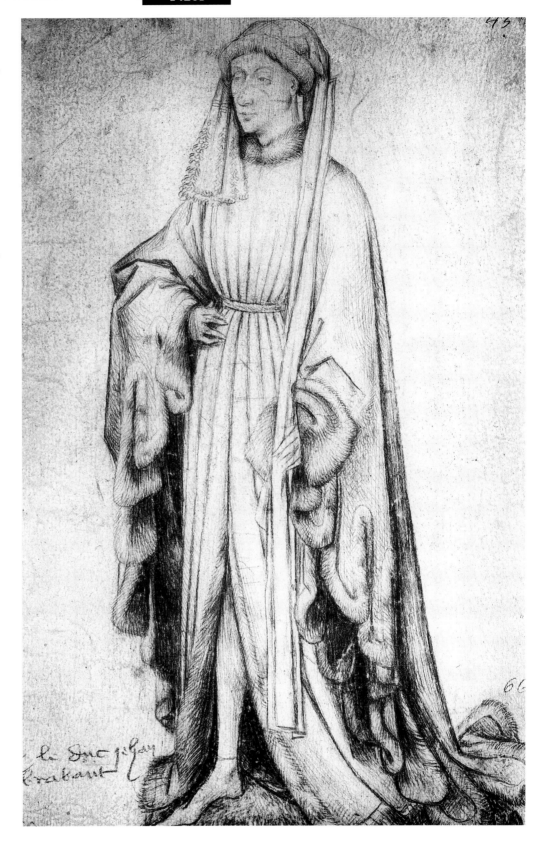

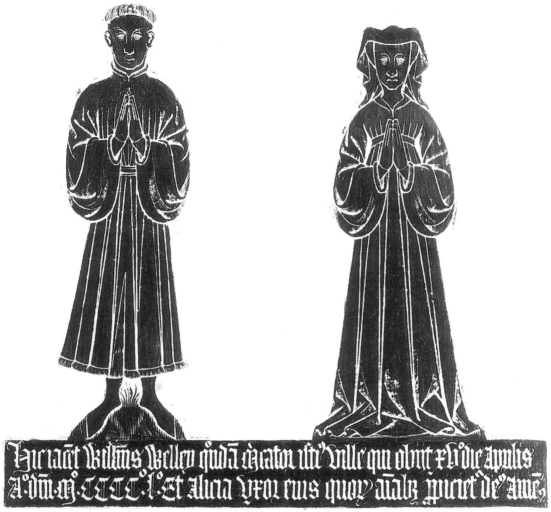

19. **William Welley, merchant, and his wife Alicia, mid-1430s (?)**
English School, brass rubbing

Note Although the brass records Welley's death in 1450, the dress suggests it was ordered or designed about 15 years earlier.

Head Welley's hair is cut extremely short. His wife wears a headdress with side projections shrinking at the base and expanding upwards to form a heart shape; there is a fluted veil arranged on top, falling onto the shoulders.

Body Both gowns have shrinking bag-shaped sleeves; the collar on the woman's gown is considerably smaller than earlier collars.

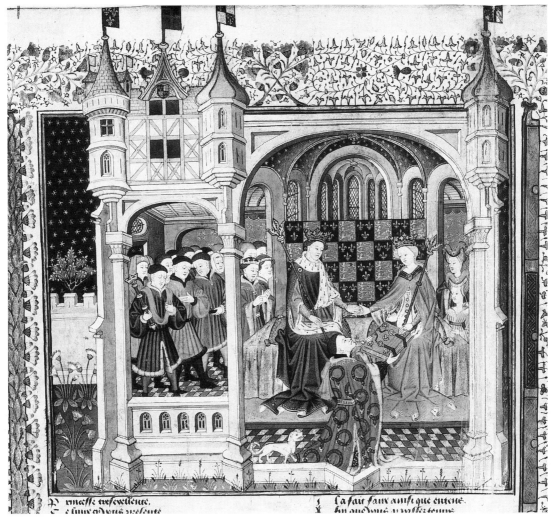

20. **Margaret of Anjou, Queen of Henry VI, receives a book from John Talbot, first Earl of Shrewsbury,** *c.* **1445**

English School, manuscript illumination

Note Shrewsbury accompanied Margaret to England for her wedding in 1445. She and the king wear ceremonial dress.

Head The men still have very short hair; their hoods have heavy *bourrelets*. The Queen's ladies wear horned headdresses with *bourrelets* on top.

Body There is a marked sense of order in the folds of the men's gowns, which are now knee-length; their sleeves have lost almost all of the bag shape. The Earl's gown is the most obvious exception to this rule, as it is his livery gown as a knight of the Order of the Garter, and its surface is duly covered with the badge of the Order. The doublet collars have squared-off front openings.

Accessories Ankle-length boots with short, pointed toes are the rule. Talbot and the man beside the King have collars of SS.

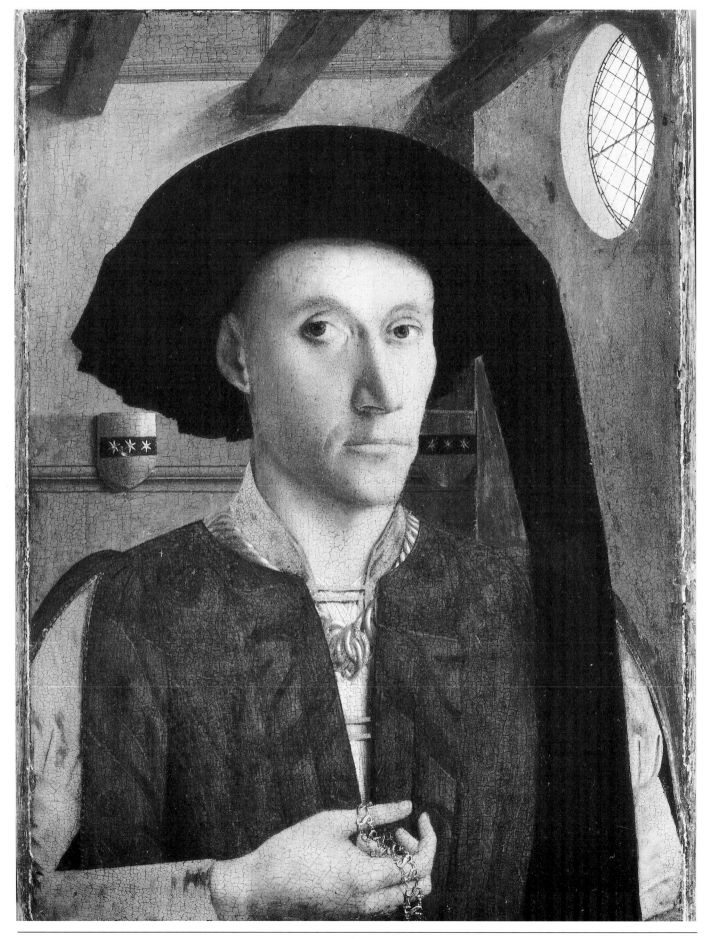

21. Edward Grimston, 1446
Petrus Christus

Note Grimston was an official of Henry VI's Household, employed as a negotiator with the Low Countries. The portrait was presumably painted on one of his visits to Flanders.

Head The *bourrelet* is now the most prominent part of the hood.

Body Three layers of clothing are visible. There is a green figured collarless gown, with vertical slits in the sleeves, through which the arms are passed. Next there is a red velvet doublet, with tight lower sleeves and puffed upper sleeves; this puffed section grows more pronounced in the next decade. The doublet is too skimpy to close across the chest, and is held as near shut as it can be by pairs of laces which emphasize the whiteness of the shirt beneath.

Accessories A collar of close-set gold links between the gown and the doublet, and a finer collar of SS held in the hand.

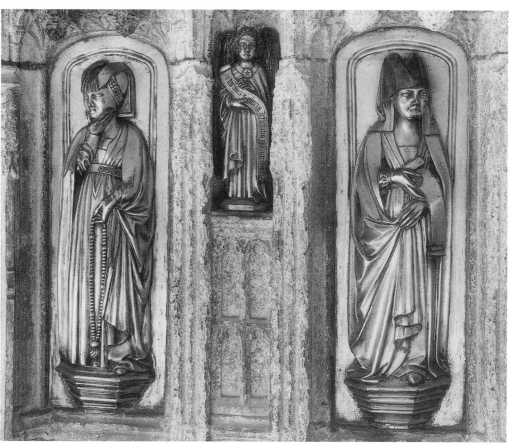

22. Two female weepers from the tomb of Richard Beauchamp, Earl of Warwick, 1452–3
John Massingham (?)

Head The headdresses have an outline of two small horns, either emphasized by a *bourrelet* with a small front flap and larger back flaps, or with a shoulder-length veil on top.

Body Under their cloaks the women have gowns with deep V-necklines. The neckline on the right is filled in with a stomacher, and that on the left by an under-collar or scarf, a low stomacher, and the top of the kirtle. The sleeves are fairly tight, especially at the wrists.

Accessories The figure on the left has a flower-studded belt, and holds a rosary; her companion, who holds a scroll, must be understood to be wearing a belt at a similar height.

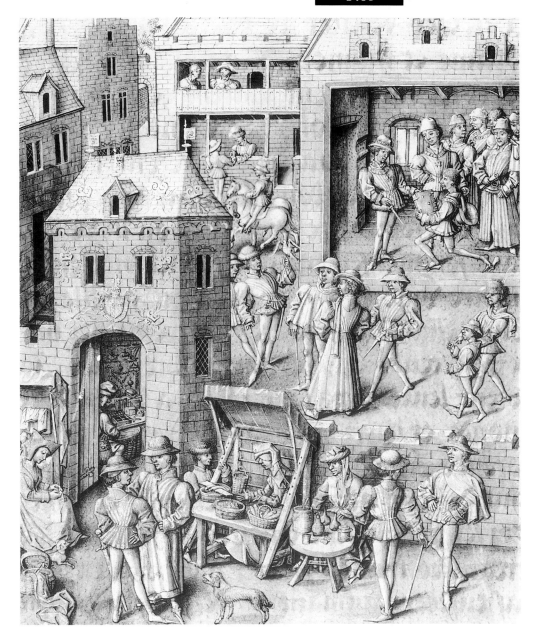

23. Flemish street scene, with presentation of a book to Philip the Good of Burgundy in the background, *c.* 1460
Jean le Tavernier

Note The curious posture of the men is Tavernier's own reaction to the effect of padding in the sleeveheads.

Head Fashionable men have abandoned the *chaperon* for hats, although some keep the *cornette* attached to these hats. Tradesmen still wear very old-fashioned *chaperons*. The working women wear *chaperons* with front flaps.

Body The pleating and padding of men's dress has given them an extremely unnatural shape, whose apparent discomfort must be increased by the too-long sleeves. The scooping out of the back neckline appears to be genuine in some cases, allowing the collar of the *pourpoint* or doublet to show, but in others it is no more than a vestige of the practice, with the standing collar being part of the *robe*. Short capes can be worn on top of short *robes*.

Accessories The hose are carefully seamed down the back of the legs, and on the feet are ankle-length boots, sometimes protected by pattens. No elegant man can afford to be without a walking stick to lean on, although a sword may provide an acceptable substitute.

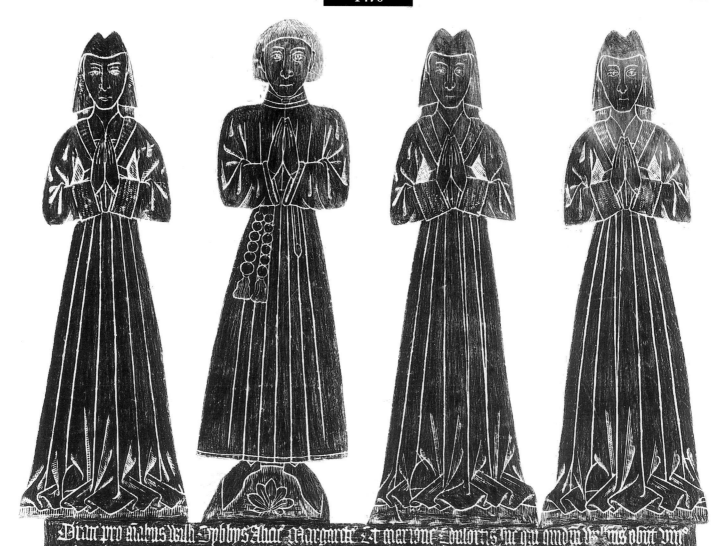

Dran pro aiabus Will Gybbys Aliac Margarete Et mervine Eueloris fue qui quidm Wills obiit viii
die mesis Januarii Anno Dowini aillimo I I I I lxxxvi Duorum animabus purcat de Amen

24. **William Gybbys and his wives, Alice, Margaret and Marion,** *c.* 1470
English School, brass rubbing

Note Gybbys died in 1485, but the dress does not tally with this
date. The wives' outfits are almost identical and are presumably
from a standard pattern: their sleeves suggest a date *c.* 1450, and
the bodices perhaps *c.* 1460. Gybbys's appearance belongs *c.*
1470.

Head Gybbys wears his hair cut in a fringe and over his ears.

Body Gybbys's gown has the diminishing pleating of the years
around 1470, and the concomitant levelling of the shoulder-line.
The gown, however, retains the drawn-in waist at this date, and
it is ankle-length because of the formality of the situation.

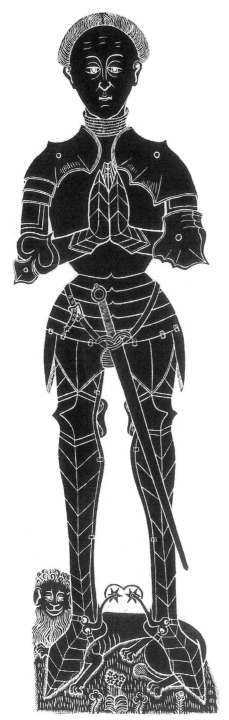

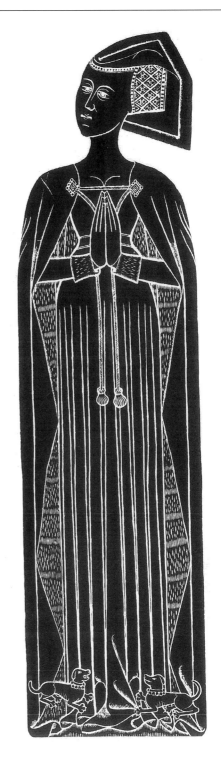

25. **Sir John and Lady Joan Curzon,** *c.* 1472
English School, brass rubbing

Note Sir John's armour is spiky enough for a date *c.* 1470, although his hair is very short. His wife's dress is also consistent with this date.

Head Lady Curzon wears a lozenge-patterned pill-box cap at the back of her head, with a short veil drawn back from the forehead into small 'wings'.

Body The cords of the fur-lined cloak obscure most of the details of the neckline, but it appears that the breasts are pushed up by the very tight bodice. The 'waist' is high and narrow, and the skirt flares from the hips.

26. Henry Stathum, his wives Anne and Elizabeth, and his widow Margaret, *c.* 1481

English School, brass rubbing

Note This brass is probably datable to the time of Henry's death in 1481 and is interesting because it shows an attempt to portray the two wives who predeceased him in by now old-fashioned dress, such as they might have worn in their lifetimes. The availability of such images to the brass engraver could well explain why so many brasses refuse to fit neatly into a logical sequence of changes in fashion.

Head The widow wears a long veil and pleated wimple, while the wives (on the right) wear the headdresses of the 1440s.

Body The wives' gowns are marked as old-fashioned by their baggy sleeves and loose cuffs. Although widows were not really meant to observe fashion, and her gown has the less fashionable belted waistline, the widow has been unable to avoid the long mitten-like cuffs of fashionable dress, here turned back to show the praying gesture of her hands.

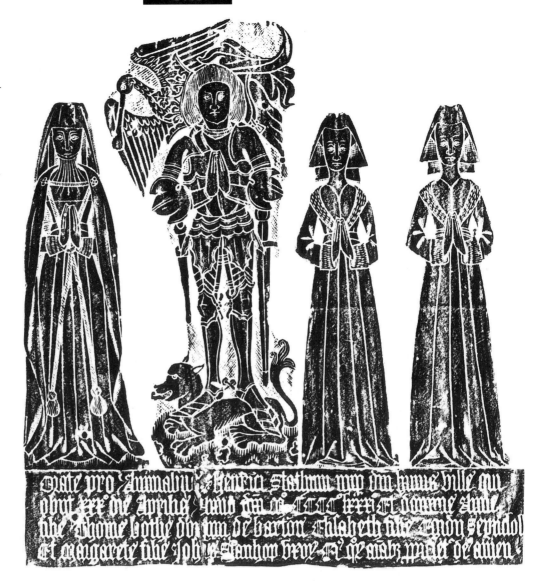

II **Lady Donnne and her daughter**
c. 1477

Hans Memlinc
Colour illustration, between pages 128 and 129

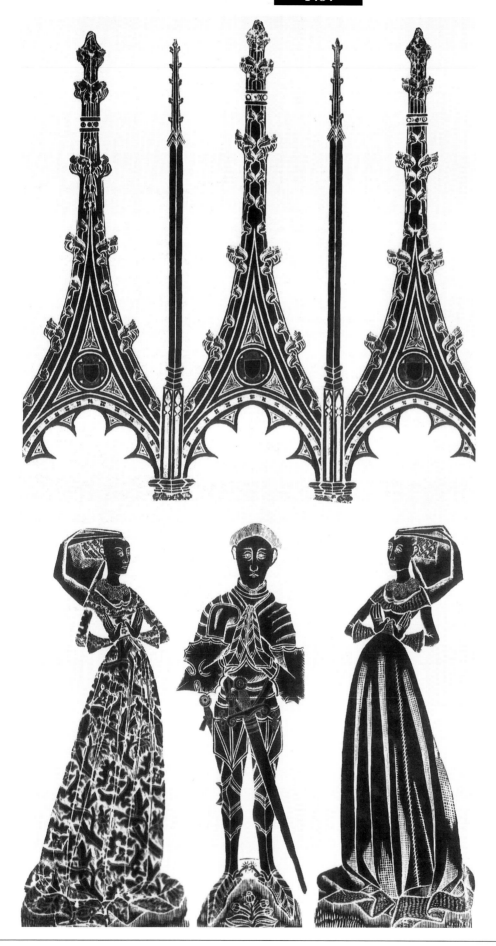

27. Sir Thomas Peyton and his two wives, both called Margaret, *c.* 1484
English School, brass rubbing

Note The necklines are consistent with the date of Sir Thomas's death, 1484, despite the shortness of his hair.

Head Both women wear the fully developed 'butterfly' headdress, consisting of a veil held out on wires over a pillbox cap set on the back of the head.

Body The necklines of the gowns show a peculiarly English feature at this date, the upward point of the collar and the stomacher at the cleavage. It is increasingly usual to turn back the cuffs, though the retention of the belt under the bust is slightly old-fashioned. The gown on the left is remarkable for its textile, which is in a standard cloth of gold pattern, and instead of having the more usual fur collar, cuffs and hem of the other gown, these areas are made of another patterned textile, perhaps figured velvet.

Accessories Both women have necklaces composed of a series of large leaf shapes, such as came into fashion *c.* 1480.

28. The Lover greets the God of Love, early 1490s

Flemish School, manuscript illumination

Note This manuscript is made particularly interesting by the attempts of the illuminator to produce old-fashioned dress for the Lover, whom he dresses, as here, in fringing to suggest the dagging in vogue at the start of the century, and to whom he gives a belt with pendant pieces of metalwork, also derived from the earlier period. The illustration is from the *Roman de la Rose* (*c.* 1240–*c.* 1280) which by this time is a venerable classic and as such worthy of some historical research in dress.

Head Both men have fashionably long hair, with the God of Love wearing a flat cap with turned-up side flaps.

Body The God of Love has a very loose *robe* with long tubular sleeves, slit to allow the arms through at a convenient height. It is lined and trimmed with velvet at the lapels and 'cuff', and is pulled across the body in the fashionably casual manner. Beneath he has a velvet garment which completely hides the *chemise*.

Accessories The God of Love's shoes have the new rounded toes; the Lover's right shoe has an old-fashioned pointed toe, but the artist seems to have failed to remember this 'historical' detail and has given the left shoe a rounded toe.

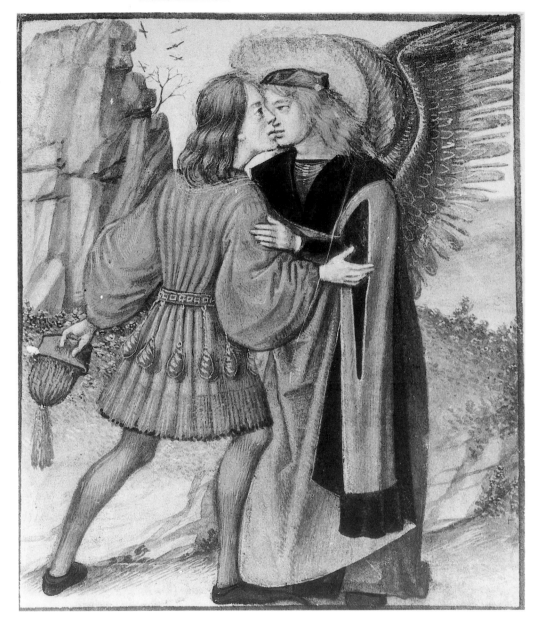

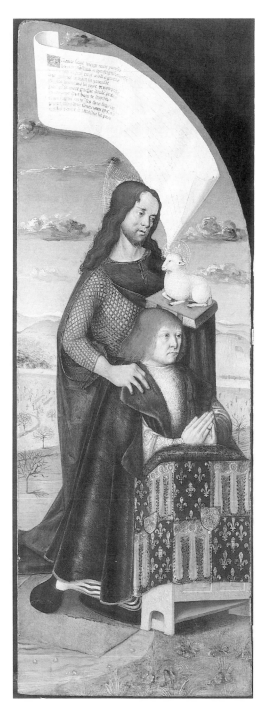

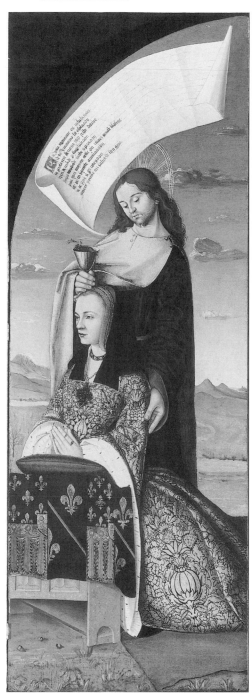

29. Jean and Jeanne, Comte and Comtesse de la Tour d'Auvergne, with St John the Baptist and St John the Evangelist, 1495–8

The Master of the de la Tour d'Auvergne Triptych

Head The Comte's hair is of fashionable length and texture. The Comtesse wears a version of the French hood, with the black outer layer moved back on the head to reveal two bands of crimped gauze on the front of the undercap; the black cloth falls on to the shoulders while the inner cap stops at the base of the throat.

Body The outer layer of the Comte's costume is a garment which has the lapels and vertical armhole slit of a *robe*, but the shape of a cloak which is at least semi-circular. Underneath is a cloth of gold *cote* (?) with baggy upper sleeves and more fitted lower sleeves.

The Comtesse's cloth of gold *robe* has the new side fastening at her right side, and the sleeves have very rapidly developed into huge funnel shapes which have to be turned back to near the elbows if the hands are to be used. The *pièce* or stomacher has a fairly wide neckline, and under it is still worn a linen scarf.

Accessories The Comte has high-fronted shoes with bulbous toes, and stockings or tights in two layers: a dark, inner one and a paler outer layer which is cut into narrow vertical strips for most of its length.

The Comtesse wears a collar of enamelled (?) flowers at the base of the neck, and a large cruciform pendant with hanging pearls is suspended from a chain.

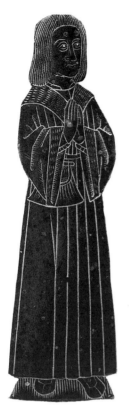

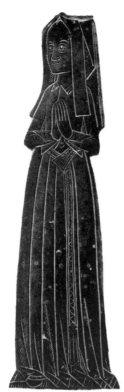

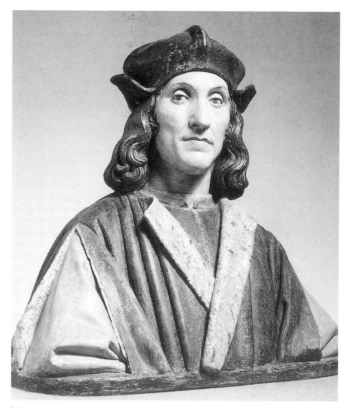

30. Robert Serche and his wife Anne, c. 1502
English School, brass rubbing

31. Henry VII, 1508–9
Pietro Torrigiano

Note Robert Serche died in January 1501 (1502 new style).

Head The most important feature is Anne's headdress, which is an early version of the 'gable' headdress worn by English women into the 1530s and sometimes later. It is split vertically at the shoulders into a frontlet and a longer veil at the back.

Body Robert's gown with its furry lapels and cuff is moderately fashionable, but Anne's dress is less so; she does not wear the wide sleeves or the square neckline of current high fashion, but prefers to split her cuffs and turn them back, and to force her neckline up in an inverted V above the centre-front closing.

Accessories Anne has a very long, loosely buckled belt.

Note The rather austere, undecorated dress worn by Henry VII was in marked contrast to that worn by his flamboyant son, Henry VIII.

Head The cap is made of blocked felt with a ridged crown at front and back, and a turned-up brim at sides and back. Shoulder-length hair is worn brushed under.

Body The standing collar of a front-fastened doublet projects above the collarless gown. The sleeves of the gown are left open to show the ermine fur lining, and the same lining forms revers that are crossed over in the front. The heavy, gathered folds of the gown fall from the shoulder seams.

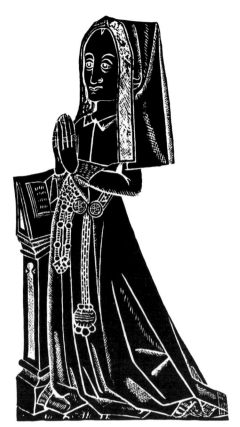

32. J. Wyddowsoun, 1513
English School, brass rubbing

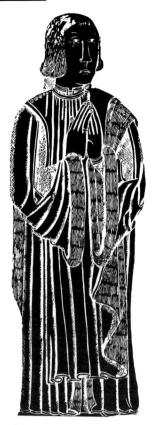
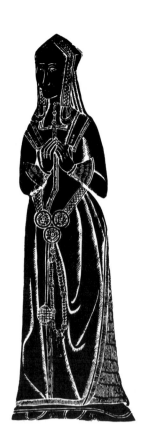

33. J. Marsham and wife, 1525
English School, brass rubbing

Head A linen hood with hanging lappets frames the face. Such a hood, if worn over an understructure, could be turned into a gable head-dress.

Body The bodice of this gown fits closely to the waist and then falls in ample folds to a fur-bordered hem. The narrow sleeves end in matching fur cuffs.

Accessories The belt around the waist is weighted down with a large double clasp, and with the purse and rosary beads which are suspended from it.

Note Neither is wearing fashionable dress, but that of a period some 20 years earlier, a misleading feature found in other brasses. It is possible that the man's mantle and gown signify the ceremonial dress of a mayor.

Head The woman's hood is a transitional style between gable headdress and English hood. Its decorated lappets hang short of the turned-out lappets of the undercap to which it is attached. The man's hair reaches the nape of his neck; he wears a fringe and is clean-shaven.

Body The square neckline of the woman's fur-lined gown is filled in with a buttoned partlet. Ornamental bands define the join between bodice and the close-fitting sleeves with fur cuffs. The gown is fitted to below waist level and then falls in folds; the trained skirt is caught up at the back and arranged so that the fur lining is visible. The small standing collar of the man's shirt is seen above the round neckline of his sleeveless mantle which is buttoned on the right shoulder. The lining is turned back over the other shoulder and falls in soft folds. The gown sleeves are full and widen towards the wrist where they form pendulous fur cuffs.

Accessories The woman wears a low-slung belt with triple clasps, a pomander, rosary beads and a crucifix.

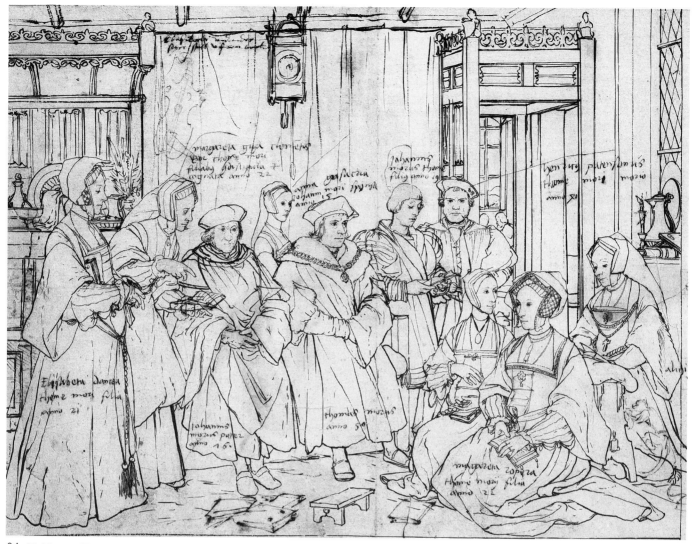

34. Sir Thomas More and his family, 1526
Hans Holbein

Note Holbein's drawing is a unique record of the dress worn by members of an influential and well-to-do family. There is a marked contrast between the fashionable dress of the younger men and the conservative dress of their elders. The collar of linked SS signified the allegiance of the wearer to the Crown; it appears in many portraits of members of Henry VIII's court.

Head 1, 2, 9 and 10 (numbering the figures from left to right) wear a later form of the English hood, in which one or both lappets are pinned up with crossed bands of striped material concealing the hair. The back section of fabric could either be left free (2, 10) or be pinned-up (1, 9). The two younger girls (4, 8) wear a rounder linen head-dress fastened under the chin. The older men wear caps of the old-fashioned square style, but the younger man (7) wears a bonnet tilted at a fashionable angle.

Body The women (except 8) wear square-necked kirtles under their gowns; the necklines filled in with buttoned partlets and necklaces. Their front-fastening gowns have heavy, slightly trained skirts (number 2 has her gown caught up). The bell-shaped sleeves of their gowns are turned back into deep cuffs and reveal full quilted undersleeves open along the back seam to display puffs of chemise. The man's short gown worn by number 6 has a standing collar and braid-trimmed sleeves cut with extra fullness to the elbow before narrowing to the wrist. The gown worn by number 7 has its bulky fullness gathered onto a yoke and straight sleeves from elbow to wrist. Sir Thomas's father (3) wears a judge's mantle with the bulk of the cloth drawn over his right arm, with a judge's robe beneath. Sir Thomas wears a gown with broad fur revers and short slit sleeves from which emerge undersleeves.

Accessories The women wear low-slung sash-like girdles, one of which ends in tassels (1). Sir Thomas wears a collar of linked SS, and holds a muff, as does his father.

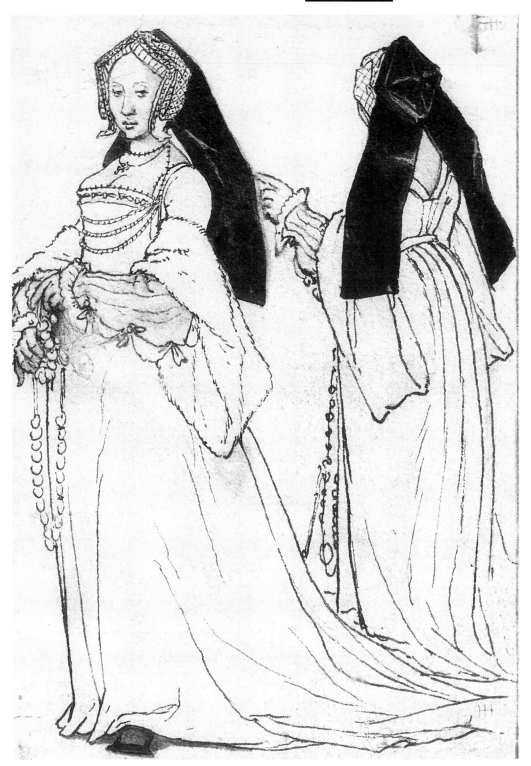

35. An unknown English lady, *c.* 1535
Hans Holbein

Note Holbein not only meticulously delineated the details of dress but also recorded contemporary stance and posture. The complex cut of the sleeves was appreciated best when the wearer clasped her hands together at waist level.

Head The English hood is of the later style in which the lappets are pinned up on top and the hair is concealed by crossed bands; a linen undercap curves onto the face. The back view shows the hood had evolved into a distinctive box-like shape to which are attached two tubular sections of fabric.

Body The low square-cut neckline and the bodice are covered with a profusion of chains and strings of tiny beads. The bodice fits closely to the upper half of the body and then swells out in full folds from the waistline. The back view shows how the pleats in the V-necked bodice lead to the fullness of the trained skirt. The bodice sleeves are turned-back into cuffs to show their lining, and the undersleeves are open along the back seam and held with ties, so that puffs of chemise can be pulled through.

Accessories A rosary is held in the hands.

36. Henry VIII, 1536
After Hans Holbein

Note Male dress was intended to enhance and exaggerate the wearer's masculinity; this was achieved by creating a massive chest and wide shoulders. Henry adopts the aggressive and dominant stance that was an essential part of this image.

Head The halo brim of the bonnet is decorated with jewels, trimmed with an ostrich feather and worn at a jaunty angle.

Body The narrow frill of the shirt is turned down over the small standing collar of the doublet. The gold brocade doublet is slashed at regular intervals to disclose puffs of the shirt below; the puffs are caught with square-cut jewels. The matching sleeves of the doublet are decorated in a similar way and finished with a wrist frill. Over the doublet is a jerkin with a wide U-opening to the waist; its full, deep skirts hide the hose. A prominent codpiece has been decorated to match the doublet. The upper garment is a short gown, bordered and lined with fur. The excessively broad shoulders are enhanced by the full, elbow-length upper section of the sleeve; the lower section hangs free. Bands of interlaced cord decoration on the gown's sleeves are repeated as a border on the hem.

Accessories A sash has been tied around the waist, and a second, lower sash has a dagger suspended from it. A pearl-studded collar is worn across the chest over a longer chain with a pendant gold medallion. The garter of the Order of the Garter is worn round the left knee. The shoes are square-toed with slashed uppers.

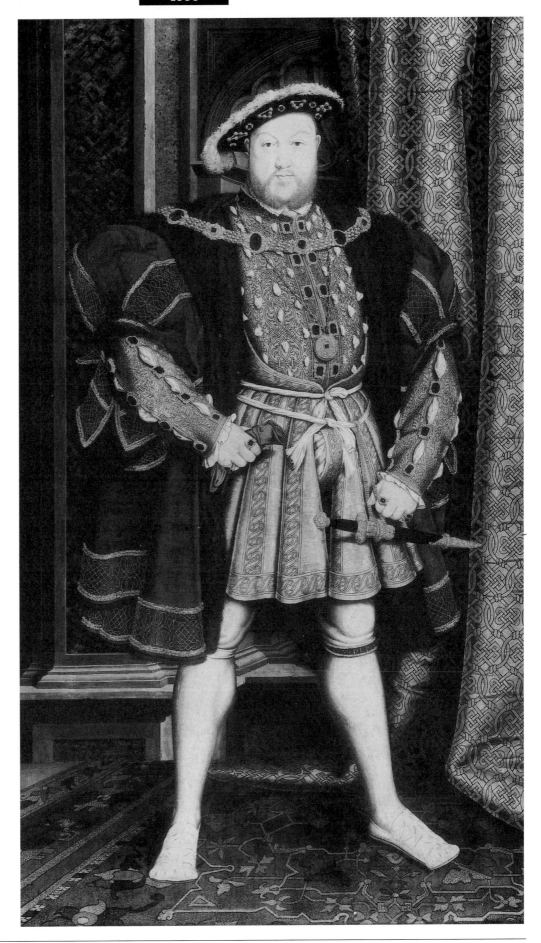

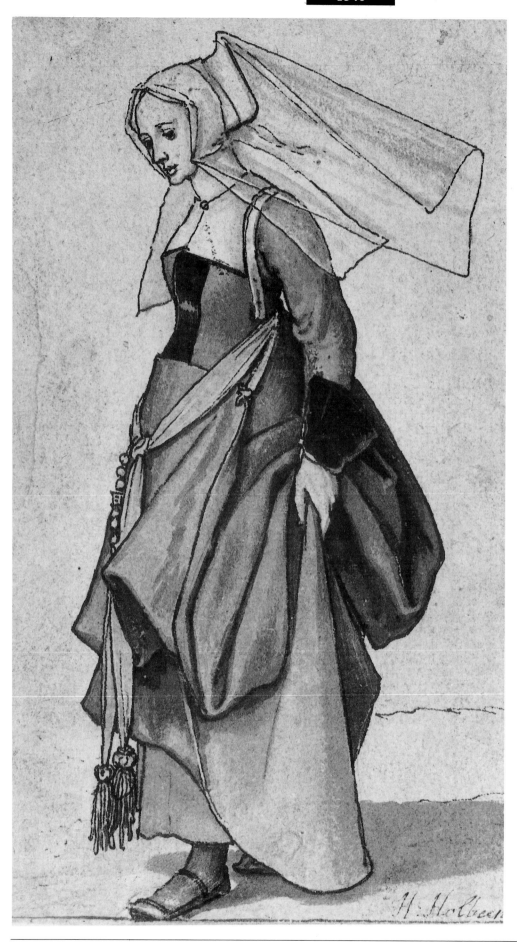

37. An English lady walking, c. 1540
Hans Holbein

Note A well-to-do, middle-class woman bunches up her gown to avoid the dirt of the streets. Her clothes are plain, but fashionably cut, the main point of emphasis being the head-dress.

Head The hair is completely hidden by a linen cap on a frame understructure, with a fine linen veil pinned at the sides and billowing out at the back.

Body A linen partlet, similar in transparency to the veil, is pinned with a brooch. The gown fits closely to the upper half of the body; its square neckline curves upwards slightly. The sleeves are cut tightly and are worn with a turned-back velvet cuff. The skirt is pinned up to the waist girdle revealing a kirtle also pinned up at the front.

Accessories Woollen or linen hose are worn with square-toed shoes that are cut low at the front and sides and fastened with a strap.

38. Lady of the Bodenham family (?), c. 1540–5
John Bettes (attr.)

Note This portrait gives a strong impression of the contrast that was created when blackwork embroidery was set against a dark background of velvet and satin.

Head In this English version of the French hood, the top of the crown is flattened across the head to curve wide of the temples and then turned in at an angle to end over the ears; it has upper and lower bands of decoration called billiments. The hair puffs out slightly from a distinct centre parting.

Body The bodice collar is turned outwards to display its lining of blackwork embroidery and narrow, attached frill. The tight-fitting bodice of satin with a velvet yoke ends in a deep V on the figured velvet forepart and smooth black satin overskirt. The trumpet-shaped sleeve, closely fitted to the elbow, has its lower fullness turned back to display a velvet lining; a full satin undersleeve is cut to reveal a chemise sleeve embroidered with a stylized honeysuckle motif, the wrist frill embroidered with a design similar to the collar.

Accessories A simple chain is worn around the neck. A pendant pinned to the yoke depicts a seated female figure with a lute and the words 'Praise the Lord for evermore'. A ribbon girdle, entwined with a chain, hangs at the centre-front of the skirt.

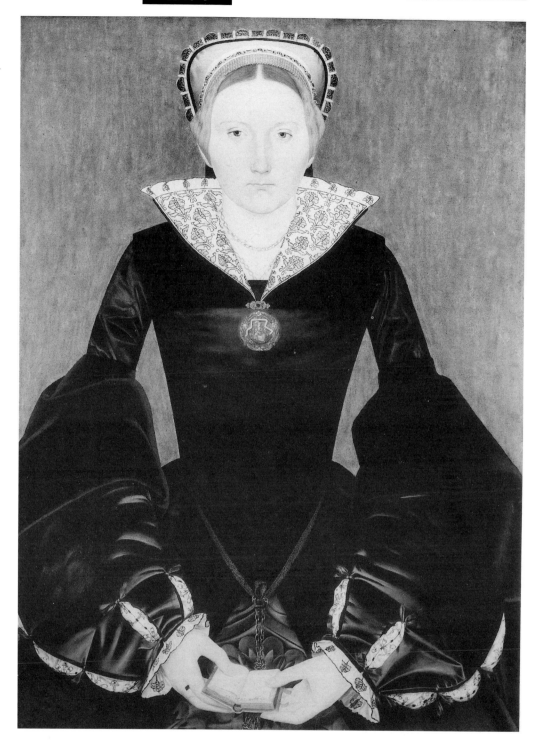

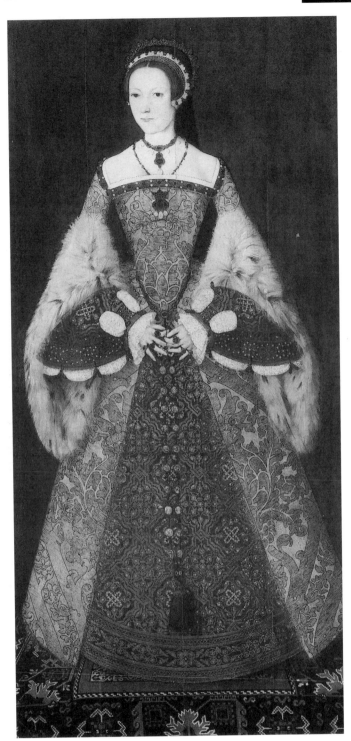

39. Lady Jane Grey, *c.* 1545
Master John (attr.)

Note This full-length portrait reveals that a new silhouette has evolved. The triangular shape of the bodice is balanced by the inverted triangular appearance of the lower part of the body, the stiff, smooth lines of which are dictated by the recently introduced Spanish farthingale worn beneath.

Head Lady Jane wears a French hood with elaborate upper and nether billiments of gold and pearl with a crimped border.

Body The low-cut and slightly curved neckline of the silver brocade bodice extends into a V-shape below the waist. The funnel-shaped sleeves, attached to the bodice, are turned back to reveal the lining of lynx fur, and undersleeves of crimson and gold brocade decorated with pearls and gold braid. The undersleeve is cut with a deep, lower curve from elbow to wrist, and the edge is caught together at intervals with aglets. The embroidered chemise sleeve has been drawn through these gaps, and is edged with a wrist frill. The silver brocade overskirt is lined, like the sleeves, with lynx fur; it is worn with a forepart that matches the undersleeves.

Accessories A necklace with pearl drops and a large pendant hangs round the neck, and a narrower jewelled chain disappears into the bodice. From a jewelled girdle placed around the lower edge of the bodice hangs a chain of antique cameos with a red tassel at the end.

40. Unknown man, c. 1548

Anon.

Note The brilliant red of the main garments forms a foil to the bold black embroidery on the white shirt. Shoulders had attained their most exaggerated size and shape by this date.

Head The flat bonnet has a broader brim held down on one side with an elaborate medallion; an ostrich feather has been pinned to the other side. The hair is worn short.

Body The high-necked shirt has an attached frill which is embroidered with blackwork. The same pattern is continued as a border to the front opening of the shirt. Voluminous slashed sleeves of red satin, secured with aglets, emerge from the shoulders of the short gown to end in a scalloped edge above the flared frill of the shirt sleeves. Under the gown is a matching jerkin that has a low standing collar, slightly protruding belly and full, overlapping skirts, the borders of which are slashed. The upper hose have been slashed to display their darker-coloured lining. Matching codpiece and hose complete the outfit.

Accessories The narrow leather belt with dagger and tassel attached, and the sword-belt, draw attention to the slightly lower waistline. The shoes are closed to the ankle and have rounded toes which have been slashed diagonally and studded with tiny jewels.

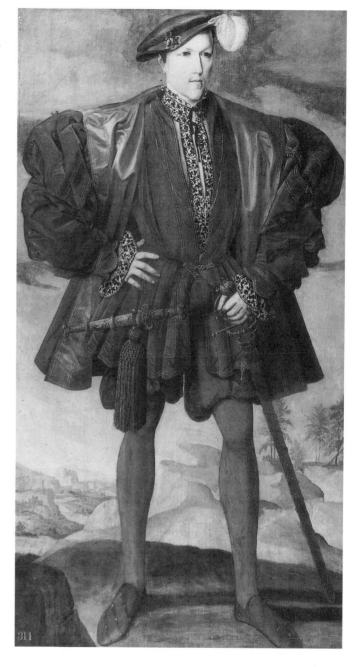

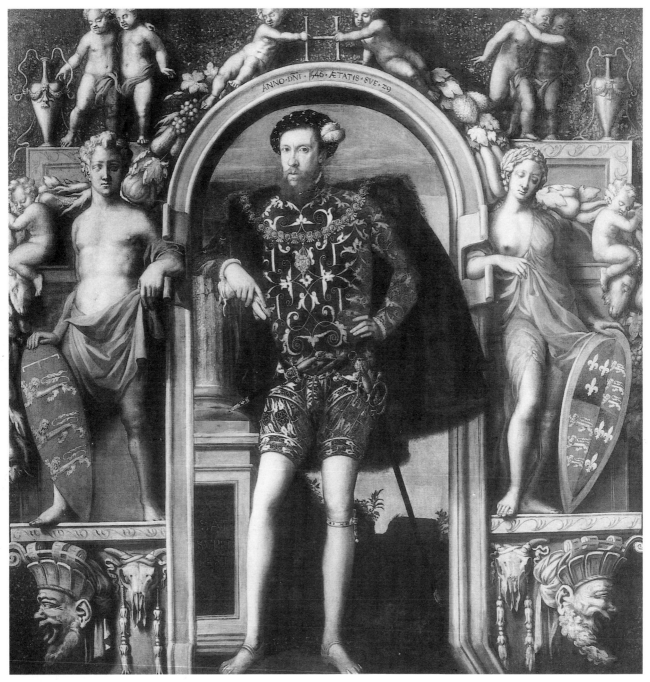

41. The Earl of Surrey, c. 1550
William Scrots

Note Surrey was renowned for his extravagant taste in dress; he wears an Italian fashion and adopts an Italianate pose. One of the charges at his trial in 1547 was that he wore foreign dress. He was found guilty of treason and executed. This spectacular collar of the Garter was worn by Edward VI at his coronation in 1547. This commemorative portrait of Surrey was painted a few years after his death.

Head The halo brim of the bonnet is decorated with small aglets and is topped with an ostrich feather. The Earl wears a moustache and full beard.

Body The fur collar of a full, sleeved cloak rests across the shoulders. Fitting closely around the neck is the gathered shirt frill. A doublet with a much lower waistline, a slightly swollen appearance and very short skirts has straight sleeves worn with wrist frills. It surface is decorated with an intricate pattern of gold braid that encircles areas of velvet appliqué. The codpiece is in the same material as the early form of trunkhose, distended in an oval shape at the top of the leg and held at mid-thigh with two bands of matching material.

Accessories He wears the collar of the Order of the Garter across the chest and the garter of the Order is fastened below his left knee. He also wears a belt with a dagger attached, and a sword-belt. Gloves with a pendant decoration are held in the right hand. The shoes have slightly splayed out and slashed uppers, and a shaped heel is just discernible.

42. Mary I, c. 1550–5
Hans Eworth

Note From about 1545 to 1550 the one-piece gown worn over the kirtle became less important, though it was retained as an overgarment. Female dress now consists of two distinct parts – a stiffened bodice and a skirt, the rigid shape of which was dictated by the farthingale worn beneath.

Head Mary wears the English version of the French hood.

Body The face is framed by a gathered frill attached to the embroidered standing collar which is closed by a jewelled carcanet. It is difficult to see whether this collar is attached to the chemise or the partlet, as both were worn to fill in the V-shaped opening of the high-necked bodice. The yoke of the black velvet bodice has an upstanding collar, lined with white satin and trimmed with cutwork, and worn half-opened and slightly turned back. The black satin sleeves, fitting closely to the upper arm, widen and are turned back to form the pendant cuffs of black velvet. The red satin undersleeves are trimmed along the bottom edge with gold cutwork and pairs of aglets and are gathered into a jewelled band around the wrist, where a cutwork frill flares out over the embroidered frill of the chemise sleeve. A matching black skirt, worn over a Spanish farthingale, is open over a red satin forepart.

Accessories A large medallion is pinned to the yoke of the bodice, and a Book of Hours is suspended from the chain girdle.

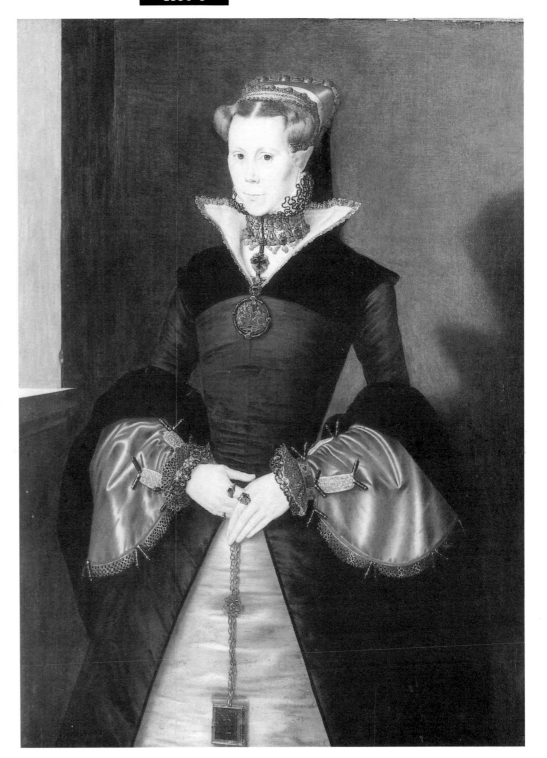

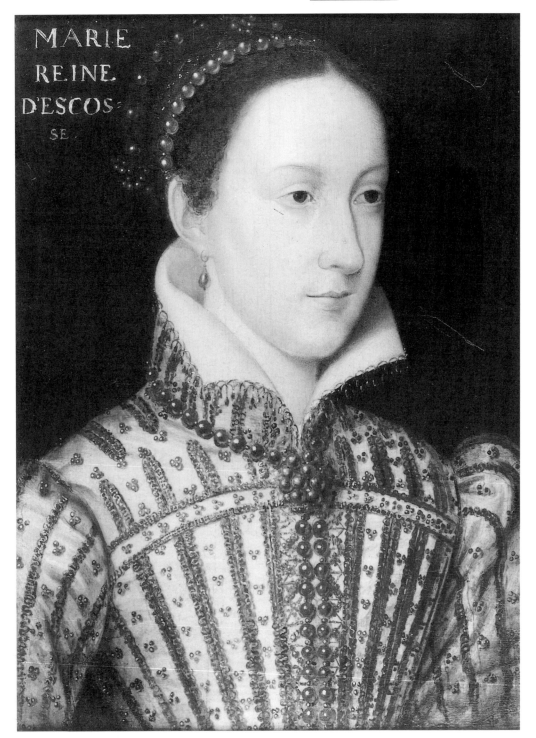

MARIE
REINE
D'ESCOS·
SE·

43. Mary, Queen of Scots, 1560–1
School of Jean Clouet

Note This portrait, probably painted prior to Mary's departure to Scotland from France, shows her wearing the sophisticated and elegant style of the French court. Her pearls 'like that of black muscat grapes' were a prized possession. When she was forced to sell them in 1567, Queen Elizabeth bought them secretly for £3600, and is seen proudly wearing them in William Segar's *Ermine* portrait, painted in 1585, now in Hatfield House.

Head A caul of dull black mesh with silver loops, edged with pearls, covers the back hair.

Body The high collar of the bodice is turned back to show its white lining; the edges of the collar are trimmed with silver thread from which hang oval, black spangles. The yoked bodice and sleeves of pinky-red satin are covered with vertical double rows of silver braid, with groups of three tiny silver beads set closely in the intermediate spaces.

Accessories She wears pendant pearl earrings; her rope of famous black pearls is knotted around her neck.

44. Sir Nicholas Throckmorton, *c.*1562

Anon

Note Although trunkhose and breeches were usually made with pockets for handkerchiefs and other accessories, Sir Nicholas has chosen to wear a separate purse to accommodate his carefully arranged handkerchief.

Head He wears a bonnet with a curved brim. His moustache and pointed beard are neatly trimmed.

Body An embroidered ruff is edged with bobbin lace. The doublet has a small standing collar and is buttoned centrally to a low waistline, its deep skirt masking the hose. Matching sleeves emerge from wings on the shoulders and are decorated with alternate pinked bands that create a striped effect. Three buttons and wrist ruffs add emphasis to the bottom of the sleeves. A cloak is worn across the shoulders.

Accessories A pendant on a fine gold chain hangs around the neck. The elaborate purse containing the handkerchief is attached to the belt, and a sword-belt is also worn.

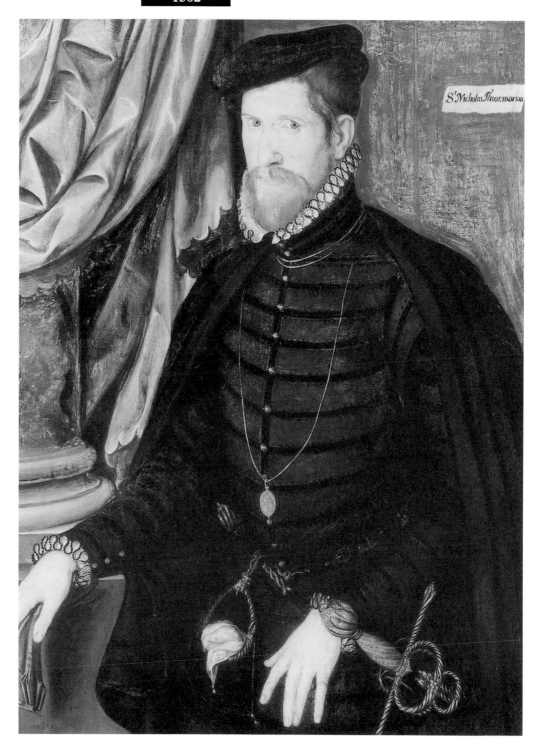

Sr. Nicholas Throcmorton

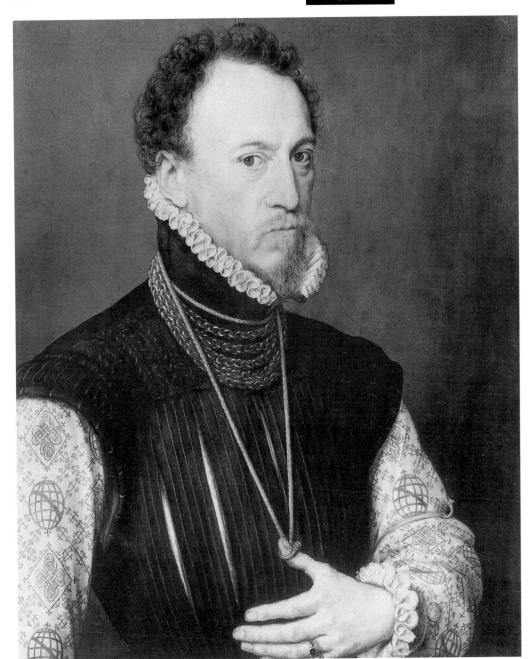

45. Sir Henry Lee, 1568
Antonio Mor

Note Sir Henry was the Queen's Champion and, in that capacity, arranged many spectacular tournaments and other festivities to entertain her. The curious devices on his sleeves and the rings attached to his clothes are probably associated with this role.

Head The closely cropped hair is balanced by a small, pointed beard and neat moustache.

Body The ruff has been left undone. The sleeveless jerkin has a high standing collar and pinked yoke; its body is paned from chest to waist. Shirt sleeves, embroidered with a design of interlaced knots and armillary spheres, emerge from the pinked and slashed jerkin wings.

Accessories Thick chains are wound around the neck. One ring is suspended on a cord around the neck, another is tied round the elbow, while the third is tied round his wrist.

||| Unknown girl, *c.* 1569
Master of the Countess of Warwick (attr.)
Colour illustration, between pages 128 and 129

46. Four Englishwomen. From left to right: a London citizen's wife; a rich citizen's wife; the daughter of the first woman; a country-woman, *c.* 1570
Lucas de Heere

Note Choice of dress was governed by status in society as well as financial circumstances. This illustration comes from a history of the English, written and drawn by a Flemish refugee who had observed the distinctive styles of dress worn by a group of London women.

Head The first woman wears a linen coif under a cap that has been wired into a curved shape. The second wears a cap which widens out above the ears and is set on the back of the head. The third wears a coif and linen cap with a fuller crown, and the fourth, a countrywoman, has a chin-clout across her mouth and a high-crowned felt hat.

Body The first and fourth women wear their ruffs closed, but the second and third have theirs undone. All of them, except for the last, wear high collared chemises and close-bodied gowns with turned-down collars and straight sleeves. Their gowns are guarded with velvet and worn over bodices and skirts. The richest (the second) wears a brocade petticoat under her gown. The countrywoman has a kirtle with a front-fastening bodice kerchief or tippet, and long apron.

Accessories All the women wear or carry a pair of gloves.

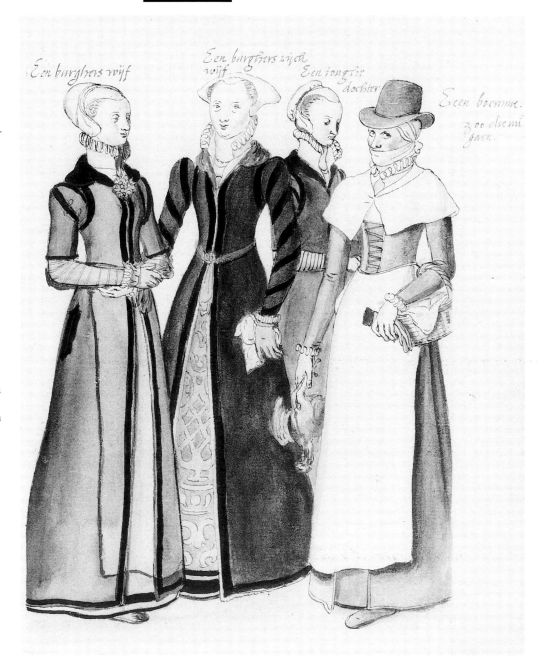

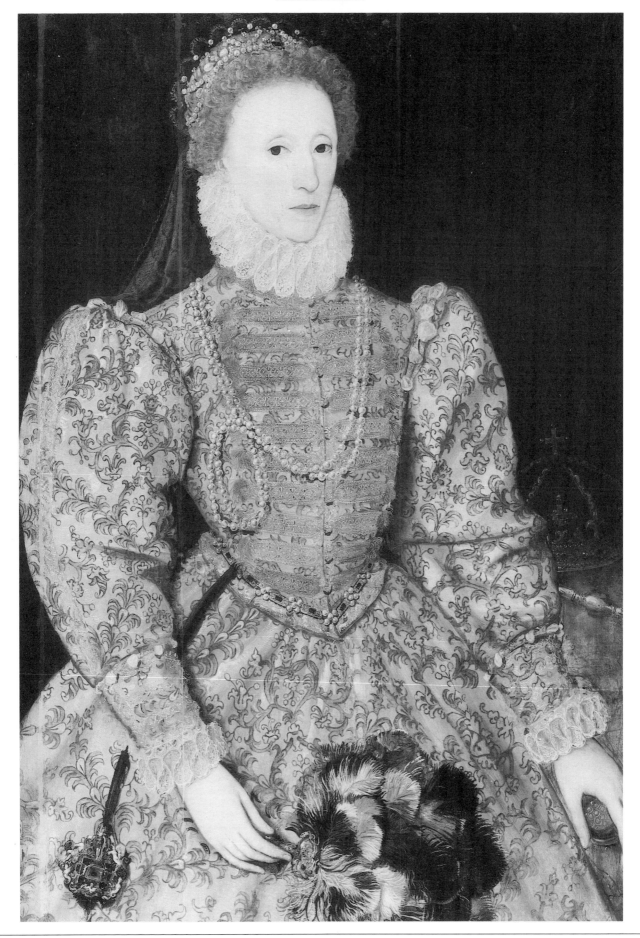

47. Queen Elizabeth I, *c.* 1575
Anon.

Note The Queen's bodice has been cut like a man's doublet, with a centre fastening, high collar and narrow tabbed basque. The jewellery is a relatively discreet arrangement of pearls which do not overwhelm the rich silk brocade of bodice and skirt.

Head A pearl billiment with a transparent veil attached is arranged on the top of tightly curled hair.

Body The neck is encircled by a deep figure-of-eight ruff. The matching sleeves, bodice and skirt are made of white silk brocaded with a gold thread in a floral scroll design. The bodice is fastened at the front with buttons which are flanked by frogging of gold and rose-coloured silk ending in fluffy tassels. The slightly pointed waistline has a narrow, tabbed basque. The fullness of the skirt is arranged in evenly spaced pleats over the Spanish farthingale worn below it.

Accessories The jewelled girdle has an elaborate pendant on a black riband suspended from it. The ropes of pearls worn round the neck are held in an asymmetrical loop on the bodice. In her right hand Elizabeth holds a fan of natural-coloured ostrich feathers.

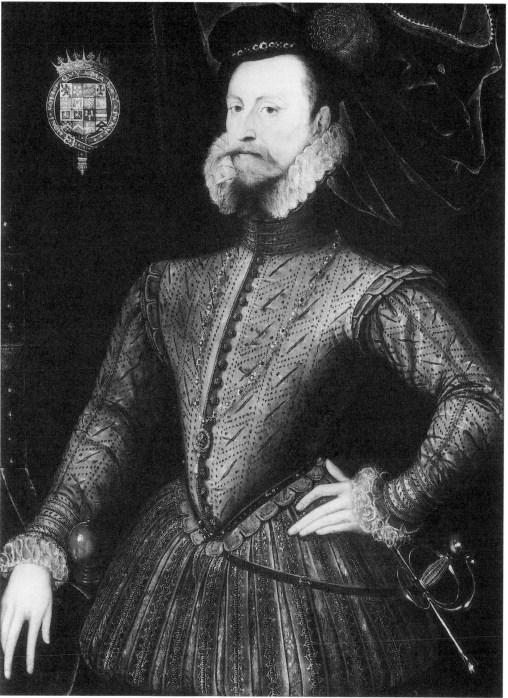

48. Robert Dudley, Earl of Leicester, *c.* 1575
Anon.

Note The Earl's intense love of finery earned him a respected position as an arbiter of taste amongst the fashionable men at Elizabeth's court. Knights of the Order of the Garter had the option of wearing either the Great George with the elaborate collar of the Order (*see* 41) or, as in this instance, the Lesser George on a lighter chain.

Head The small bonnet has a narrow jewelled band and an ostrich feather. The long, pointed beard and full moustache are carefully groomed.

Body The high, standing collar of the doublet, edged with a pickadil border, supports a lace-trimmed figure-of-eight ruff. The slashed and pinked surface of the salmon-pink doublet buttons down the front over a slight peascod belly. The matching sleeves emerge from double wings embroidered with gold braid. The tabs around the doublet waist and the cuffs are treated in the same way. The paned trunkhose are also embroidered with gold braid, and the lining of a similar coloured brocade is visible between the panes. The codpiece has almost disappeared.

Accessories In addition to the Lesser George he wears a belt and a sword-belt.

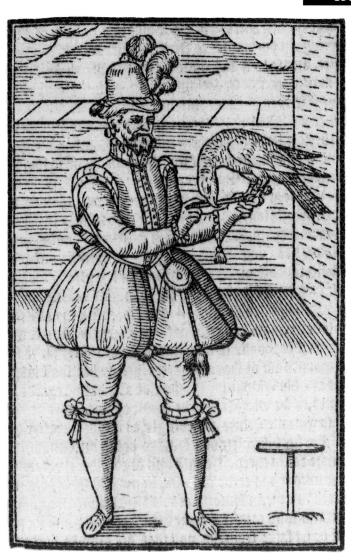

49. The Falconer

Anon. engraving from *The Book of Falconrie*, 1575

Note Falconry was a sport enjoyed by gentlemen, and this man wears appropriately fashionable and expensive dress.

Head The hat has a tallish, pinked crown, and is trimmed with a distinctive hatband and a bunch of ostrich feathers.

Body The standing collar of the doublet is worn undone. There is a small ruff and matching wrist ruffs. The slightly padded doublet curves into the waistband; it has straight sleeves and double wings at the shoulder. One side of the very full, paned trunkhose is masked by a large, tasselled pouch; canions are worn with the hose and the stockings are secured by garters.

Accessories A gauntlet glove, trimmed with a small tassel, is worn on the left hand to protect it from the hawk's claws. The high-fronted shoes have decoratively slashed uppers.

50. Sir Philip Sidney, *c.* 1577
Anon.

Note A metal gorget could only be worn with fashionable dress if the wearer had been on military service. Men's dress, by this date, is distinctly curvilinear in shape.

Head Sir Philip is bare-headed and clean-shaven.

Body His ruff, composed of a vertical figure-of-eight in one layer, is worn above the gilt-engraved gorget, and has matching wrist ruffs. The white leather doublet buttons down the front into a peascod belly, and has almost no basque. Decorating the doublet are alternate lines of vertical, serrated slashes, and horizontal lines of pinking. The exaggerated trunkhose are heavily padded, swelling out from the waist to turn in on the thigh. The black panes of the hose are embroidered with a striking strapwork pattern executed in gold braid.

Accessories The black belt, and sword-belt – the latter threaded through the panes of the hose – are outlined with gold braid.

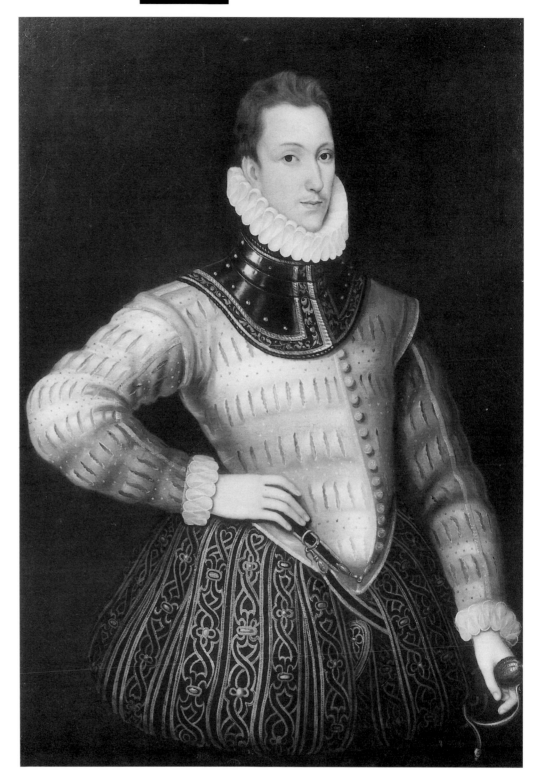

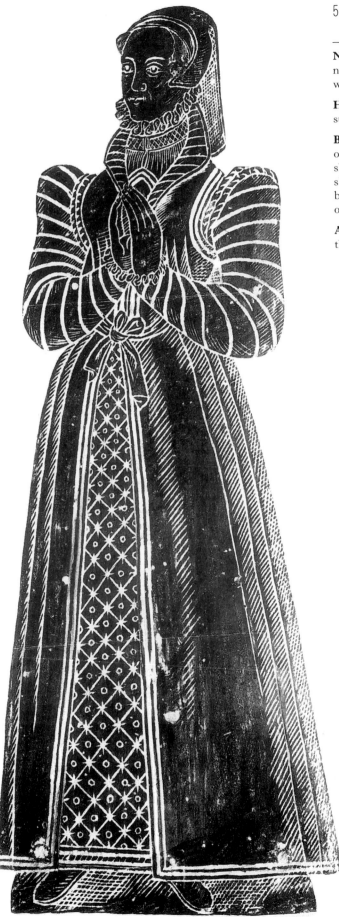

51. Jane Bradbuirye, 1578
English School, brass rubbing

Note A common feature of memorial brasses is the old-fashioned nature of the subject's dress. By the late 1570s most fashionable women were wearing an exaggerated style of ruff and farthingale.

Head The plain French hood has a short panel of material suspended from it.

Body She wears a ruff above a partlet. The turned-down collar of the gown rises up behind her head. The narrow wings on the shoulders of the gown add emphasis to the top of the puffed sleeves which taper to a narrow wrist edged with small ruffs. The bulky pleats above the waistline indicate that the gown is a loose one. It is worn over a patterned skirt.

Accessories A sash is tied in a crude bow at the centre-front of the gown.

52. Sir Christopher Hatton, *c.* 1585

After Cornelius Ketel (?)

Note Another, full-length version of this portrait shows Hatton wearing red and gold canions, white, patterned stockings and black pantofles.

Head The black velvet bonnet has a row of gold and gemstone ornaments around the brim, and an ornate pin or brooch securing the white ostrich feather. His hair is slightly fuller and longer over the ears, but his beard and moustache are neatly trimmed close to the face.

Body The white satin doublet and straight sleeves have braidings of red and gold, interspersed with rows of pinking. A cloak of black velvet is draped across the shoulders, its surface covered with pearls set into groups of gold leaves. The doublet, buttoned at the front, curves into a low waistline, its basque a mere padded roll of fabric. The trunkhose match the cloak.

Accessories A cameo of Queen Elizabeth, set in a gold mount, is suspended from the three, thick, long chains of gold worn round the neck.

IV **Sir Jerome Bowes, *c.* 1584**
Anon.
Colour illustration, between pages 128 and 129

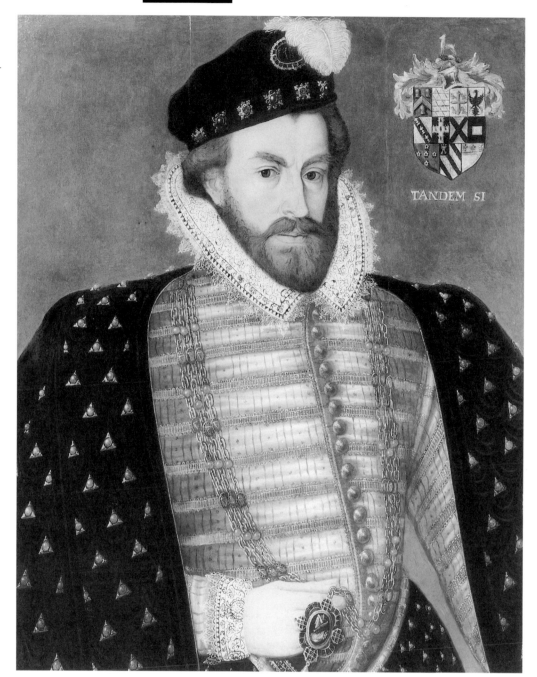

TANDEM SI

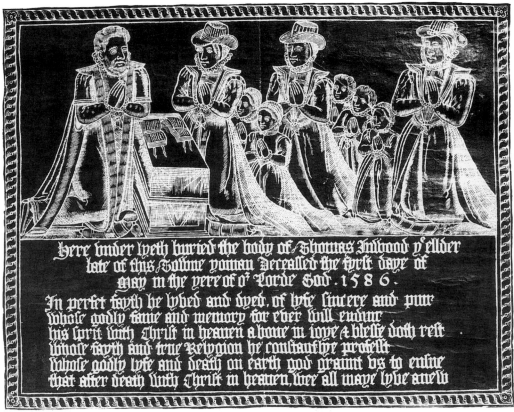

53. Thomas Inwood, his three wives and children, 1586
English School, brass rubbing

Note The conservative and old-fashioned dress worn by this family is typical of fairly well-to-do people living in the country. The style of hat shown here was popular with countrywomen and appears in many other brass rubbings of this period.

Head The wives wear low-crowned hats with upwardly curving brims over closely-fitting caps; the young girls wear cauls.

Body Both children and adults wear small, close ruffs and matching wrist-ruffs, the wives with gathered partlets, the girls with the standing collar of their bodices. Inwood has a long, fur-lined gown, short-sleeved, but with long, tubular, hanging sleeves. The wives' gowns are caught in at the waist with narrow sashes; the collars are turned down, and the sleeves are plain. Underneath they wear bodices and trained skirts, but without farthingales. The girls wear bodices with pointed waistlines and very full skirts; the two boys have long-skirted gowns.

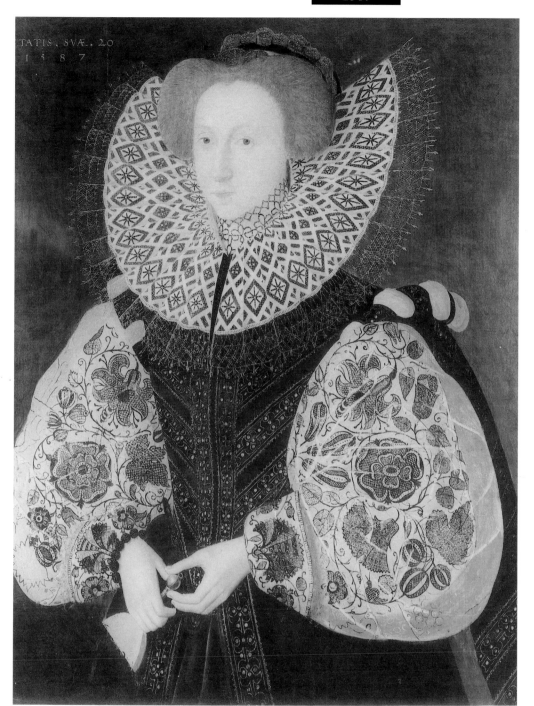

54. Unknown girl, 1587
John Bettes II

Note This portrait demonstrates the discomfort that the fashionable woman must have endured when the sleeves and ruff reached such extreme proportions. Similar examples of large scale, naturalistic patterns of embroidery can be found in many other portraits of the 1580s and 1590s; a sleeve-panel of blackwork with an almost identical pattern is in the Royal Scottish Museum in Edinburgh.

Head The girl's hair has been arranged over pads in order to produce a broad curve that dips in the centre of the head. Upper and nether billiments of pearls decorate the back of the head.

Body Her neck is encircled by a cutwork ruff that has been tilted up at the back to afford the best possible view of its geometric pattern. On the shoulders the wings are paned with puffs of the chemise pulled through. These wings and the tubular hanging sleeves are embroidered with narrow braid and spangles. The huge 'trunk' sleeves are covered with large-scale blackwork embroidery and encased in fine gauze. The bodice fits closely and is finished in an extended V-shape, its surface embellished with converging lines of braid and spangles. The matching overskirt is parted to reveal a plain underskirt.

Accessories An intricate jet-bead carcanet is worn around the throat. A black bead bracelet encircles the wrist of her right hand, in which she holds a feather fan.

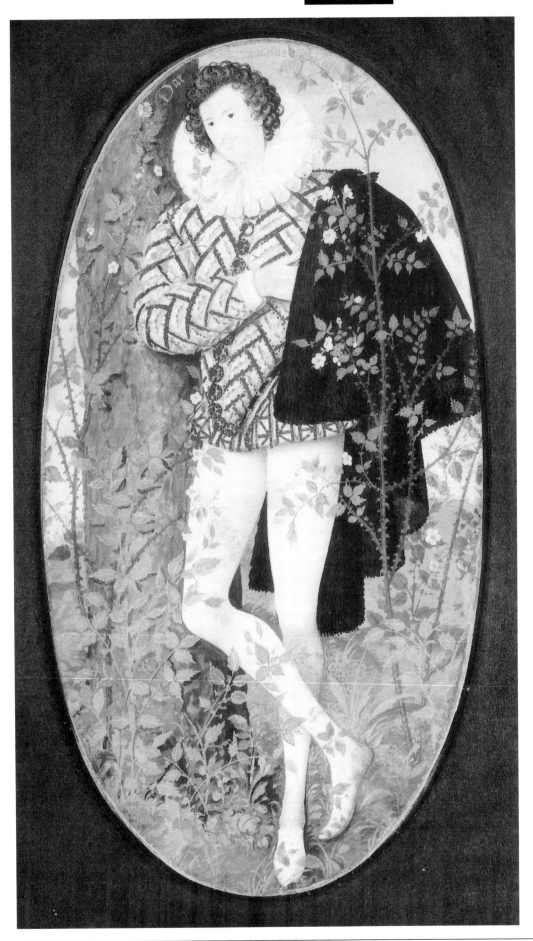

55. Unknown man, 1588
Nicholas Hilliard

Note It is thought that this elegant young man, dressed in the height of fashion, and in the Queen's colours of black and white, is the Earl of Essex.

Head His hair is fairly long, and he is clean-shaven apart from a delicate, almost imperceptible moustache.

Body The closely gathered pleats of a cartwheel ruff radiate around his neck. Nonchalantly thrown over his left shoulder is a short, fur-lined cloak with fur revers. The doublet that swells into a peascod belly shape is made from interlocking bands of serrated black and white fabric, and fastened down the front with ornamented buttons. The sleeves have been padded to produce a fashionably swollen appearance, and they are finished with plain cuffs. Very brief trunkhose and white stockings complete the outfit.

Accessories A narrow belt is just visible above the hose. The white shoes have long, pointed toes and pinked uppers.

56. Mary Huddye, 1589
English School, brass rubbing

Note This woman wears a very modified version of fashionable dress. Neither her stomacher, nor her farthingale, nor yet her ruff have the exaggerated proportions that would be required in fashionable circles.

Head She wears a bongrace over a French hood.

Body Around her neck is a closed cartwheel ruff of modest size. Her bodice is worn with a striped stomacher front and trellis-patterned sleeves that swell at the shoulder and then taper to plain cuffs. The material of the sleeves may be quilted. A small French farthingale is worn under the skirt.

Accessories Her shoes are thick-soled and closed at the ankles.

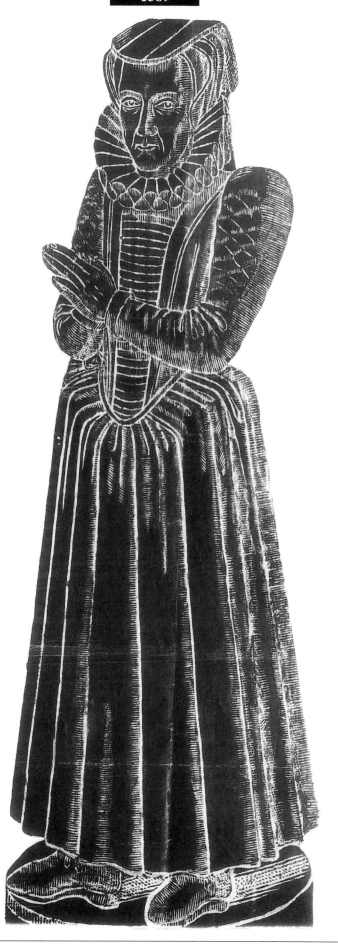

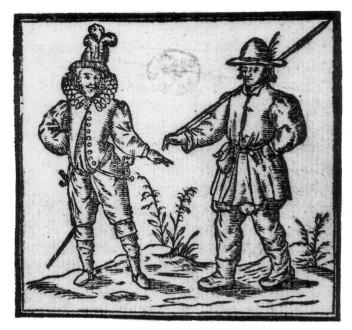

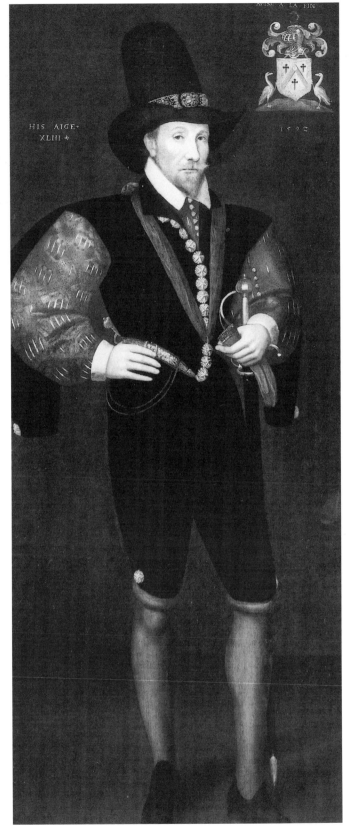

57. A courtier and a countryman, 1592

Frontispiece (anonymous woodcut) to *A Quip for an upstart courtier*

Note The text of the pamphlet from which this illustration is taken criticized courtiers for wearing expensive imported fabrics and styles while the countryman was content with simple, homespun clothes and a corresponding set of moral values.

Head The courtier wears a tall-crowned hat with ostrich feather trimming. His beard has been cut in the pickdevant style and is worn with the customary moustache. The countryman's hat, probably made of straw, has a wide flat brim.

Body The exaggerated clothes worn by the courtier consist of an undone cartwheel ruff, peascod belly doublet unbuttoned to reveal folds of the shirt beneath, and baggy breeches buttoned just above the knee. The country man wears a loose coat with a tiny collar, baggy hose and loose leggings.

Accessories The countryman's accessories are functional – a pouch attached to his belt and study startups. The courtier wears a belt, sword-belt and spurred boots turned down at the knee.

58. Thomas Kennedy of Culzean, 1592
Anon.

Note This stylish 43-year-old man wears a style of breeches called Venetians; various styles of breeches and trunkhose were fashionable in the last decade of the century.

Head Kennedy wears a Copotain hat, its brim turned up on each side, and trimmed with a richly embroidered hatband. His pointed moustache is worn with a pickdevant beard.

Body A plain falling band has been turned down over a sleeveless jerkin with hanging sleeves. The jerkin curves into a peascod belly, the line of which is followed by ornamental buttons. Underneath the jerkin is a doublet that buttons up to the neck, and trunk sleeves that have been decorated with regular lines of pinking and slashing. The buttoned slit in the left sleeve was used as a pocket. The Venetians fit smoothly to above the knee, with stockings fastened over them.

Accessories A riband worn around the neck has a ring threaded through it. He wears a belt with a narrow looped chain and holds a glove with a fringed cuff in his left hand. Shoes without fastenings fit closely around his ankles.

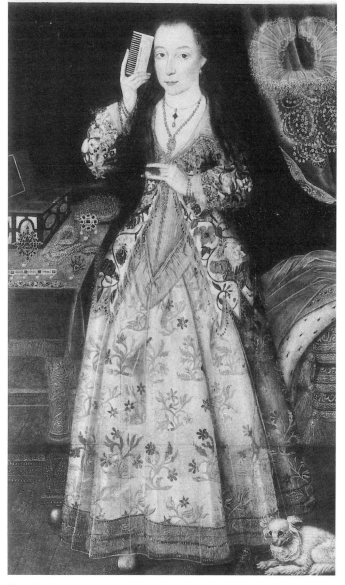

59. Elizabeth Vernon, Countess of Southampton, 1595–1600
Anon.

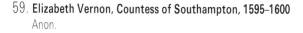

Note Embroidered jackets, also called waistcoats, could be bought ready-made in milliners' shops by the end of the 16th century. They were worn in the privacy of the home, as shown in this unique portrait of a young woman caught in a moment of intimacy in her dressing-room.

Head The countess combs her loose hair with an ivory comb.

Body The back seam of her jacket sleeve is undone and has been tied together with a series of pink bows. The jacket, embroidered in vivid colours with a design of flowers and insects, with its bow ties undone, is complemented by a turned-back lace collar and matching cuffs. The jacket hem is cut in points and edged with pendant spangles. The pink underbodice or stays end in a deep

V, with front lacing. A gauze apron is attached. The white satin underskirt has been embroidered with sprigs of blue flowers, and its hem is bordered with lines of spangles.

Accessories She wears a small pendant on a thin gold chain and a knotted rope of pearls around the neck. The mules on her stocking-clad feet are studded with pearls. Displayed on the curtain is a circular ruff with gauze ruching; beneath it there is a decoration for a stomacher designed as a circling pattern of enamelled white flowers interspersed with black and red gemstones set in gold. Her ermine-lined red mantle rests on a cushion, and her other jewels and pin cushion are beside the jewel case.

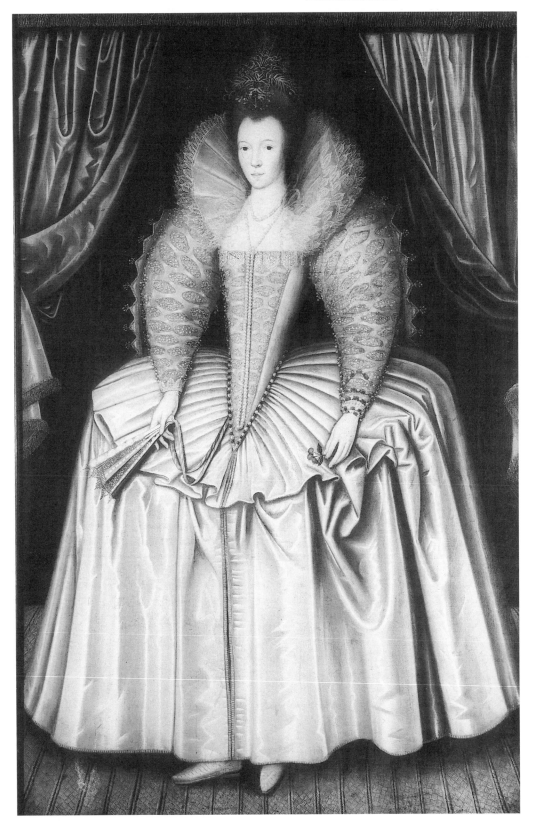

60. Lady Elizabeth Southwell, *c.* 1599
Marcus Gheeraerts the Younger (attr.)

Note Elizabeth was sent to court at the end of 1599 to become a maid of honour to the Queen. In this portrait she wears her court dress, certain features of which – the spiky headdress, serrated hanging sleeves, open fan-shaped ruff, and a colour scheme of white and silver – appear in other portraits of the Queen's maids of honour in the last decade of the reign.

Head Her headdress consists of silver fern-like leaves scattered with diamonds and other gemstones, and surmounted by a feather; it is worn atop swept-up hair.

Body Her open fan-shaped ruff is composed of multiple layers each of which is trimmed with points of lace. The join between the ruff and the bodice has been masked by ruched gauze. Trunk sleeves of white satin have been decorated with clusters of pearls on wire stems set in oval compartments. They are framed by hanging sleeves that fall behind the skirt; their outer and possibly inner edges have been serrated and stiffened with wire to carry projecting ornaments of pearls in groups of three. The stomacher matches the sleeves and is attached to a bodice with a square-cut neckline. Her plain white satin skirt has been arranged so that the pleats radiate out from the waistline, to be folded under and around the rim of the wheel farthingale so that a flounced effect is created. A narrow line of braid edges the central opening of the skirt.

Accessories A long rope of pearls is knotted in the middle. The narrow jewelled girdle has a folding fan attached to it. Her pointed white leather shoes have pinked uppers.

61. Sir Walter Ralegh and his son, 1602

Anon.

Note The early-17th-century delight in decoration – pinking, embroidery, applied braid and lace – is amply demonstrated in this double portrait.

Head Short hair worn with a neat moustache and spade beard was usual for mature men. The round-brimmed hat, trimmed with an aigrette, is tipped at a fashionable angle.

Body Shallow ruffs and falling bands were equally fashionable, matched by appropriate cuffs. Sir Walter's jerkin is fastened at the waist only, to display the doublet beneath. Shorter, rounder trunkhose are worn with plain canions, with the stockings rolled above the knee and held by tight garters. The younger Ralegh wears an alternative fashion of doublet and matching breeches.

Accessories The boy's gloves have embroidered tabs. Both father and son wear swords. Although Ralegh senior was a soldier, the carrying of a sword is equally associated with gentlemanly rank, and is thus appropriate for a boy. Swords were worn throughout the first half of the century, less so in the second half.

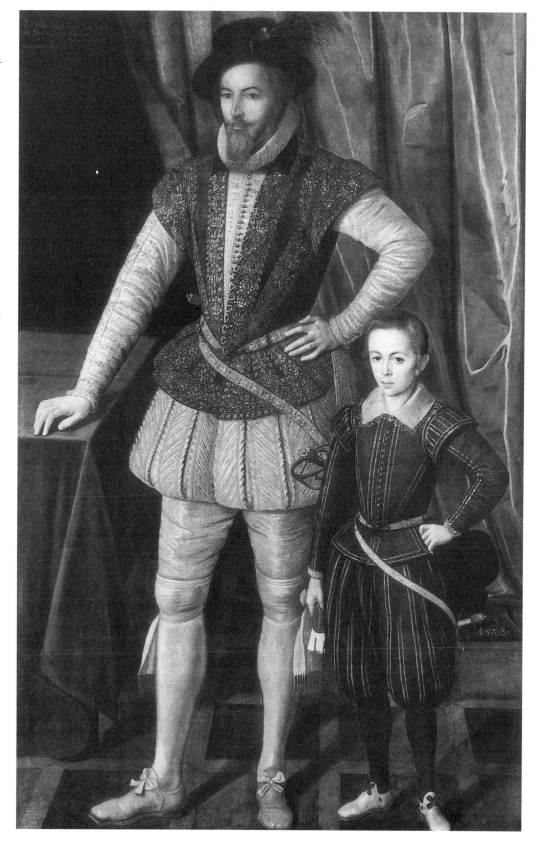

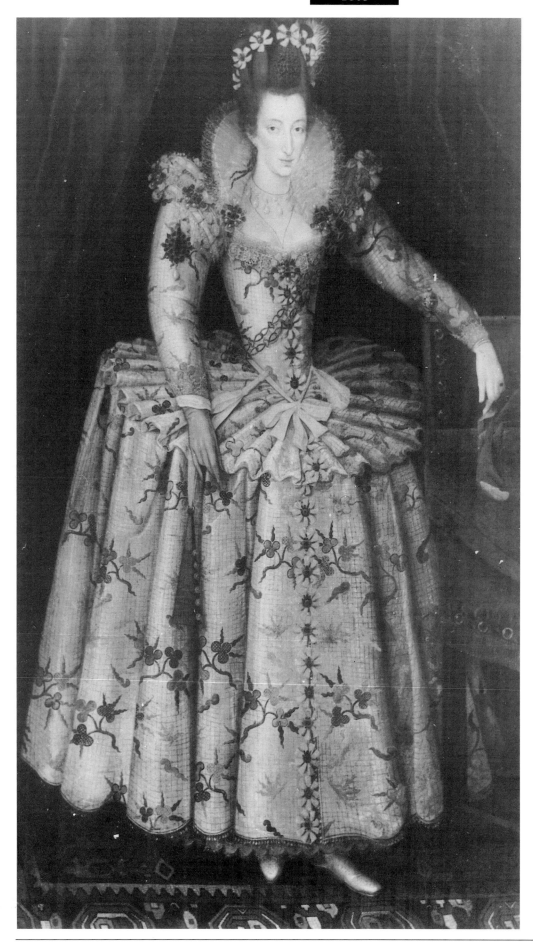

62. Anne Vavasour, *c.* 1605
Marcus Gheeraerts the Younger

Note This style of dress was expected at court. Queen Anne, like Queen Elizabeth, admired the formality of the farthingale.

Head An upswept, formal hairstyle, its structured braids elaborately decorated, marks a temporary elongation of the female appearance.

Body A small halo ruff sits between ornately trimmed shoulder wings. The stiffened bodice, worn over stays, has a more rounded décolletage. A wheel farthingale is worn under the skirt, the open front of which is held by rosettes, but reveals something of the scallop-edged petticoat beneath. The gathered upper panel of the skirt gives the illusion of a long basque from the bodice, its folds both defining the size but blurring the edge of the farthingale.

Accessories Rich jewels, lavish and unusual embroidery, ribbons and lace trimmings, and a fan suspended from the waist, provide suitable embellishments for a formal style of dress.

63. Mary, Lady Scudamore, 1614–15

Marcus Gheeraerts the Younger

Note Informal dress was easily as rich in appearance as the formal dress worn by women, although less constricting.

Head The hair, full at the sides but flatter on the crown, allows the cap of wired linen and lace to fit forward over the head and brow. Deep cuffs match the cap, but a plain ruff, with tasselled tie-strings, creates a break between patterned cap and dress.

Body A full-length gown is worn loose, but its buttons and loops could fasten. The blackwork embroidery of the linen jacket has a sinuous design complemented by the bolder pattern on the petticoat.

Accessories The black ribbon bracelet is a use of ribbon found much among jewellery at this date. Plain gloves with contrasting cuffs were popular with both men and women.

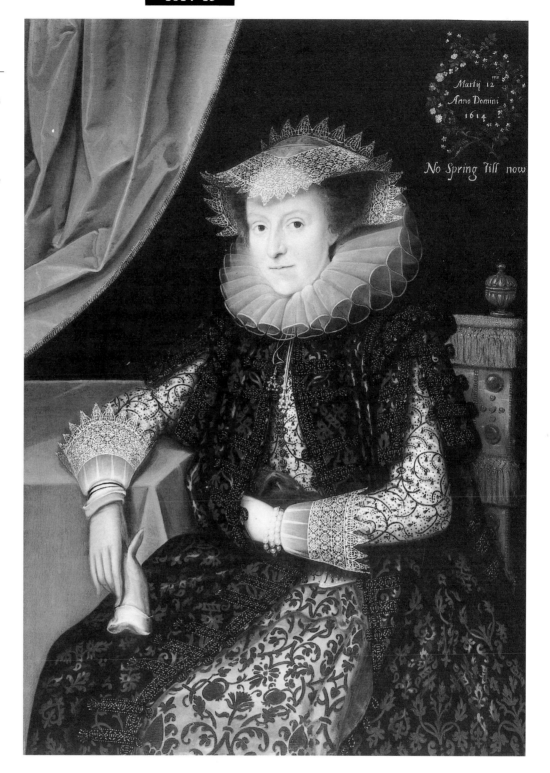

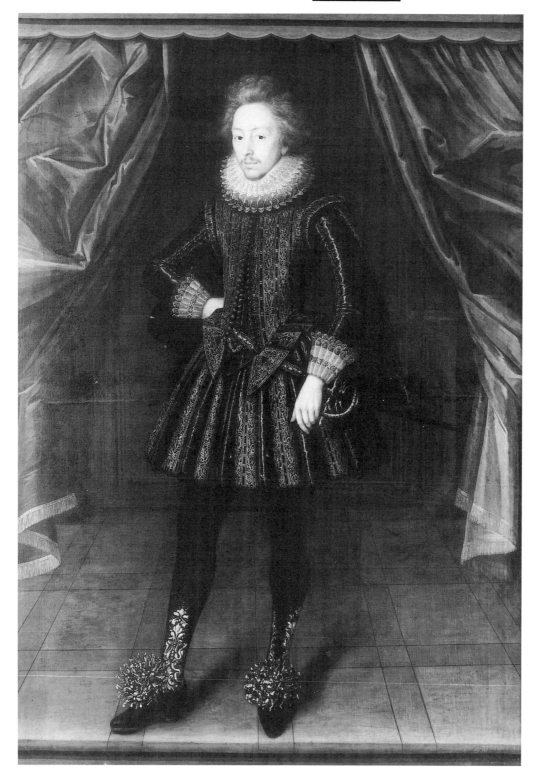

64. Dudley, 3rd Baron North, 1614–15
Anon.

Note A glittering young courtier combining the elegance and brashness which characterized the fashionable world.

Head The softly waving, fuller hairstyle echoes that of women at this date.

Body The small, densely pleated ruff was still fashionable; the choice between styles of neckwear was left to individual taste. An embroidered jerkin with false, hanging sleeves matches the stiff trunkhose; both are worn with a plain doublet. Deep cuffs mirror the decoration and pleating of the ruff. The stockings are magnificently embroidered with rich clocks at both sides of each leg.

Accessories Low-heeled shoes are dwarfed by huge, sparkling rosettes of spangled ribbon. The high-crowned hat is a plain beaver.

65. Anne Cecil, Countess of Stamford, *c.* 1615
William Larkin

Note An unusual use of material provides a focus of attention for this transitional fashion, which occurred between the formal court style of the farthingale, and a more naturalistic line.

Body Hanging sleeves billow out around the main sleeve, but are attached and turned back at the elbow to reveal the lining silk. The skirt has a flattering, natural line, but the smooth pattern of applied embroidery and slashing on the bodice and side skirts is given a three-dimensional quality on the hanging sleeves and central area of the skirt by skilful pattern realignment and extravagant use of material.

Accessories The ribbon bracelets – one attached to a ring, the rope of pearls and plain fan appear secondary to the large, lace-edged handkerchief which is an expensive accessory rather than a functional necessity.

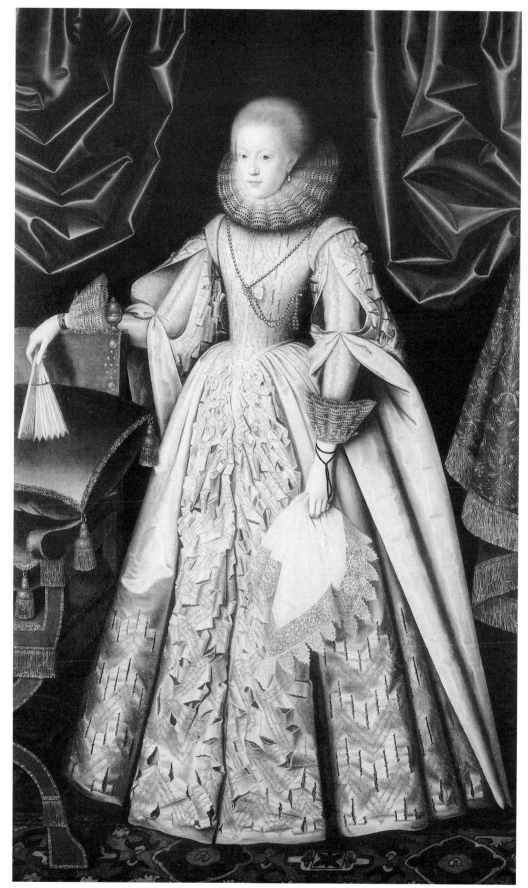

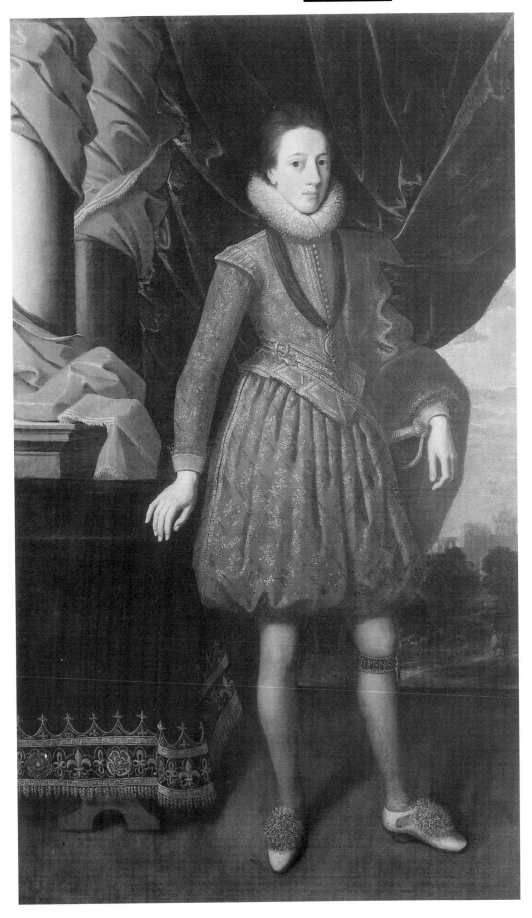

66. Charles, Prince of Wales, 1617–18
Abraham van Blijenberch (attr.)

Note A restrained example of the triangular evolution of men's fashions at this date.

Head Short hair and a smooth, beardless face are encompassed by a fashionable layered ruff which, in this instance, has some similarity to the shoe rosettes.

Body The high-waisted doublet suits a young man's figure, as do the matching, fuller breeches. The brocaded silk has been slashed to enhance rather than detract from the sprig motifs, and the applied braid provides an elongation of line to balance the bulkiness of the lower torso. The fur-lined shoulder cape is pushed up the arm to reveal the delicate lace of the cuffs. The prince wears the Lesser George of the Order of the Garter on a broad blue ribbon around his neck, and the actual garter is worn on the left leg.

67. Lady Elizabeth Grey, Countess of Kent, *c.* 1619
Paul van Somer

Note Queen Anne died in 1619 and this portrait is of one of her ladies in mourning dress. Black was not synonymous with mourning, but the details of dress confirm, in this instance, that she is in mourning.

Head The hairdressing is of the formal, earlier style associated with Court dress, and is surmounted by a small cap trimmed with feathers.

Body The standing ruff and deep, matching cuffs are also of traditional size and construction. A high waistline draws extra attention to the low décolletage, but an elongated line is created by the additional length of skirt and the long, hanging oversleeves.

Accessories The ebony beads are held in position by ties on the shoulders and by the central rosette. A signet ring is tied around one wrist through a silk ribbon point; the brooch on the left bosom contains the emblem of Queen Anne.

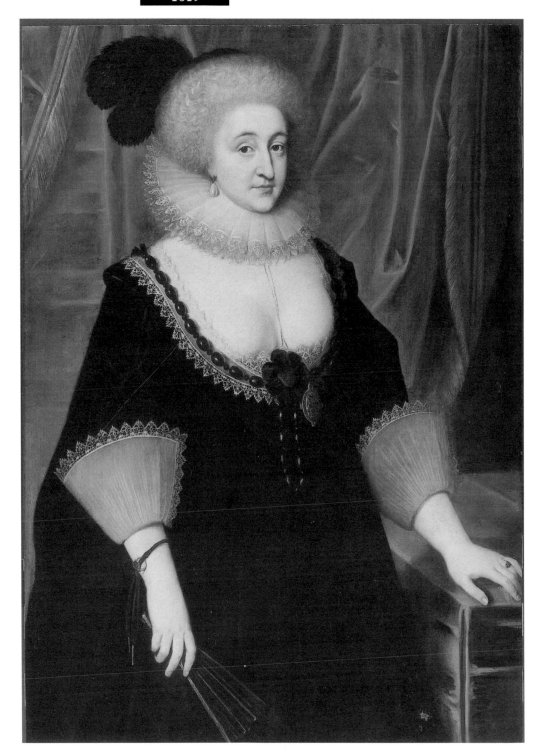

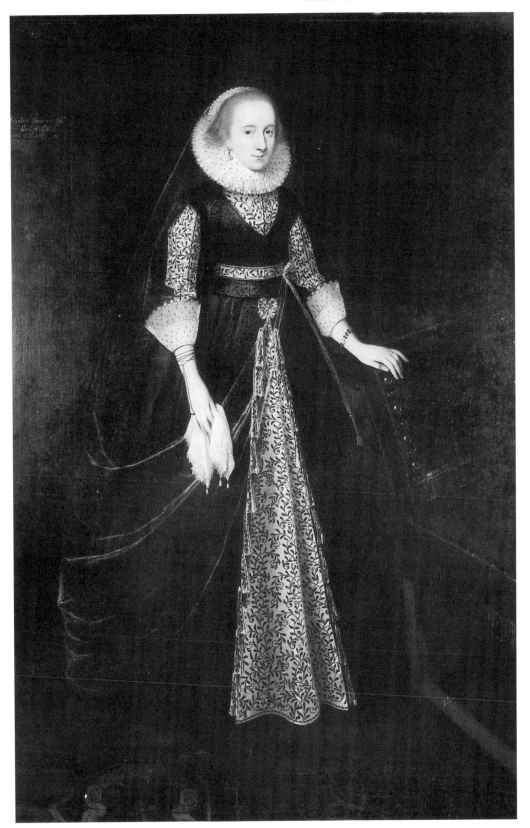

68. Elizabeth Howard, Countess of Banbury, 1619–20
Daniel Mytens

Note A restrained elegance characterizes the dress of this fashionable young aristocrat.

Head The straggling hairstyle is in curious contrast to the neat headdress and embroidered linen ruff.

Body The dress is in two distinguishable layers, an embroidered jacket and petticoat worn under a tabbed jerkin with hanging sleeves and matching skirt. The two materials are similarly embroidered, and the use of a pale belt, decorative loops on the skirt, and rosettes on the sleeves creates a harmonious unity between light and dark fabrics. The narrower line of the dress is heightened by the transparent gauze veil which is brought from the headdress to the waist of the skirt.

Accessories A dark feather fan and white handkerchief continue the theme of contrasts, and the jewellery is a delicate mixture of pearls and gemstones.

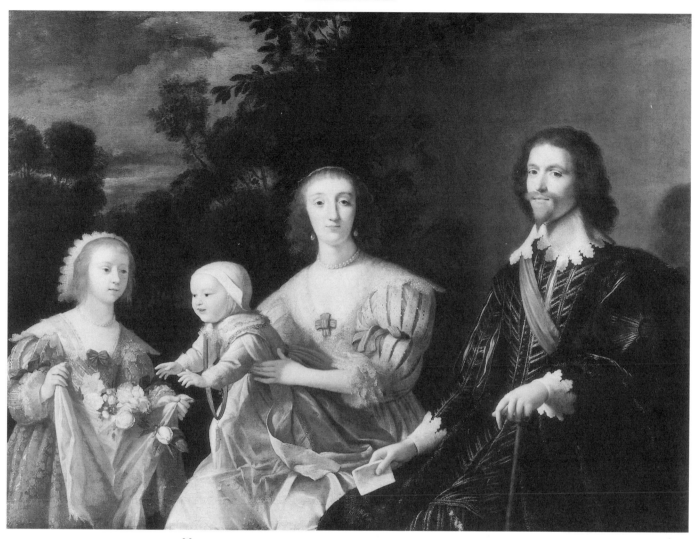

69. George Villiers, 1st Duke of Buckingham and his family, 1628
Gerard Honthorst

Note An influential and wealthy family dressed in keeping with their important role in the fashionable world.

Head The similarity between male and female hairstyles is apparent – long, softly waving, full at the shoulder, although the Duchess's has a slight fringe and a knot of longer hair behind.

Body Her deep lace collar is wide over the shoulder with matching tiered cuffs. The high-waisted bodice and skirt are of satin, embroidered in part with spangles and metal thread; a new style of sleeve consists of elbow-length panes in two tiers held by ribbons. The Duke wears a small falling band of lace over a paned doublet with unusually long tabs and with matching breeches. His fur-lined shoulder cape carries a Garter star, as decreed by Charles I in 1627.

Accessories The Duchess's pearls set the mood for the simpler jewellery which was fashionable from the 1620s.

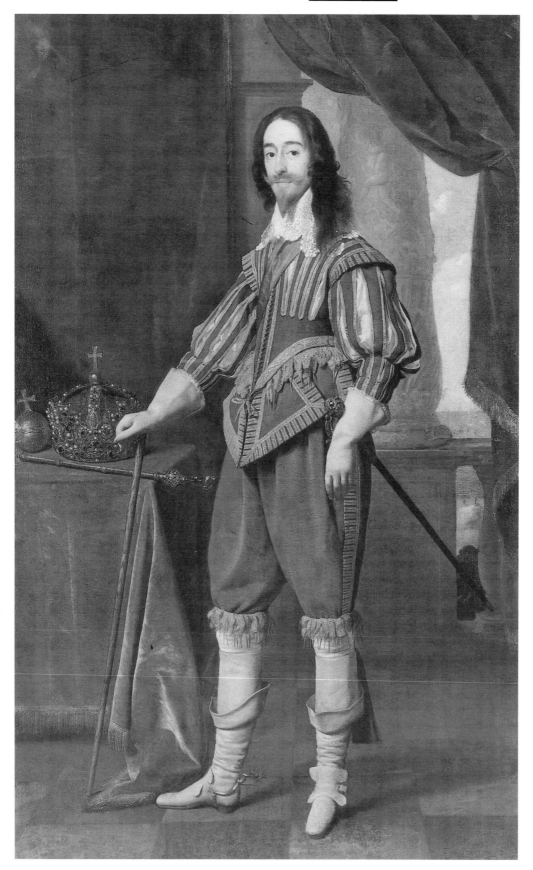

70. Charles I, 1631
Daniel Mytens

Note The King was the epitome of restrained masculine elegance, and his wardrobe accounts demonstrate a genuine but not extravagant interest in fashion.

Head The softly waving hair, longer at one side, is complemented by a pointed beard and an upward curling moustache.

Body The lace of the collar is a dominant feature, providing curving, sinuous lines in contrast to the elongated line of the doublet and breeches. A three-dimensional quality is given to the doublet by full sleeves, lines of metal braid and decorative points, with similar points at the knees of the moderately full breeches.

Accessories A glimpse of stocking is visible above the tightly fitting boots which are folded back into deep tops. The front flap of the boots provided a handsome strap to which spurs could be fastened.

71. Queen Henrietta Maria, 1634–5

After Sir Anthony Van Dyck

Note The Queen wears hunting dress and is accompanied by her dwarf, whose dress is a perfect miniature of contemporary male fashions.

Head The full, softly curling hair with a lock arranged over one shoulder mirrors the male hairstyles of this date, as does the low-crowned, wide-brimmed hat and deep lace collar fastened at the neck.

Body The bodice collar is taken down to the waist and held by the looped belt or sash. The bodice has deep side tabs and a central stiffened stomacher. Skirt and bodice are of matching material which has been pinked. Narrow rows of braid create the impression of a slimmer vertical line, although the skirt is full, worn over hip pads. The cuffs are of tightly gathered layers of linen.

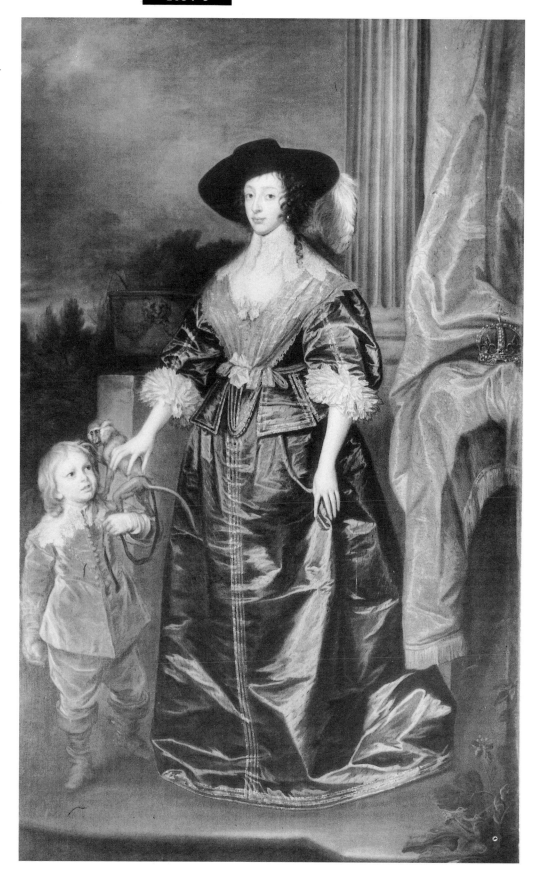

∨ **Queen Henrietta Maria, 1633–5**
Anon.
Colour illustration, between pages 128 and 129

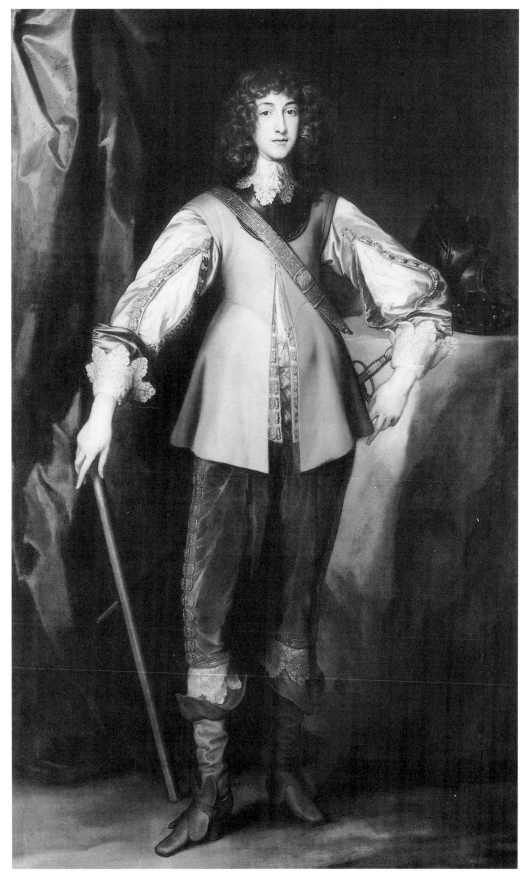

72. Prince Rupert, *c.* 1637
Studio of Sir Anthony Van Dyck

Note A young prince with both British and continental European connexions adapting his taste to suit the English court.

Head Full curls, fashionably long, and a cleanly shaven face were usual for young courtiers in their teens.

Body A small collar, tied with a flourish of loops, reveals most of the gorget under which a buff jerkin is partly laced. The doublet is also open displaying the shirt. The decorative buttons and loops on the doublet front and open sleeves could be fastened if required. The sleeves have a contrasting turnback cuff. Longer, looser breeches are similarly decorated and have discreet ribbon loops at the waist.

Accessories The soft boots are developing the baggy creases and full tops favoured at European courts.

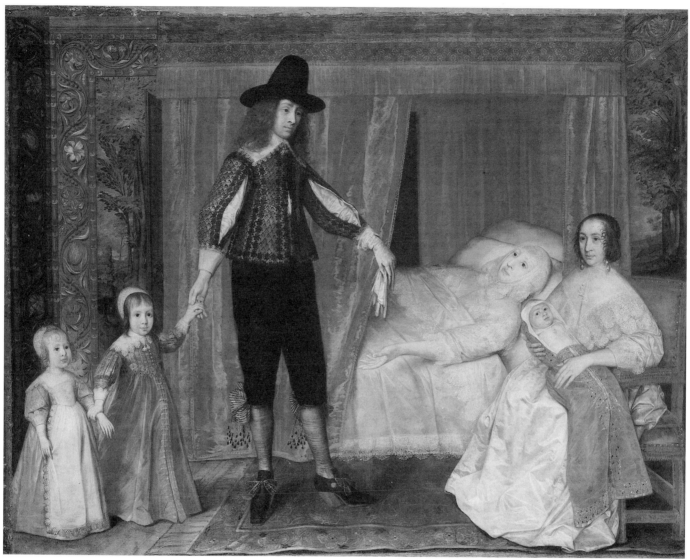

73. **The Saltonstall family,** *c.* 1641
David des Granges

Note A provincial family group with money to spend on good clothes, but not in step with the newest fashions.

Head The man wears the newly fashionable high-crowned hat over his shoulder-length hair, and is clean shaven. The seated woman has tightly curled hair worn closer to the sides of the head than was found in the 1630s.

Body His collar is of moderate size, with the narrowest of lace edging. The high waistline of the open fronted doublet and the fuller sleeves follow the fashionable line, but the breeches are not so full and short as would be seen in London. The seated woman's bodice has the more tubular sleeves of the early 1640s but her lace-edged collar is closed modestly across the low décolletage which was usual at court.

Accessories The shoes are tied with a ribbon rather than a rosette, a change of the 1640s. As is usual with children under the age of seven, at first glance their sex is indeterminate, but the taller child is a boy – with a doublet-style bodice and no apron.

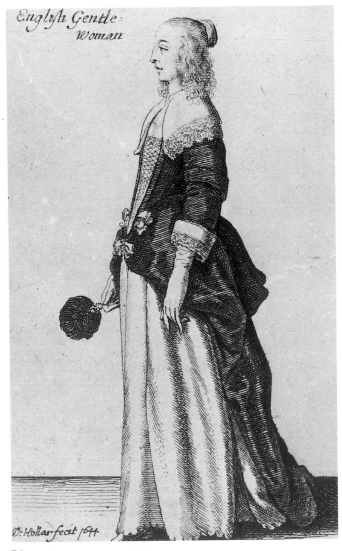

English Gentle-woman

V: Hollar feat 1644

74. English noblewoman, 1644
Wenceslas Hollar

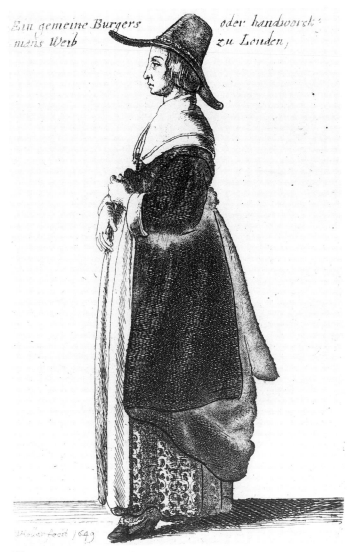

Ein gemeine Burgers mens Weib   oder handwerck: zu London,

Hollar feat 1649

75. Merchant's wife, 1649
Wenceslas Hollar

Note The dress of the mid-1640s has evolved a distinctive line which retains some features from the 1630s.

Head The hair is smooth at the temples and the longer side hair falls in loose curls, with a tight knot at the back of the head.

Body A square kerchief, folded triangularly, but shallower than earlier ones, is worn above a square-necked bodice with a long, stiffened stomacher. The two-tier sleeves have shallow horizontal cuffs above gloved hands. The softer, less bulky skirt is looped back to reveal a scallop-edged petticoat.

Accessories The round feather fan is the accessory of a fashionable young aristocrat.

Note Subtle distinctions in dress between social classes were carefully observed in the seventeenth century, and the more decorative accessories found in higher social groups (74) are missing from this woman's dress.

Head The hair is taken back smoothly over the ears under the curving brim of the high-crowned beaver hat.

Body A plain linen kerchief is worn over the shoulders and fastened at the throat. Much of the bodice is masked, but the sleeves are in one piece, fairly full, but with plain cuffs. The patterned – possibly embroidered – petticoat is revealed by the looped-up skirt but partly hidden by the apron.

Accessories The high-heeled shoes are trimmed with modest rosettes.

76. The execution of Charles I, *c.* 1649

Anon., detail from a Dutch engraving

Note This rather grim scene provides evidence of the dress of ordinary London citizens in the late 1640s.

Head Headwear varies between skull caps and high-crowned hats with shallow brims, some with ribbon bands, others with jaunty feathers; all are worn over straggling shoulder-length hair.

Body There are several styles of dress, with some men in deep collared capes, others in jerkins and doublets with full breeches. The woman in the foreground wears the type of dress depicted by Hollar (75). The executioner on the right, holding the King's head, and the royal servant, second from the left, wear fashionable loose-fitting tubular breeches.

Accessories In the foreground the men wear low-heeled shoes with simple tie fastenings, but the platform group mostly prefer wide-topped boots.

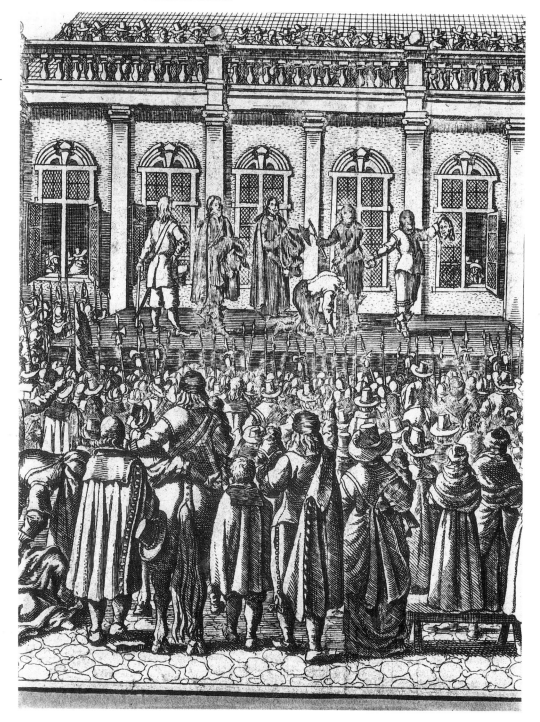

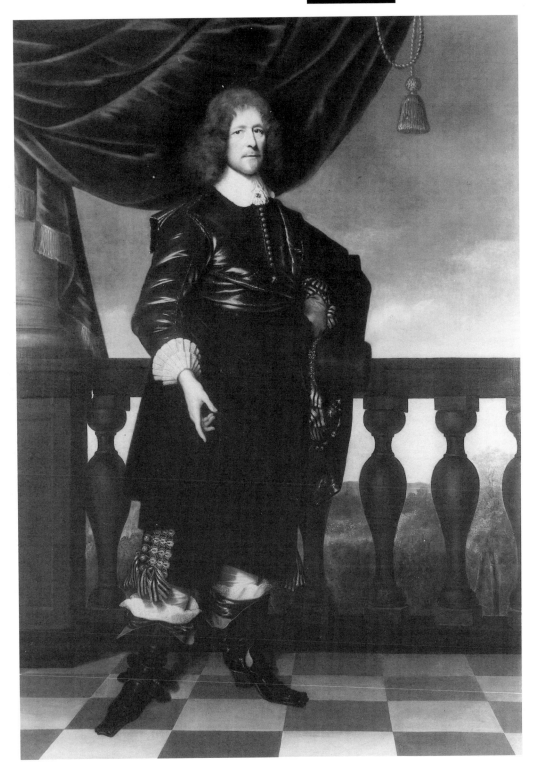

77. Oliver St John, 1651
Pieter Nason

Note The severely vertical appearance of menswear became more extreme in the 1650s as the traditional doublet and breeches changed in form.

Head St John has the carefully groomed and somewhat shorter and fuller hairstyle of the early 1650s, accompanied by a neatly trimmed beard and moustache.

Body His doublet is a traditional closed one, the sleeves edged with crisp double-tier lace cuffs. The lining of his cape matches the doublet, but the breeches are wide and tubular, very much in line with high fashion, and decorated with braided button fastenings and ribbons.

Accessories Matching ribbons add symmetry to his hat and gloves. The soft boots have elongated toes and high, sloping heels, and the boot tops use swathes of both silk and lace to provide width to the lower leg.

78. Mrs Elizabeth Claypole, 1658
John Michael Wright

Note As daughter of the Lord Protector, Oliver Cromwell, Mrs Claypole is dressed in a manner befitting a virtual princess – in a breastplate and surrounded by allegorical symbols.

Head The position of the knot of hair can be seen at the back of the head with some of the side curls pinned away from the face up to the knot.

Body A loosely held cloak reveals the edge of the smock and the full, layered ruffles around the sleeves. The skirt is held up, partly obscuring the central band of decoration but showing the braid at the hem and the lining beneath.

Accessories The jewellery is a traditional mixture of pearls and gemstone clasps.

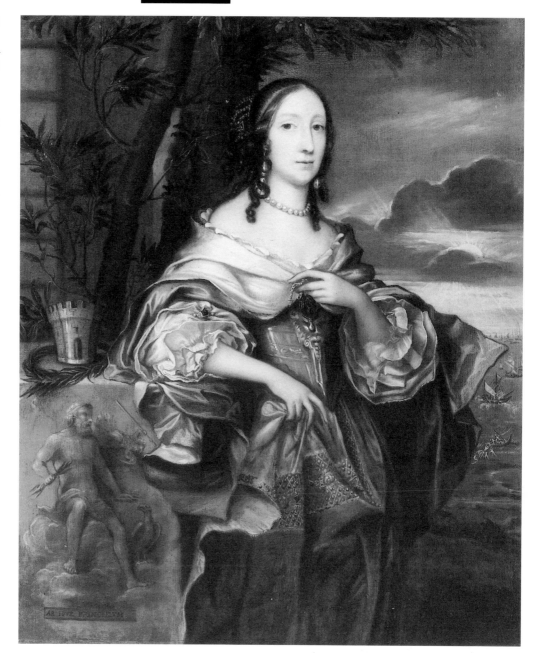

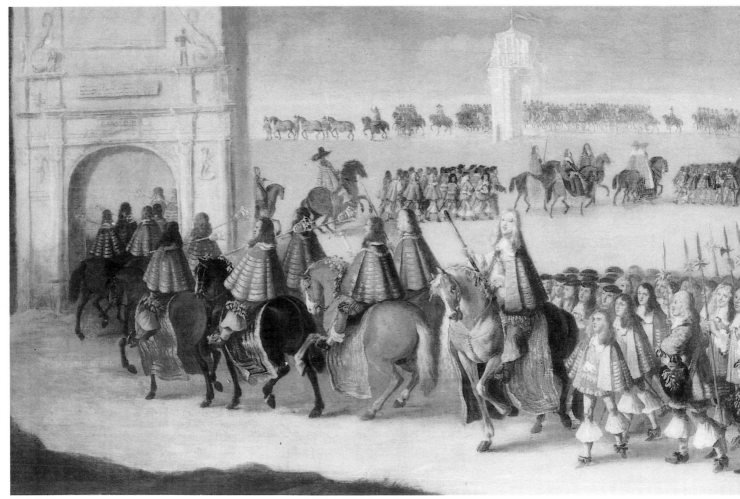

79. Charles II entering the City of London, 1661
Dirck Stoop

Note Although many of the men are wearing ceremonial uniforms, the group around the King are dressed in the height of fashion.

Head The long, full, centrally parted hair may, by this date, be enhanced with pieces of false hair.

Body Shaped collars with ornate tassels are worn over loosely fitting short jackets with open sleeves, caught at the wrist and edged with loops of ribbon. The wide 'petticoat' breeches are worn above the knee, and braided or edged at the waist and bottom edge with ribbons.

Accessories Deep falls of linen are a new, exuberant style of garter. High-heeled shoes with long, narrow toes are tied with soft bows and the tall beaver hats are decorated with feathers and more ribbons.

80. Unknown couple, *c.* 1667
Anon.

Note In a pastoral setting a fashionable young couple wear clothes which reflect her passive and his active pursuits.

Head The woman's hairstyle is very full at the sides of the head, with the ringlets suspended away from the face. The man wears a full, curled wig under a broad beaver hat.

Body The woman's dress has a long, stiffened bodice, a soft scarf round the neck and the shorter sleeves of the mid-to-late 1660s; the skirt is pushed back to reveal a decorated petticoat. The man's coat is semi-fitted, in the manner of the new style for menswear which evolved in the mid-1660s, with buttons fastened to the waist, deep-cuffed full sleeves and a knot of ribbons on the right shoulder.

Accessories The woman's flat straw hat protected her complexion from sunshine, and the fan was both functional and decorative. Below the man's full breeches his riding boots still have the wide tops of an earlier fashion.

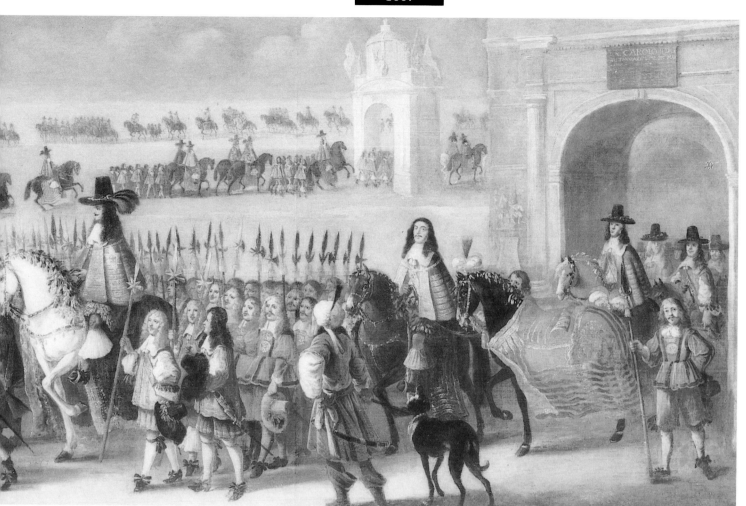

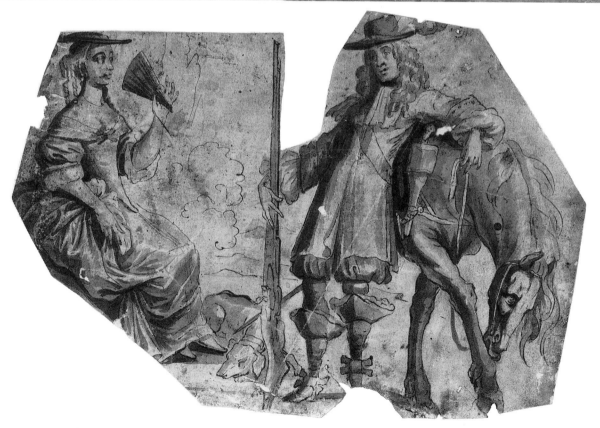

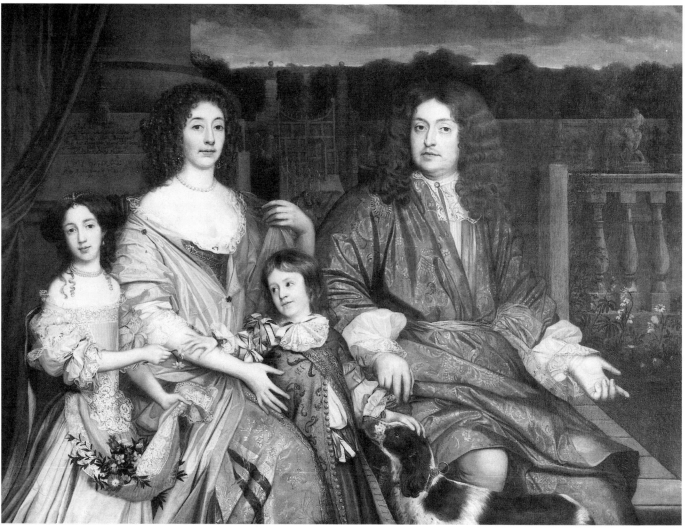

81. **The family of Sir Robert Vyner, 1673**
John Michael Wright

Note This group illustrates the importance of children in late-17th-century portraiture; their dress often reflects current fashions more accurately than their informally dressed elders.

Head Lady Vyner's hair is dressed in a mass of curls and ringlets which add width to her head. Sir Robert's wig is long, but equally full at the sides of the head.

Body Both adults wear loose gowns; hers is held by one clasp, partly revealing the stiffened bodice and striped silk brocade of her skirt; his is sashed loosely round the body, and worn over a linen shirt with rich lace collar and cuffs. The girl's dress has the formal fashionable elements of wide neckline, flat stiff bodice and short sleeves over full, tiered smock sleeves. The lace is delicate and complementary to the pale silk. The boy wears a loose-fitting vest (or coat) with short, ribbon-bedecked sleeves, with matching ribbons at the waist.

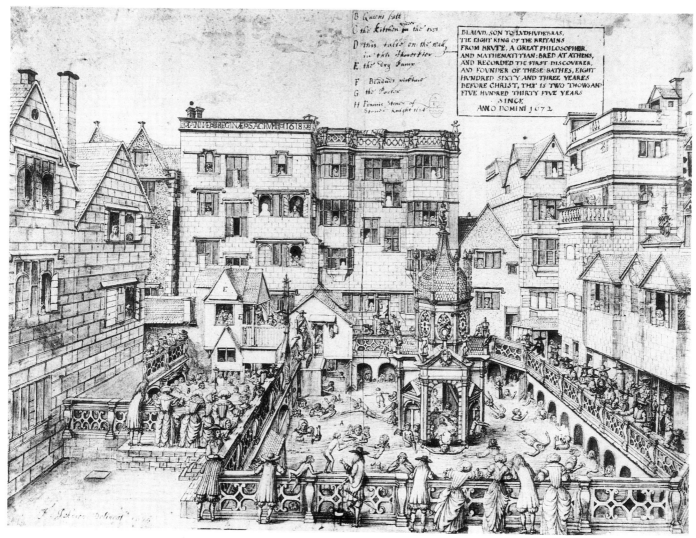

82. The baths at Bath, 1675

Thomas Johnson

Note Drinking the waters or bathing at spas was popular with men and women of all social classes in the late 17th century.

Head The majority of men wear wide-brimmed hats over their hair which ranges from the natural, straggling variety to full, long wigs. All of the women wear hoods.

Body The rather shapeless, inelegant line of early men's coats is well illustrated by the rows of figures watching the bathing. Breeches vary between the wide, tubular style edged with ribbon loops and the closer-fitting style with a knee-band. The short-sleeved, fitted bodices of the women are cut in one piece with the skirt in the mantua style, and all of the skirts are pinned or taken up and back to display the petticoats beneath, many of which would be of a rich, contrasting material or lavishly decorated with braid or fringe.

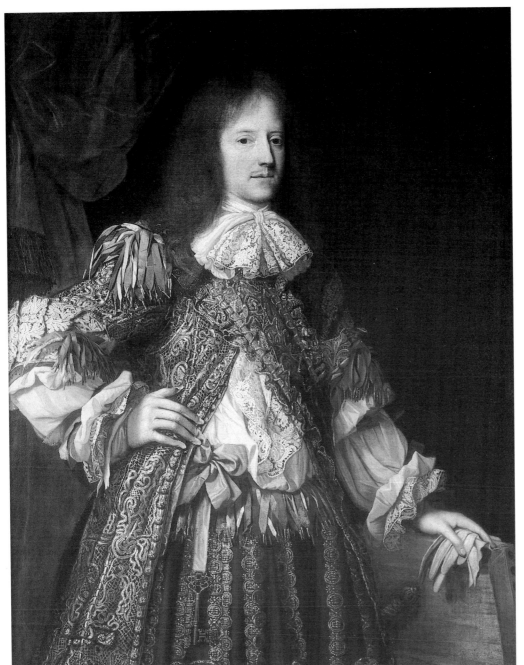

83. The 1st Earl of Bath, 1676
John Michael Wright

Note The sitter was Master of the Wardrobe to Charles II, and an influential and fashionable courtier.

Head The long, smooth wig and narrow moustache are insignificant foils to the grandeur of the Earl's dress.

Body The tiered cravat is composed of layers of fine linen overlaid with lace. His richly embroidered coat, with its deeply cuffed sleeves, is so ornately decorated that the loose, inelegant line of its cut is barely noticeable. No waistcoat distracts attention from the lace-edged shirt front, or from the wide petticoat breeches with their ribbon points at the waist. Matching ribbons decorate the cuffs and form a shoulder knot.

Accessories The broad embroidered sash, *en suite* with the coat, acts as a sword hanger; the Earl's key of office is suspended from the rosette at his waist.

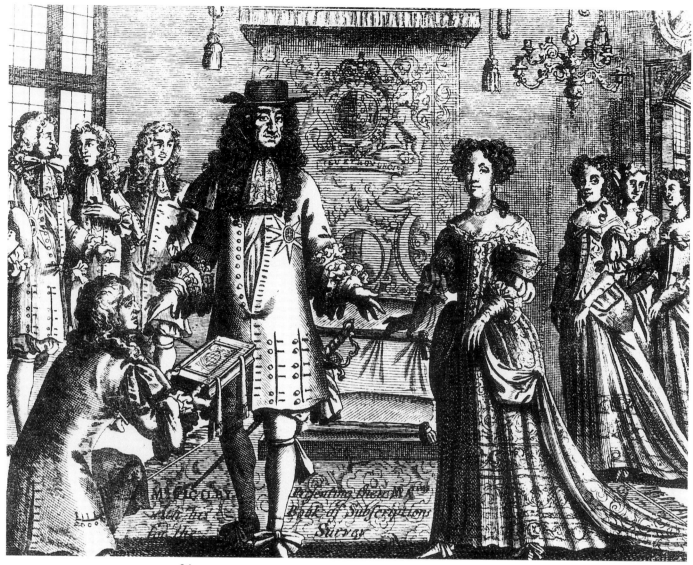

84. Charles II and Queen Catherine

Engraved frontispiece from Ogilby and Morgan's *Map of London*, 1682

Note A private presentation at court, with all of the figures in semi-formal dress.

Head All of the men, with the exception of Ogilby (kneeling), wear curled wigs, but only the King wears a hat. The universal fashion of wearing hats indoors disappeared around 1680. The broad, tightly curled hairstyles of the ladies echo the shape, if not the length, of the male styles.

Body Softly gathered cravats, full shirts with ruffled cuffs, and full breeches are worn with the ubiquitous loose coats with their assemblage of buttons. Coat sleeves are longer, but retain wide cuffs. Stiff long-fronted bodices are worn with looped-up trained skirts over patterned petticoats.

Accessories All of the women wear elbow-length gloves and pearl jewellery. Their narrow-toed shoes are similar in style to those of the men.

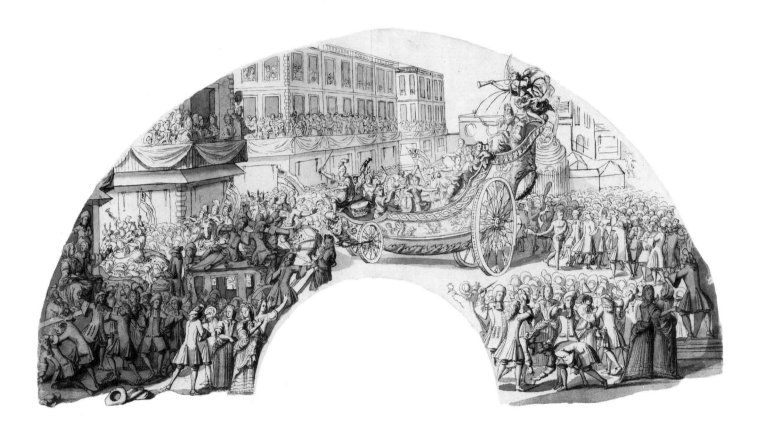

85. The Chariot of the Virgin Queen, Lord Mayor's Pageant, 1686
Anon.

Note A festive outdoor event, affording a lively but unusual London street scene.

Head A sea of men's hats with up-turned brims, worn over wigs and shorter natural hair, is leavened by female hoods over upswept hair, and one high-crowned woman's hat (right).

Body The change in men's coat design is carefully recorded; the upper body is more fitted, the skirt width absorbed into full pleats at sides and back. Pockets vary between vertical and horizontal slits, with some horizontal flaps in evidence. Stockings are rolled over the knees of the closer fitting breeches. The women wear short-sleeved mantuas, with the skirts swagged back over the hips to display one or more petticoats.

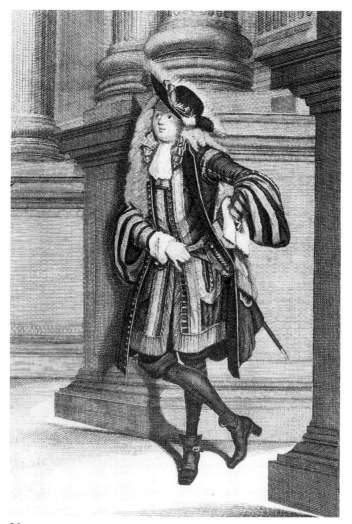

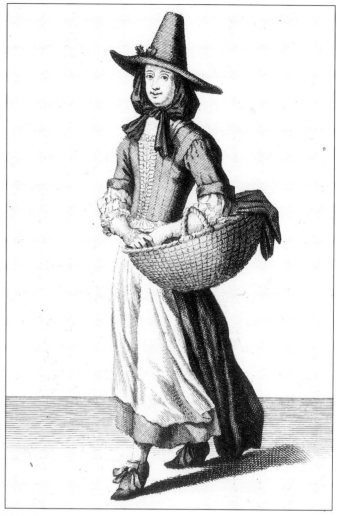

86. 'Homme de qualité . . .', 1687
J.D. de St Jean

87. 'Old Satten, Old Taffety or Velvet'
Marcellus Laroon I, *Cries of London*, 1688

Note This young exquisite embodies the decorative flamboyance which could be superimposed on the fairly severe lines of men's dress.

Head The very full wig is probably powdered; its width allied to fashionable impulse dictates the rakish angle of the ornately trimmed hat.

Body A semi-fitted, long-sleeved waistcoat is worn with the coat; both garments are lavishly decorated with bands of applied metal lace and bullion fringe. Broad, pendant coat cuffs acted as a frame for waistcoat sleeves or, in other circumstances, the billow of shirt sleeves and ruffles. Moderately full breeches are worn to the knee.

Accessories The waterfall effect of the cravat over the knot of ribbons is echoed by the fringed gloves, with the weighted bullion decoration falling gracefully over the hand.

Note There was an important secondhand market in materials in the 17th century, reflecting the high cost of the luxurious imported silk textiles.

Head The street seller wears the traditional conical crowned, wide-brimmed hat of the lower classes over her plain hood.

Body Her dress is a modest version of the mantua. The pleating of the material to fit the torso and to sit smoothly over the shoulders, and the set of the short sleeves are easier to see than in the highly decorative mantuas found in French fashion plates. Her skirt is floor-length and does not require careful arrangement of folds, but hangs free and is only a little longer than the petticoat. The linen apron complements the crisp simplicity of the modestly ruffled smock sleeves.

Accessories The shoes are plain, not exaggeratedly long-fronted, as was fashionable, but tied with ribbons, perhaps from the seller's own stock.

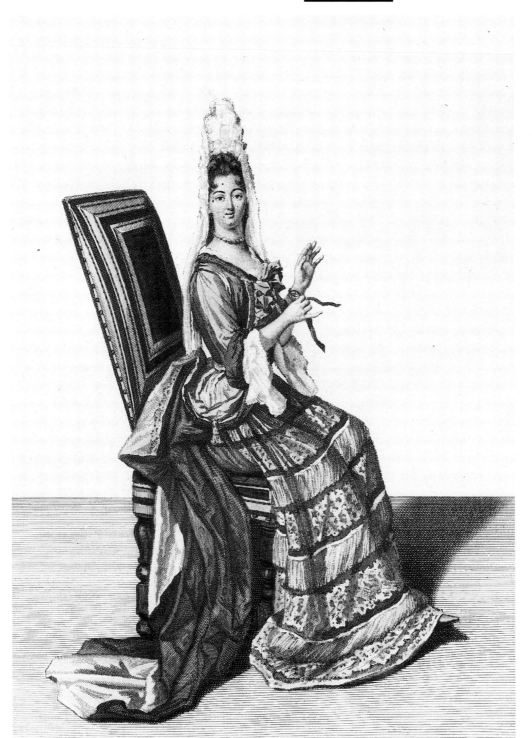

88. **'Dame de la plus haute qualité', 1693**
J.D. de St Jean

Note A young noblewoman dressed in the richest fashions of the early 1690s.

Head Above upswept hair the lace commode has four tiers, decreasing in width. Lace streamers or lappets fall from the sides of the cap, edging the face and extending to the middle of the back.

Body The silk mantua has loosely fitting elbow-length sleeves and a stomacher decorated with *échelles*. The skirt is looped back and folded to display the contrasting lining and the border embroidery. The striped, brocaded silk petticoat is further enriched with applied bands of metal fringe.

Accessories In addition to the usual pearl necklace and earrings, a locket or miniature is tied onto the left wrist.

VI **'Homme de qualité en habit garny de rubans . . .', 1689**
J.D. de St. Jean
Colour illustration, between pages 128 and 129

89. John Dryden, 1696–7
James Maubert

Note A rare full-length portrait of a man informally dressed.

Head The long wig appears somewhat disordered, as if in need of the ministrations of its maker; the pyramids of hair above the temples are disarranged and lop-sided.

Body A fringed linen cravat is worn with a plain shirt with unadorned cuffs. The comfortable bulk of the satin robe, with its wide sleeves, wrapover front and warm, ankle-length are clearly visible.

Accessories Dryden wears mules on his feet, low-heeled for ease of movement, but bullion-fringed to indicate taste and expense. These indoor slippers were popular; they followed the prevailing shape of shoe fronts but were more comfortable to relax in.

VII **Prince James Stuart with his sister, 1695**
Nicholas de Largillierre
Colour illustration, between pages 128 and 129

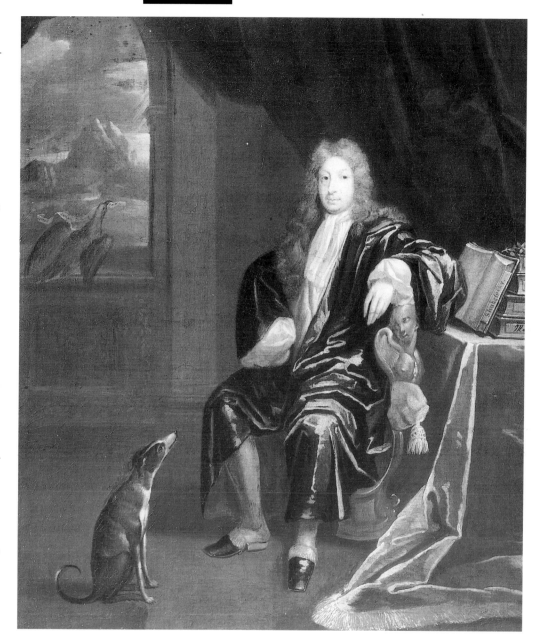

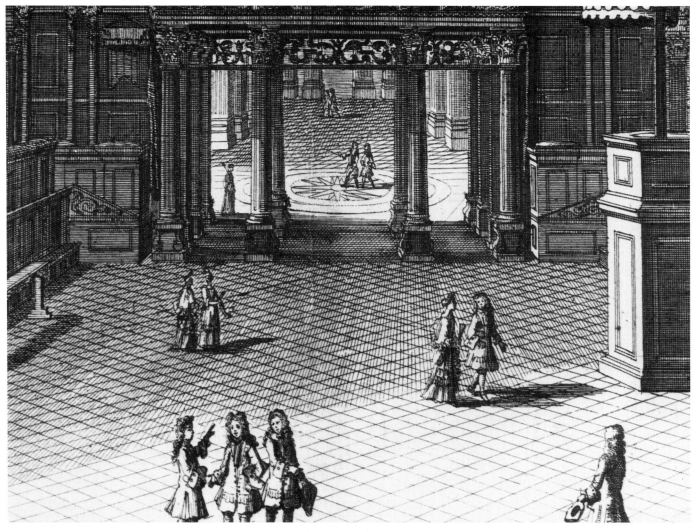

90. **The interior of St Paul's Cathedral (detail), 1698–1700**
Anon. engraving

Note By the end of the century men's and women's dress had evolved into the elegant but easy styles which were modified, refined but not dramatically changed until the late eighteenth century.

Head All of the men wear the full, broad wigs of the turn of the century, with the considerable length pushed back over their shoulders. The women's commodes are diminishing in size, with the height falling forward over the forehead.

Body The men's coats have the wider sleeves and proportionately shallower cuffs from which only the sleeve ruffles emerge. The stiffly pleated coat skirts were interlined to achieve this rigid silhouette. All of the pockets are horizontal, with flaps. The women's mantuas have fuller sleeves and their petticoats are widening and developing a tiered, somewhat frilly line.

Accessories Tricorne hats were now the most popular form of headwear for fashionable men.

Chaucer reciting before an elegant audience *c.*1400

English School, manuscript illumination

Note The splendid impracticality of the costume suggests that here we see the royal court.

Head The men who are not bare-headed wear hoods flat on top of their heads as if they were caps, with the capes and tippets twisted into fantastic shapes. The women wear their hair arranged in little bundles above the ears, and decorated in front with curved gold bands.

Body Both men and women wear gowns with high collars and trailing sleeves; the woman at the bottom left cannot get her hands out of hers. Sleeves like this provoked much adverse criticism, on account of their impractical size and the expense of the fabric. In 1402 Parliament petitioned the king to prohibit their use, along with gowns which reached the ground, by anyone below the rank of knight banneret.

Accessories There is a profusion of gold belts and chains, some of which are decorated with small bells.

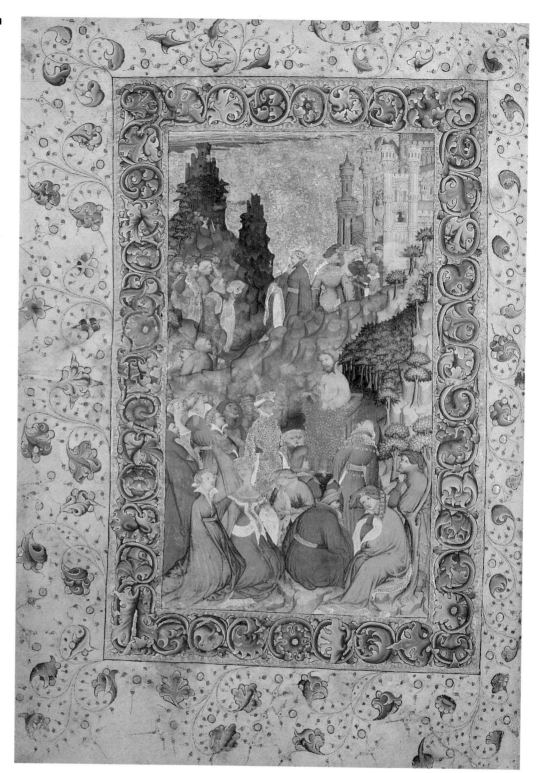

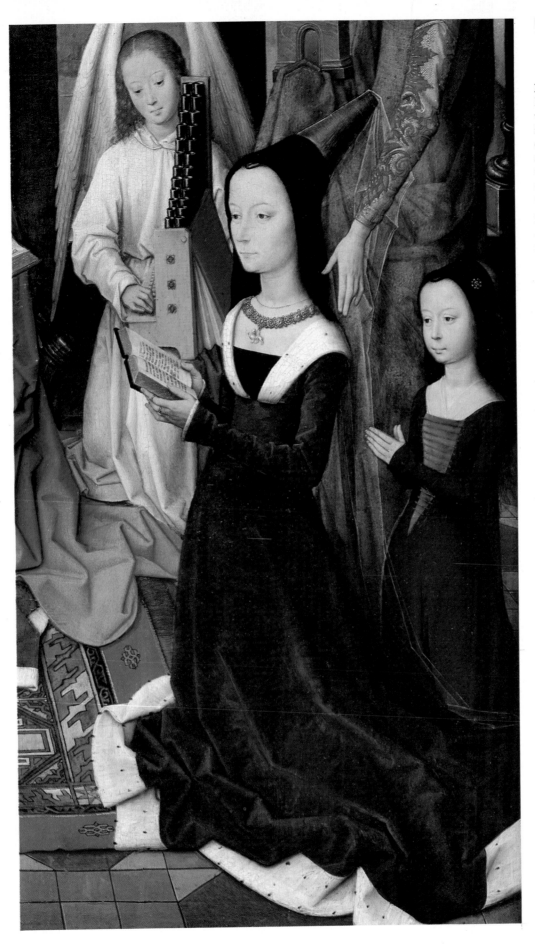

II   Lady Donne and her daughter *c.*1477

Hans Memlinc

Note It is unlikely that Lady Donne ever wore Flemish dress, which we see here, but her outfit is a good example of contemporary Flemish fashions, and her daughter's dress shows that children were not always dressed in smaller versions of their parents' clothes.

Head Lady Donne and her daughter both wear a velvet frontlet with a small loop at the front. The child is allowed the greater freedom of wearing her hair pulled through the frontlet, with no further inconveniences, but her mother's hair must be contained in the tall cone which is inserted into the back of the frontlet. On top is a transparent floor-length veil.

Body Lady Donne wears a fashionable gown, with ermine collar and hem. The front lacing on her daughter's gown can be loosened as she grows, and she is not squeezed into a tight, deep belt like her mother's.

Accessories Lady Donne wears round her neck the Yorkist livery collar of suns and roses with a heraldic lion pendant. Her daughter has a brooch pinned to her frontlet.

III Unknown girl, *c.*1569
Master of the Countess
of Warwick (attr.)

Note The late 1560s saw a
preference for brighter, fresher
colours set off by enamelled gold
jewellery, arranged in a highly
distinctive manner, gold braid
trimming and strong, naturalistic
embroidered patterns.

Head A small velvet cap,
decorated with feathers and
jewelled roses is perched on the
crown of the head, over hair
drawn back into a gold caul. A
pink, a favourite Elizabethan
flower, is tucked behind the left
ear.

Body A double-layered ruff,
embroidered in gold, is drawn in
closely around the neck; it is
complemented by matching
wrist ruffs. The partlet has a
standing collar edged with gold
braid and embroidered with the
same pattern of roses as the
sleeves. The chemise is seen
beneath the open front of partlet
and bodice. The latter has
matching raised shoulder bands
through which rounded puffs of
the chemise sleeve are pulled.
The tightly fitting bodice has a
central fastening, the piped
velvet edges of which have been
whipped over with gold thread.
Appliqué panels of gold braid on
a black ground decorate the front
of the bodice and the shoulder
bands. The skirt, matching the
plain ground of the bodice swells
out from the waistline.

Accessories A narrow sash acts
as a girdle. The emphatic
jewellery includes a pearl and
gold rope around the neck with
a pendant enamelled gold figure;
a ribbon from which an oak-leaf
pendant studded with pearls is
pinned asymmetrically to the left
breast; and a thick chain looped
up and pinned to the bodice.

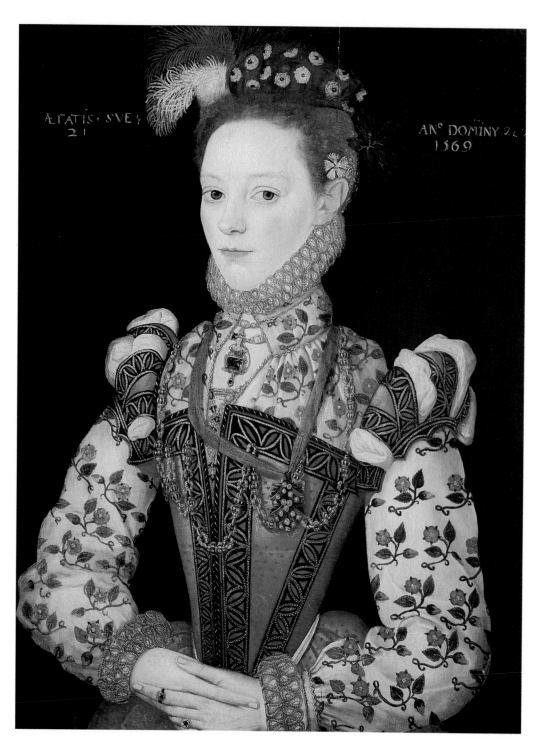

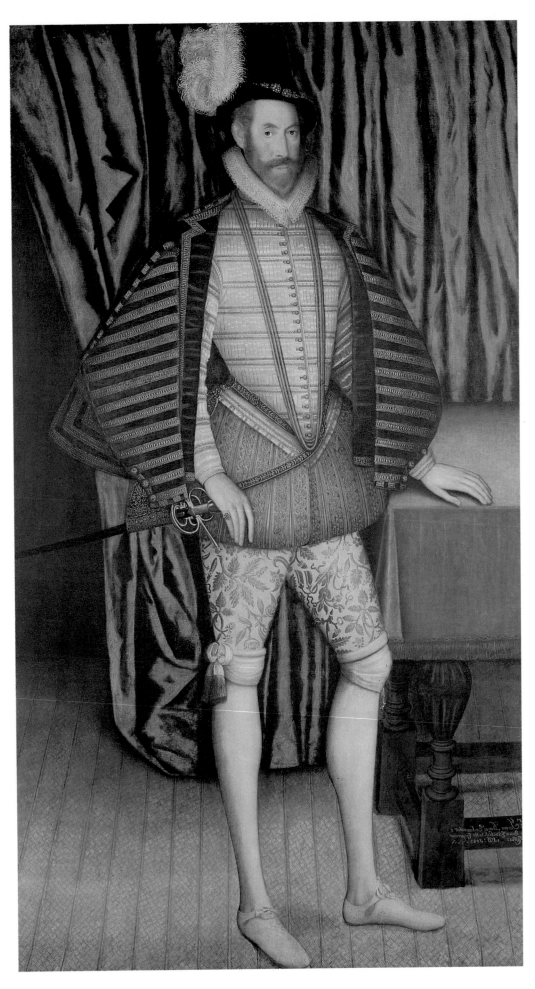

IV Sir Jerome Bowes, *c.*1584
Anon.

Note Sir Jerome was an impressive man, reputed to be 'three storeys high'. When this portrait was painted, he had just returned from a successful diplomatic mission to Russia.

Head The black tall-crowned hat is worn with a pearl hat-band and white ostrich feather.

Body The lace falling band is worn with an underpropper so that it tilts. Across the shoulders is a green velvet, sleeved cloak, heavily guarded with gold braid. The white satin doublet has a modified peascod belly; it buttons down the front and is decorated with horizontal lines of gold braid that enclose bands of vertical slashes. The panes of the pale green trunkhose are embroidered with gold. They are worn with white and gold brocade canions over which white stockings are fastened with gold-fringed garters.

Accessories Sir Jerome wears three heavy gold chains around his neck. His green belt, sword-belt and hangers are embroidered with gold. He wears shoes of the same type as Sir Walter Ralegh (see Fig. 61).

V **Queen Henrietta Maria, 1633-5**

Anon.

Note The elegance of dress associated with female fashions at the Caroline Court owed more to simplicity of decoration and richness of colour than to ease of style.

Head The Queen's hair is teased into small curls which frame the sides of the face, and the knot at the back is surmounted by a delicate pearl tiara.

Body The low-cut bodice is edged by a deep collar which partly disguises the awkward set of the bulky sleeves, but the tension on the satin created by the high waistline is evident in the creases above the curved stomacher tab. The fullness in the skirt is drawn to the back of the waist and supported on hip pads. The applied pearl decoration adds interest and elongation of line to the essentially simple construction of bodice and skirt.

Accessories Pearl earrings and necklace complement the applied decoration on bodice and skirt. The coloured fan leaf is linked to the dress by the use of matching ribbons on the bosom and at the waistline.

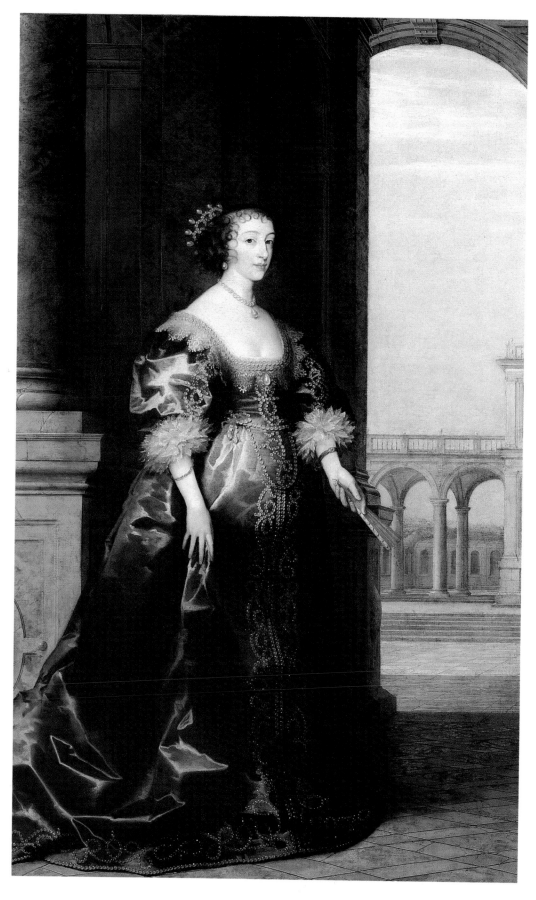

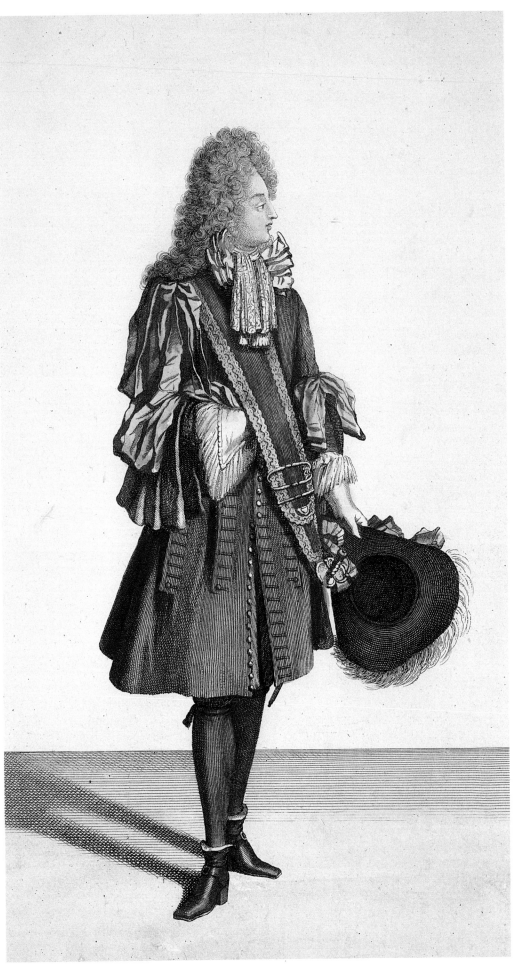

Note The exquisite grooming which French court protocol demanded from courtiers, and which to a greater or lesser extent was copied throughout Europe, is epitomized in this fashion plate.

Head The tightly curled wig is much higher above the forehead, carefully framing the face and falling back over the shoulders and away from the tiered cravat with its stiffened ribbon wings.

Body The body of the coat is fitted, with the fullness of the skirts taken into side pleats. The pleated pendant cuffs reveal a proportion of the rich brocade of the narrower waistcoat sleeves. Plain breeches, stockings and shoes do not draw attention away from the cascade of ribbons and the lace-edged sword hanger which dominate the upper half of the torso.

Accessories The hat is edged with feathers and more ribbons, and shows signs of becoming the newly fashionable tricorne shape. The gauntlet gloves are worn to show how the bullion fringe can fall – either in a line with the glove, or over the wrist.

Prince James Stuart (the 'Old Pretender') with his sister, 1695

Nicholas de Largillierre

Note Children were exquisitely dressed as miniature adults, but their portraits were less susceptible to the informal, classical or drapery styles of painting which dominated English portraiture in the late seventeenth century. French formal portraiture, as this example demonstrates, demanded a correct representation of fashionable dress.

Head The prince wears his own hair, shorter than a fashionable wig, but brushed up into peaks above the temples. The construction of his sister's commode, with its graduated tiers of lace attached to a cap, is clearly visible.

Body The lace and ribbon cravat was accepted formal wear; the studied elegance of the brocaded waistcoat with cuffs turned over the coat cuffs, the stiff-skirted coat buttoned just enough to display its fine cut, the leather shoes with contrasting tongue lining, the modified tricorne and the Garter orders and sword reflect the stylish rigidity of French Court circles. The princess's dress is a child's version (complete with leading strings) of the stiff-bodied gown which French royal ladies wore on great occasions in preference to a mantua.

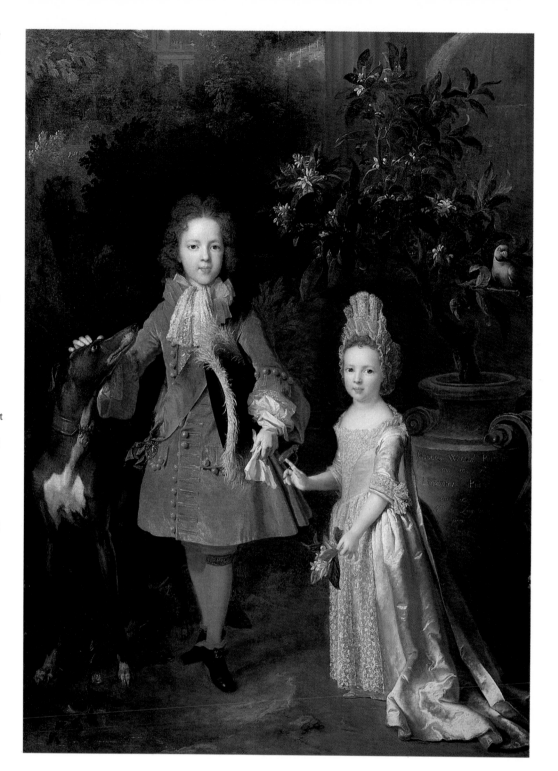

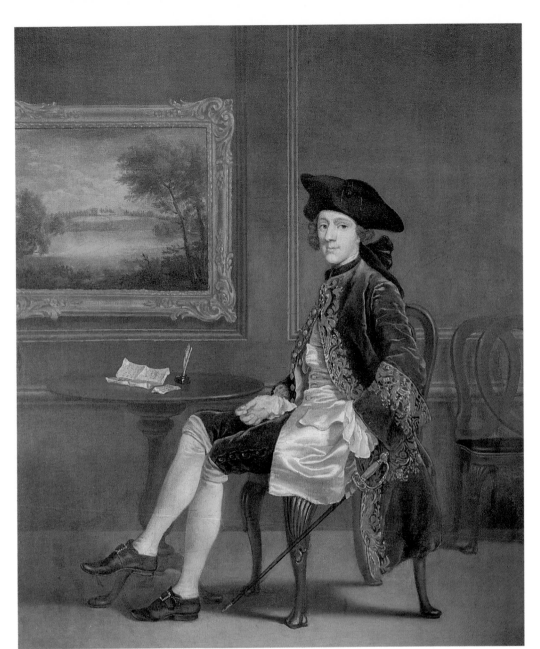

VIII **John Conyers,** *c.*1747
Francis Hayman

Head It is probably his own hair here, in loose side curls, the back hair tied into a large black silk bag, the ribbon ends of which are brought round to the front in the solitaire style.

Body The coat and breeches are of a lustrous blue silk, probably velvet; the weight and luxury of the coat are increased by the gold embroidery trimming the front edges, the cuffs and the pocket flaps. The waistcoat is of plain satin, a gap in the buttoning at mid-chest indicating the fashionable gesture of inserting the hand there.

Accessories The black three-cornered hat is trimmed with a cloth button and loop.

IX **Miss Eleanor Dixie,** *c.*1755
Henry Pickering (attr.)

Note Although traditionally known as Eleanor Dixie, the sitter is more likely to be her stepmother, the second wife of Sir Wolstan Dixie whom he married in 1753.

Head The straw hat, trimmed with blue silk ribbon, is held on the head by a similar ribbon in a bow at the nape of the neck, over the white linen cap which is just visible.

Body It is at this time that the sack becomes formal dress, with a tightening of the bodice and a regimentation of the back pleats which are sewn down from the shoulder; it is invariably worn as an open robe. The silk, possibly a Spitalfields brocade, is a delicate floral design within lattice-work compartments in white, on a white ground. The line of the bodice is long and pointed, the robings set wide apart, and a lace-edged kerchief of fine lawn is crossed over and fastened with a blue breast bow. The sleeves are tightly fitting to the elbow, with treble flounces and huge sleeve ruffles.

Accessories The girl is caught in the act of drawing on her long white silk gloves – these were an indispensable part of formal dress.

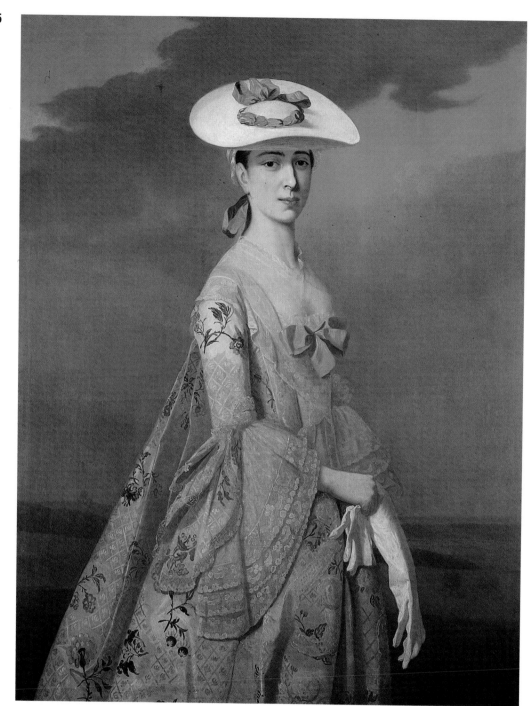

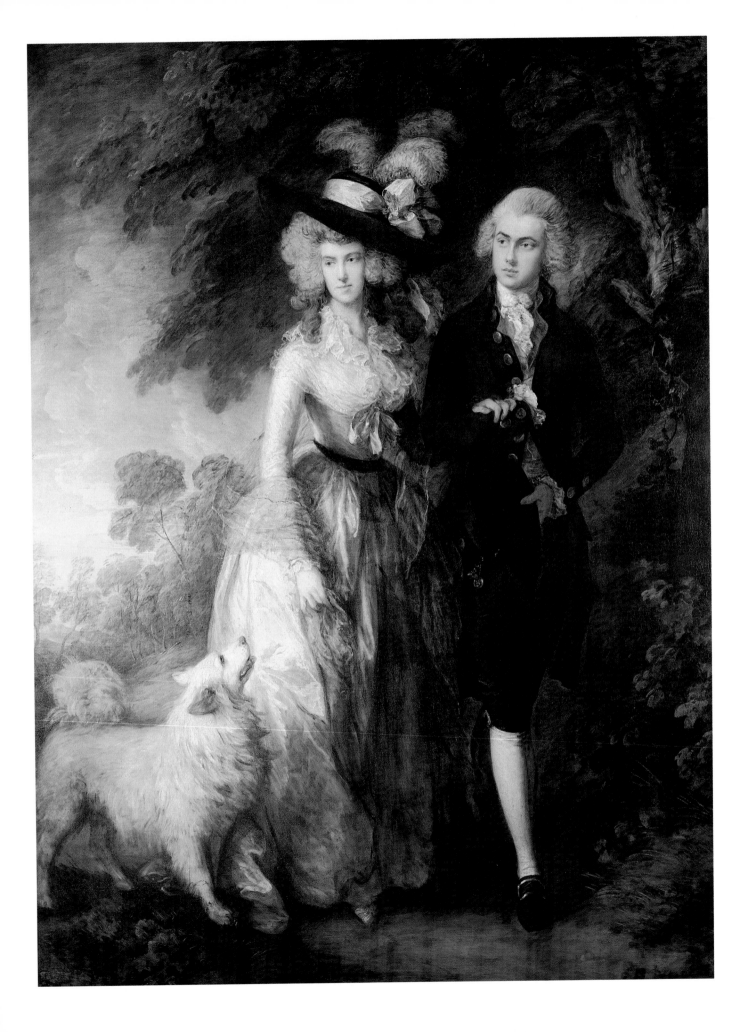

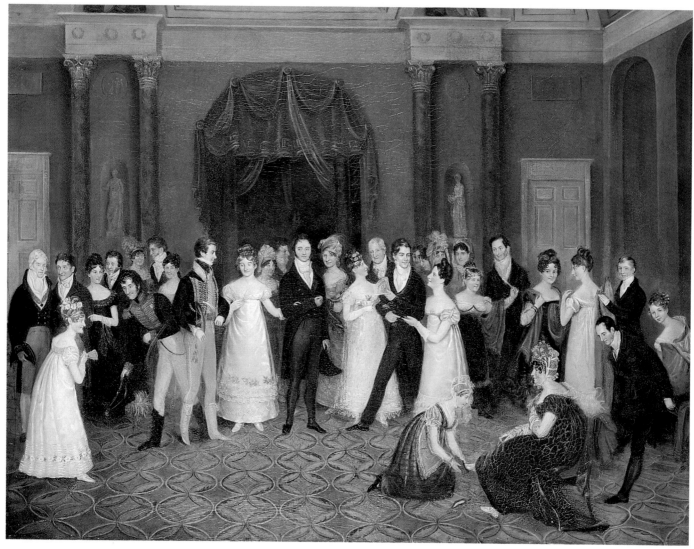

XI The Cloakroom, Clifton Assembly Rooms, 1817 (left hand page)
Rolinda Sharples

Note Fashionable ball dress is worn here.

Head The women wear their hair with bandeaux and flowers, or under silk turbans trimmed with feathers.

Body They wear dresses of light-coloured embroidered net or lace, over brightly coloured silk or satin underdresses featuring the puffed sleeves and very high waists of 1815-20. The flared skirts have deep flounced or vandyked hems, often trimmed with artificial flowers.
  The men wear white cravats and waistcoats, dark dress coats, and breeches or pantaloons.

Accessories The women's accessories include low-heeled satin shoes, long kid gloves, shawls and fans.
  The men wear lace-up pumps, except for the two on the left whose military uniforms demand hessian boots.

X The Morning Walk, *c.*1785
Thomas Gainsborough

Note This is the ideal of English fashionable dress in the 1780s, which was followed all over Europe.

Head The hairstyles of this newly married couple complement each other. William Hallett's own hair is powdered, and 'curled with irons to give the head a large, bushy appearance' (C. P. Moritz, 1782). Elizabeth Hallett's hair is frizzed out at the sides, with thick ringlets to the shoulders; her large black hat is trimmed with white ribbons and ostrich feathers.

Body The almost impressionist technique of the artist makes it difficult to discern the details of Mrs Hallett's white silk dress, which is probably an open gown, girdled with black silk around the waist. The breast is emphasized with a ribbon knot and a kerchief of fine muslin or gauze. The silk gauze stole echoes the contrived carelessness of her hair and dress.
  Her husband wears a black suit, cut to slope away at the sides; in 1782 Moritz had found that 'the English seem, in general, to prefer dark colours'.

Accessories Mr Hallett carries a black round hat trimmed with a buckled band. At his waist, seals dangle from a watch chain.

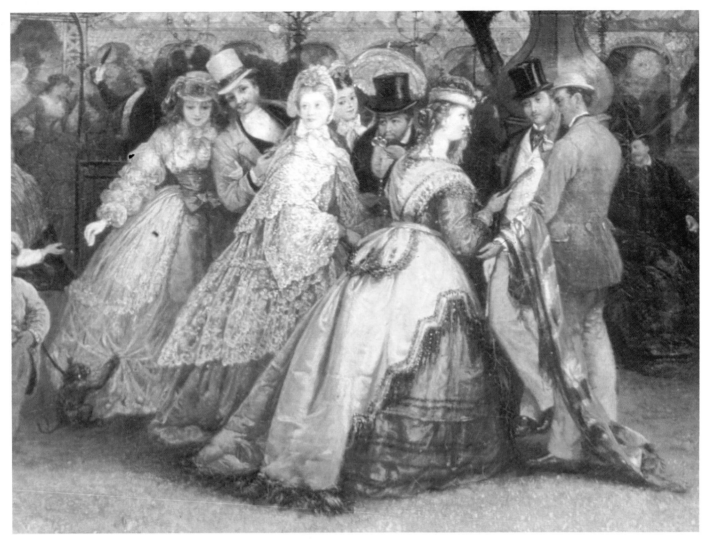

XII The Dancing Platform at Cremorne Gardens (detail), 1864
Phoebus Levin

Note Expensively dressed ladies of the town frequented such popular pleasure gardens.

Head To offset the wide crinoline skirts, headwear is small and neat, whether it is a narrow-brimmed hat (left), a popular 'spoon' bonnet (centre), or an unusual toque (right).

Body Crinolines are still very large, but with more fullness at the back; this is emphasized by the use of basques and shaped overskirts, which by 1868 will have developed into bustles and pannier skirts.

The woman in the centre wears a lace mantle with an attached cape over her silk day dress, the contrasts of dark plain silk and pale lace being particularly fashionable in this decade.

The woman on the left has a silk dress overlaid with multi-puffed sleeves and a draped overskirt of tulle. The third dress features a bodice with sash-like basques at the back, and a separate overskirt with cutaway sides.

XIII St. Martin-in-the Fields (detail), 1888
William Logsdail

Note Here we see a middle-class woman and child in fashionable winter outdoor dress. The child in the centre of the picture exemplifies by contrast the social inequality of the day.

Head The woman wears her hair in a knot under a tall, high-crowned hat, known as a 'post-boy', probably of felt or beaver, and trimmed with silk ribbon and feathers. This flower-pot-shaped hat was one of the most popular of the decade, matching the overall silhouette with its narrow, tubular forms.

Body She wears a sheath-like cloth coat (reds were popular in the 1870s and 1880s) edged with fur.

Accessories She has high-heeled shoes or boots, gloves and an umbrella.

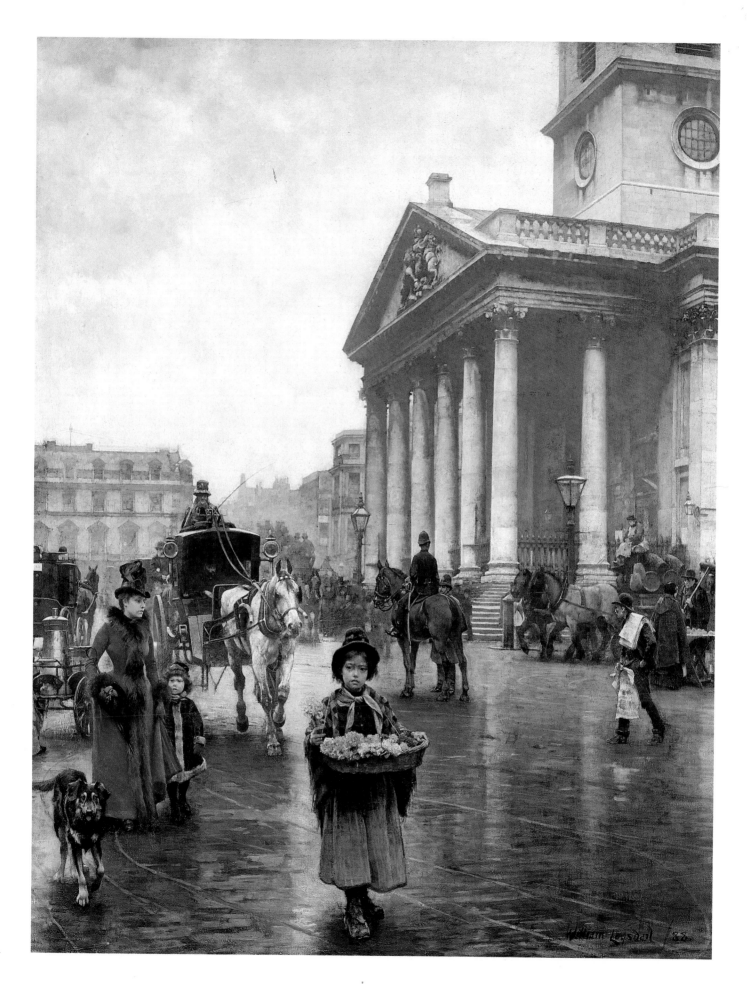

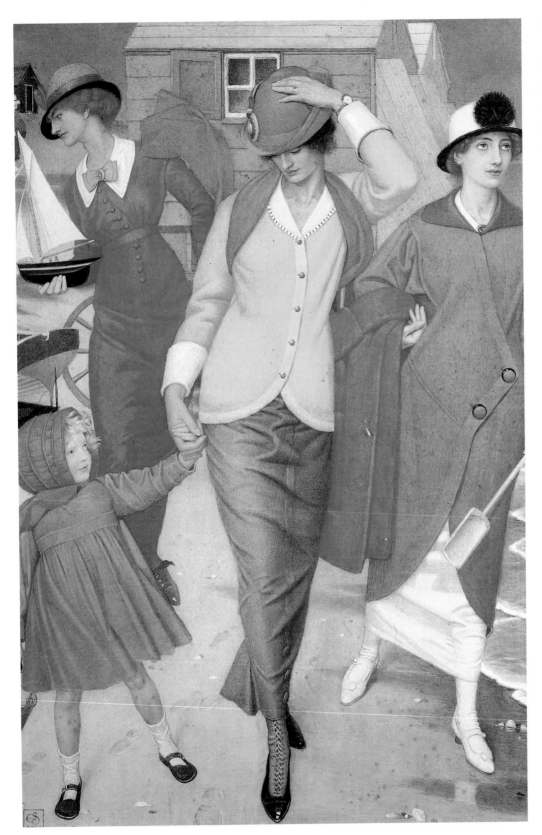

XIV 'Along the Shore', 1914
Joseph Southall

Note Although dressed for a seaside stroll, it is evident that long strides would be virtually impossible in the narrow, hobble skirts; however the hemline has begun to rise and the dress of the woman on the right is moving towards a more practical and comfortable style.

Head By 1914 hats were smaller with narrower brims; there was a fashion for turned-up brims tilted up at the back (centre). Long hair was dressed with a certain amount of volume over the ears.

Body The dress on the left has the raised waistline and narrow skirt which had been in fashion for several years. The jacket and coat of the other two women suggest a lessening of the emphasis on the high waist and a loosening of the silhouette while retaining its tubular line. The button fastenings are prominent on all three costumes. The little girl wears a short-waisted dress and sunbonnet.

Accessories Three different styles of footwear are illustrated: brown laced shoes (left); laced boots of black patent leather with grey cloth tops (centre) and white bar shoes with low heels (right). The woman in the centre wears a gold wrist watch; wrist watches began to replace pocket watches in the early years of the century.

XV La Caline

André Marty (attr.)
Gazette du Bon Ton, 1922

Note A plate from the French magazine *Gazette du Bon Ton* illustrates a woman's dress by Doeuillet and a man's jacket by Larsen.

Head The man's hair is cut very short and he is clean shaven. The woman's hair is long and drawn back over her ears.

Body The man wears a tweed sports jacket and tapered trousers with narrow turn-ups which reveal his socks. His shirt has a soft, turned-down collar and his knotted tie is diagonally striped. The general effect is neat and rather sharp – the centre crease on his trousers is pronounced. The woman wears a long, loose-fitting 'tube' or 'chemise' dress with a narrow tie belt at hip level; the fabric is geometrically patterned.

Accessories The man's socks are light-coloured and he wears laced shoes. The woman's plain court shoes have moderately high heels.

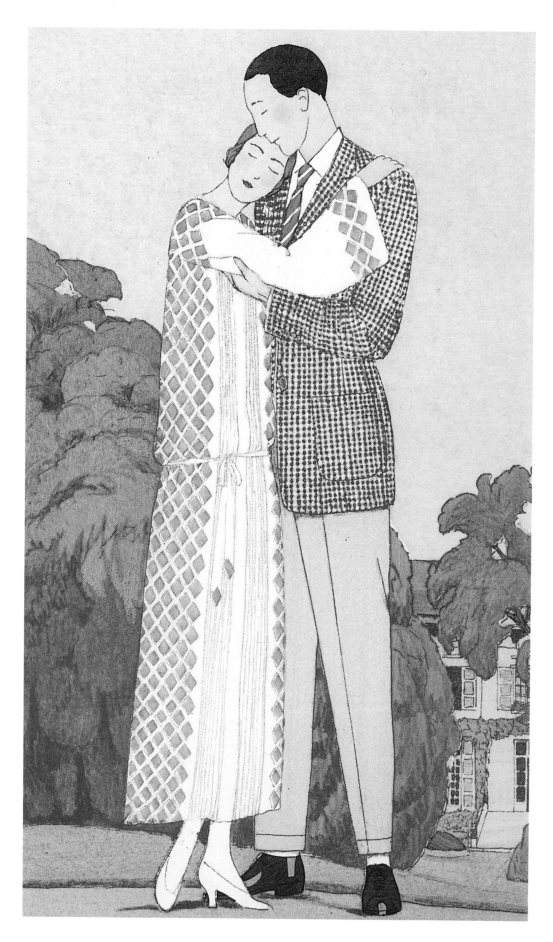

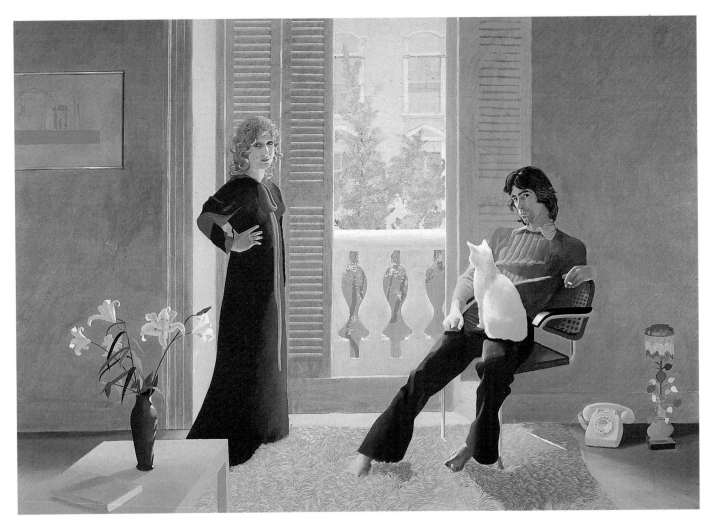

XVI **Mr and Mrs Clark and Percy, 1970-1**
   David Hockney

Note A portrait of the artist's friends – Celia Birtwell the textile designer, and her husband Ossie Clark, one of the chief dress designers for the fashion firm Quorum – in their Bayswater home. Mr. Clark's bare feet, casual pose and challenging stare seem to be deliberately flouting the established conventions of formal portraiture as does Mrs Clark's confident pose with one hand on her hip and standing, while her husband occupies the only visible chair.

Head Mrs Clark's shoulder-length hair is arranged in loose curls framing her face. Mr Clark's hair is long enough to cover most of his forehead and ears and reaches over his collar at the back.

Body Mrs Clark wears a full-length dress, high to the neck and with long sleeves; it is softly shaped to the figure and flares at the hem. Mr Clark is informally dressed in open-necked shirt, sweater and flared, corduroy jeans.

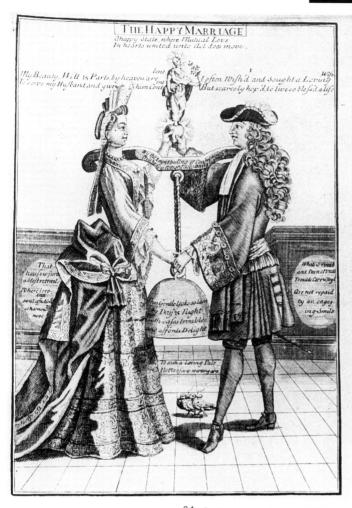

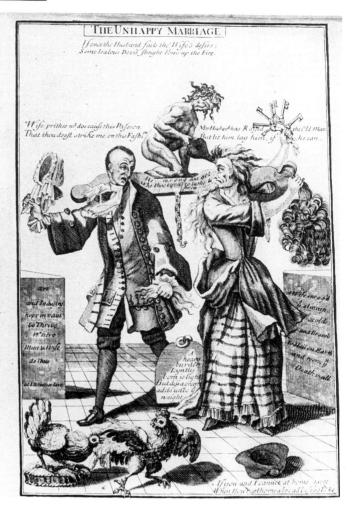

91. **Satire on marriage,** *c.* 1700
Anon. engraving

Note This shows the layers of dress, particularly in the *Unhappy Marriage* scene where the couple are probably middle-class, in contrast to the richer and more fashionably dressed pair in the *Happy Marriage*.

Head Over shaved heads the men wear full-bottomed wigs; equally elaborate in arrangement are the female headdresses or commodes, often built up with false hair – the enraged husband may be holding some of this in his hand.

Body The clothing is distinguished by heaviness and surface decoration. The men wear knee-length coats with copious side pleats and very wide sleeves; there is a last glimpse of the vertical pocket on the left. The waistcoat is as long as the coat, and both button to the hem.

Both women wear the mantua, a more formal version in the *Happy Marriage* with an embroidered tasselled train, and a plain, torn one by the unhappy wife. The horizontal patterning of the petticoat is achieved by a striped fabric on the right, and on the left by the use of applied *falbalas* of lace.

Accessories The happy husband wears a fringed sash, a quasi-military style popular since the 1670s until the beginning of the second decade of the 18th century – roughly the period of the Marlborough campaigns.

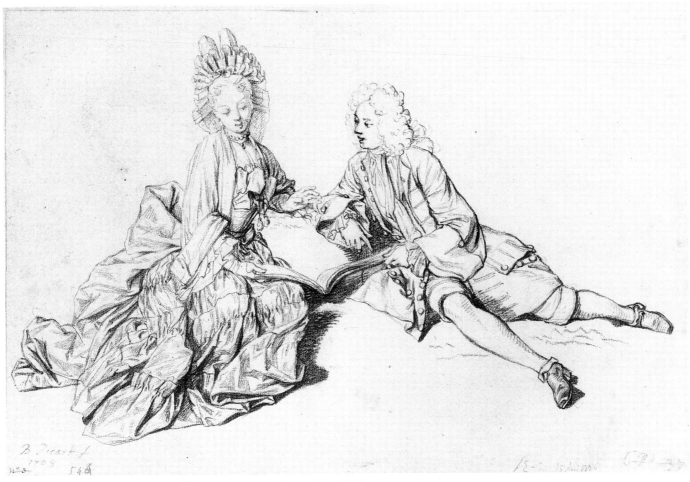

92. Two figures for a fête galante, 1708
Bernard Picart

Note These two figures who appear, slightly modified, in an engraving of 1709, *Le Grand Concert dans un Jardin*, indicate in their relaxed pose and the modified grandeur of their dress, the French taste for informality during the early 18th century.

Head The high commode headdress is replaced by the woman's softer style, consisting of a large ribbon bow placed on a frilled pinner. The full-bottomed wig (which was to remain for some years in England) has given way to a much reduced version known as a periwig, the curls being arranged in bunches at the sides and back.

Body The woman wears a mantua with soft back drapery, over a laced stomacher trimmed with a large bow, and a petticoat decorated with furbelows. The man's suit is loosely cut, with large flapped horizontal pockets on the coat. Until about the middle of the 1730s the stockings were worn rolled over the ends of the breeches at the knee.

Accessories Plain muslin forms the headdress, ruffles and cravat. In the same mood, the woman's jewellery consists of a simple string of beads, and a necklace of silk with fringed tassels.

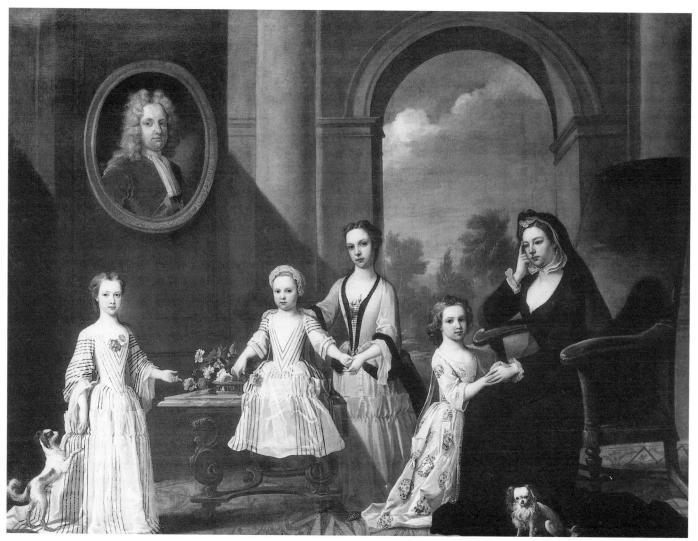

93. **Elizabeth Howland, 2nd Duchess of Bedford with her four children,**
c. 1713

Charles Jervas

Note In this group showing mourning dress, the widow wears
the deepest mourning and the children wear second mourning,
black and white. The deceased Duke's portrait hangs on the wall.

Head The Duchess wears a plain muslin pinner tying under the
chin, and with just a vestige of the top frill; over this is a crape
veil. Of the children, only the youngest son wears a baby cap of
frilled muslin.

Body The widow's black mourning dress with long tight sleeves
contrasts with the fashionable dresses worn by her two
daughters; on the left Lady Elizabeth wears a back-fastening
gown of white silk striped with black, and her elder sister Lady
Rachel wears an adult mantua of white silk edged in black over a
laced stomacher and a petticoat with one horizontal ruffle. The
youngest son, sitting on the table, wears the same dress as his
sister Elizabeth, even down to the fine muslin apron over the
furbelowed skirt. The elder boy, Wriothesley, stands at his
mother's knees in a gown of white printed silk; both the boys are
young enough to be still in leading strings.

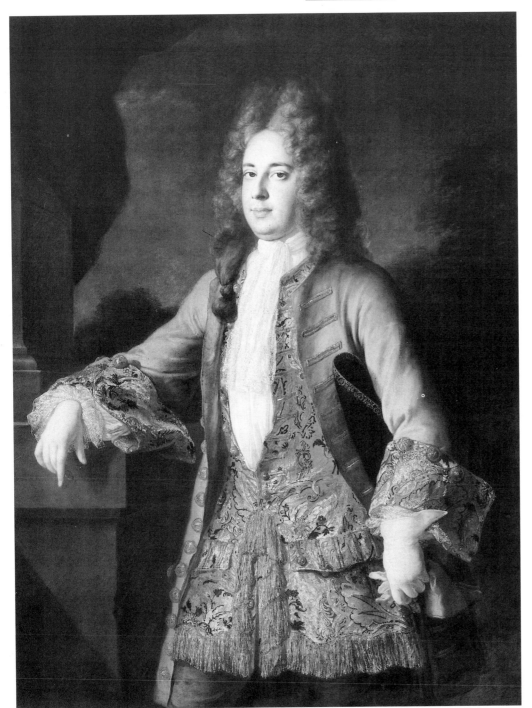

94. An unknown man, c. 1713–14
Alexis Simon Belle

Note This is the most formal, court costume.

Head The sitter (once thought to be Matthew Prior) wears a campaign wig with one end tied in a knot.

Body The suit is of a light brown silk, with button-holes and buttons of gold thread. The waistcoat is a fine example of a bizarre silk, in a design of curling, fantastic foliage on a gold ground; it is very similar to a French silk in the Victoria and Albert Museum which was used for the coronation canopy of George I (1714) and which cost £9 10 shillings a yard, very expensive in comparison to other costs in the 18th century. For court wear it was often the custom to have the waistcoat trimmed with fringe, here made of gold thread. The waistcoat buttons just above the waist, allowing the fine cambric shirt and the lace cravat to be seen.

Accessories The three-cornered black beaver hat trimmed with gold braid held under the arm is the correct wear on formal occasions. Equally elegant, and derived from the conventions of baroque portraiture, is the custom of wearing one fine kid glove and holding the other.

95. Henrietta Cavendish, Lady Huntingtower, *c.* 1715
Sir Godfrey Kneller

Note It was customary for English ladies to wear a version of the masculine suit for riding, walking and travelling.

Head She wears a short full-bottomed wig, and the fashionable male black hat trimmed with white feathers.

Body The riding habit comprises a jacket of cream-coloured camlet lined in green and trimmed with gold braid, and a matching skirt, the horizontal braiding echoing the fashionable furbelow. The wide buttoned cuffs and matching pocket flaps are prominent masculine features, as is the fine fringed linen cravat.

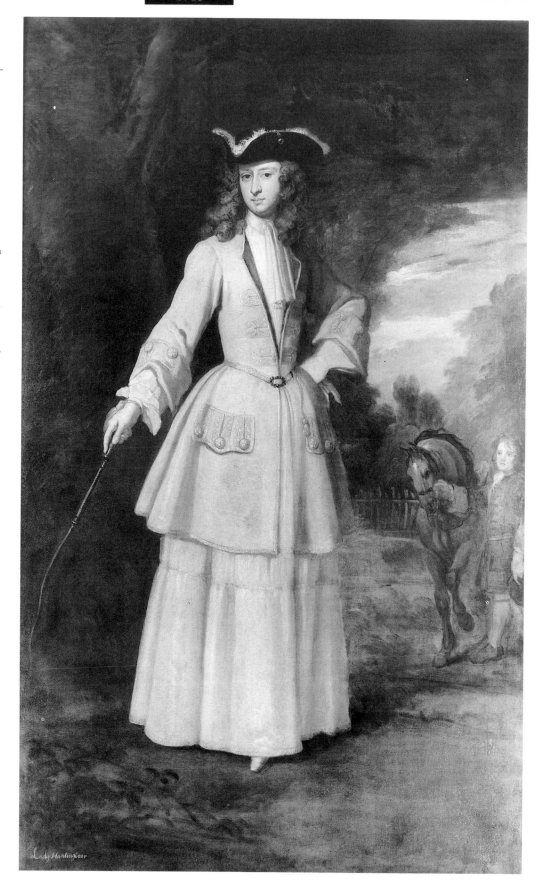

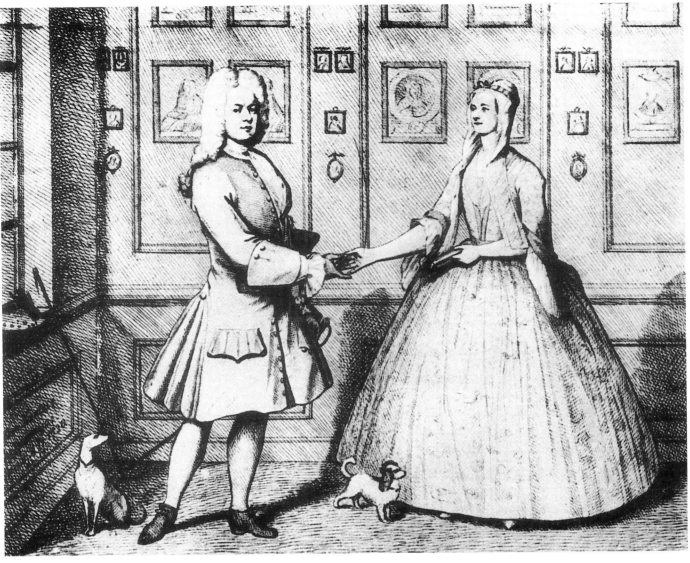

96. **George Vertue and his wife on their wedding day, 1720**
After George Vertue

Note It was customary for middle-class weddings to be relatively informal affairs, especially in the first half of the 18th century.

Head Vertue wears a campaign wig, and his wife a mob cap with double lappets of very fine linen.

Body Vertue's coat is padded to curve out over the chest, and to complement the swinging side pleats of its skirt. His wife wears a round gown with front closure over a domed hoop; a modesty piece is worn over the décolletage, and over this a fine muslin kerchief, the same material as the apron covering the central dress opening.

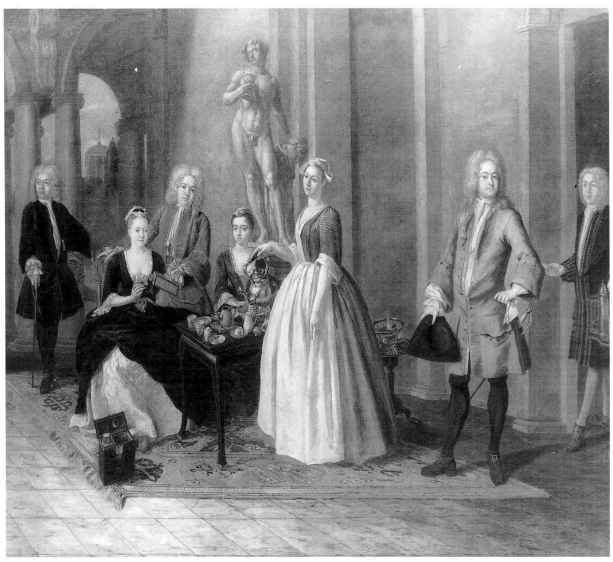

97. **An English family at tea,** *c.* 1720
Joseph van Aken

Head The men wear either short full-bottomed wigs or campaign wigs. For the women, the small lace pinner with lappets is *de rigueur*; the servant's cap is plain linen with pinned-up lappets and hides most of her hair.

Body The men wear formal, waisted suits with stiffened side pleats and large cuffs. The colours show the English preference for shades of blue and brown, the exception being the gentleman posing elegantly on the right, in a lilac coat. The servant on the far right is distinguished by his livery of blue braided with gold.

All the women wear tight-bodied gowns of the closed type; on the left a lady making tea has lifted the skirt of her black gown to reveal the white quilted petticoat beneath. Foreigners claimed in the 18th century that they found it hard to distinguish maids from mistresses; certainly the centrally posed servant is fashionably dressed in green and white striped silk.

Accessories Cravats could be worn simply knotted around the neck, or twisted with one end pushed through a buttonhole. The latter style was known as a Steinkirk and is worn by the man on the far left.

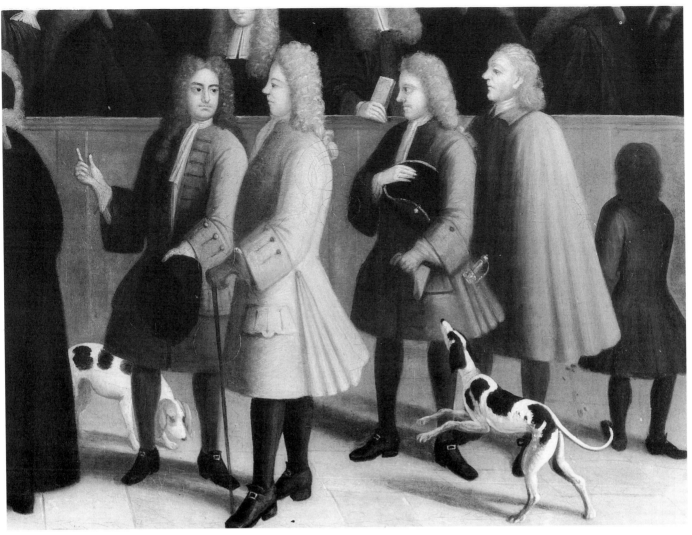

98. **The court of Chancery (detail),** *c.* 1724
Benjamin Ferrers

Head In the foreground the clients wear campaign wigs, with the exception of one man on the right who wears his own hair, rare at this date. The barristers in the background wear what Hogarth in his *Five Orders of Periwigs* (1761) called a 'Lexonic wig', i.e. a wig with two large bunches of curls and a tiny queue at the back; on the left, the serjeant-at-law wears over his wig the vestigial black coif of his office dating back to the Middle Ages.

Body The suits are sober in colour and trimming, and conservative in cut; it is likely that they would be made of the fine woollen cloth for which the English were famous, for 'they generally go plain but in the best cloths and stuffs', commented a foreign visitor in the early 1720s. On the right is a rare depiction of the cloak with small turned-down collar; this was a rather old-fashioned alternative to the greatcoat in the early 18th century.

Accessories These are also plain – brown leather gauntlet gloves, and heavy square-toed shoes in black leather with small buckles.

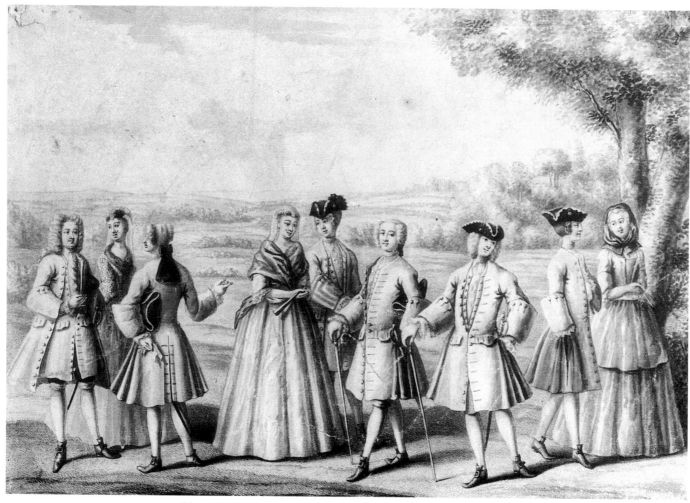

99. **A group of men and women in a landscape,** *c.* 1725
Bernard Lens III

Note It was a fashionable pastime to walk in certain public parks to show off the elegance of one's clothes and behaviour; one visitor noted, however, that English ladies 'have but little talk, and the main conversation is the flutter of their fans'.

Head The women show an increasing elaboration in headdresses, which are often made up of layers of lace with double lappets. The men's wigs include the now rather conservative campaign wig on the far left, a long bob on the right, and the most fashionable bag wigs with frizzed side curls.

Body For the men, the boot cuff – a large curving cuff reaching the elbow – reigns supreme, but there is otherwise little change in the suit; increasingly the fashionable coat is either left open or fastened only by a couple of buttons at the waist. A change in the sleeve is also noted in women's dress, where it is short and wide.

Accessories Some of the men favour the military high-cocked hats; one has a cockade. To cover the fashionable décolletage, the women adopt either a fur tippet (on the left) or a silk pelerine (a scarf with long pendants crossed over in front). On the far right we can see a caped hood worn over a lace cap.

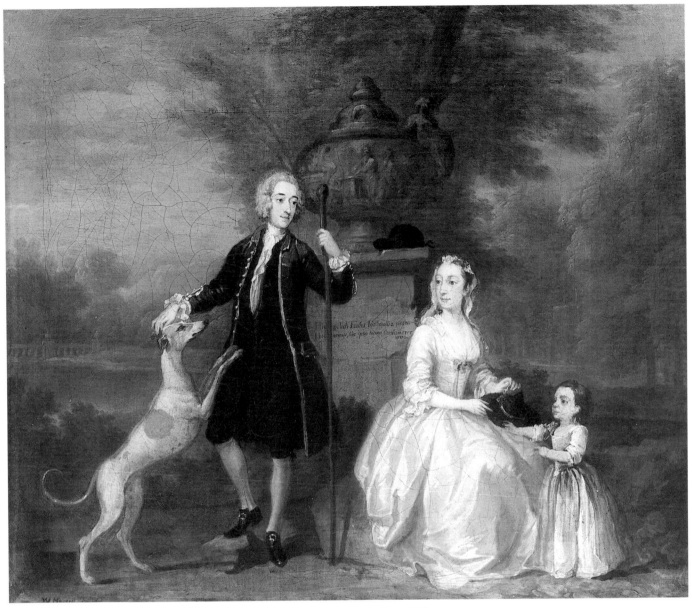

100. **Ashley Cowper with his wife and daughter, 1731**
William Hogarth

Head He wears the short powdered bob wig of the professional man (he was a barrister); his wife has a lace-edged pinner with wide lappets.

Body This is one of the earliest depictions of the frock coat, described by a German visitor at about this time as 'a close-body'd Coat without Pocketts or Plaits and with strait Sleeves'; it conspicuously lacks the large cuffs and stiffened side pleats of the formal coat. The waistcoat is considerably shorter than the coat, a trend first seen in informal country clothing of this kind. Mrs Cowper has a white silk open gown with matching petticoat. Their daughter (born in 1731 and added later by the artist) has a back-fastening stiffened bodice, and a skirt almost covered by a white apron.

Accessories Cowper's black jockey cap with peak, adopted from the racing fraternity, was worn both for riding and for country walking. His wife holds a black hat with pointed crown, a middle-class style dating from the mid-17th century, but fleetingly fashionable for country wear in the 1730s and 1740s.

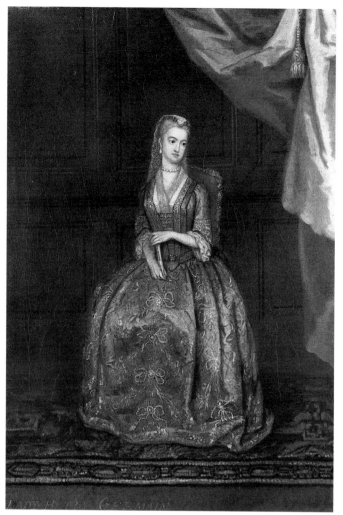

101. Lady Betty Germain, 1731
Charles Phillips

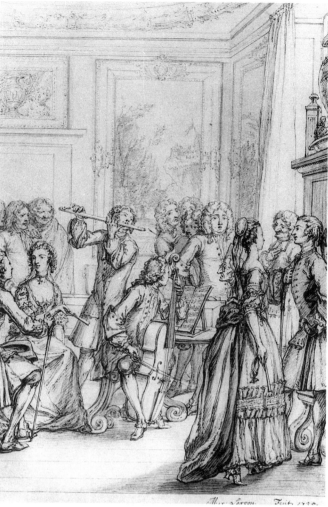

102. The Music Party, 1735
Marcellus Laroon II

Note This is a study from a large group entitled *A tea party at Lord Harrington's* (1730) in the collection of the Yale Center for British Art, New Haven. This single portrait is a rare depiction of court dress, a style of costume not often seen in English portraiture with its preference for the informal.

Head Over the lightly powdered hair is worn a lace cap with the lappets which were obligatory at court.

Body At this period court wear demanded a mantua, made here of blue silk brocaded in gold; the decoration on the dress includes silver embroidery on the robings. There are large diamond bows on the petticoat.

Accessories Attendance at court provided an opportunity for the display of jewellery, and here the sitter wears a pearl necklace and earrings, and a diamond girdle buckle.

Note This is an unidentified group which testifies to the fashion in the 1730s for musical parties; Laroon was a composer and performer himself, and depicts this concert in the manner of a *scène galante*.

Head The women's hairstyles show, on the right, a neat French swept-up coiffure with a tiny cap and pendant lappets, and on the left the curls falling to the shoulders in what was sometimes called the Dutch mode. The men have a variety of wigs, the most fashionable being the pigtail queue on the right, a contrast to the bob wig worn by the clergyman standing next to him.

Body On the right the mantua is increasingly reserved for very formal occasions, but the horizontal flounce is old-fashioned by this time – this may be a case of the artist using a drawing made some years previously.

The men's coats are still long-waisted and with side fullness; variety appears in the cuffs, with a slit cuff on the far left, an open cuff worn by the flautist, and the round boot cuff of the cellist. By this time the breeches are often buckled over the stockings.

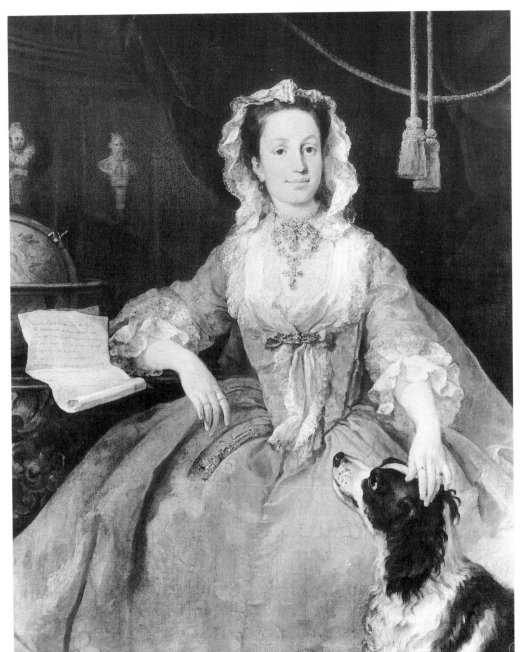

103. Mary Edwards, 1742
William Hogarth

Note Mary Edwards was a slightly eccentric heiress depicted here in the kind of rich and jewelled magnificence which is rarely seen in English portraiture.

Head The headdress is a mob cap, with ostentatiously wide lappets, and frames the face.

Body The same lace edges the kerchief and forms the chemise ruffles. Fine Flemish lace was an essential and expensive part of the fashionable wardrobe during the first half of the 18th century; Mrs Delany records in 1743 paying nearly £50 for a 'suit' of Brussels lace, comprising headdress, ruffles and tucker. The dress is a brilliant red damask closed sack worn over a large bell-shaped hoop.

Accessories The jewellery consists of an impressive necklace of pearls and diamonds (ribbon bows and the pendant cross were popular designs), diamond bodice buckle and diamond drop earrings; at her waist is a gold watch in an elaborately chased case.

104. Memorial to James Cooper and his wife, *c.* 1743

British School, effigy

Note Cooper died in 1743; the date of his wife's death is not known. This is a rare example of a funeral monument depicting a middle-class couple without sentimental or classical connotations.

Head He wears either his own hair or a wig in a long bob; his wife has a pinner with the lappets pinned up under a scarf hood.

Body The clothing is plain and rather old-fashioned; the sobriety of his untrimmed suit is matched by her simple closed robe and laced stomacher.

Accessories Mrs Cooper wears a long scarf over her shoulders. It is also worth noting the wedding ring that she wears, for this was not usual in fashionable circles until well into the second half of the century.

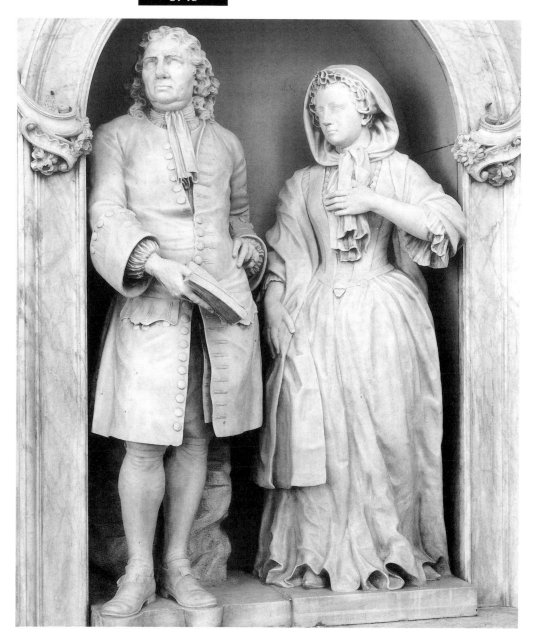

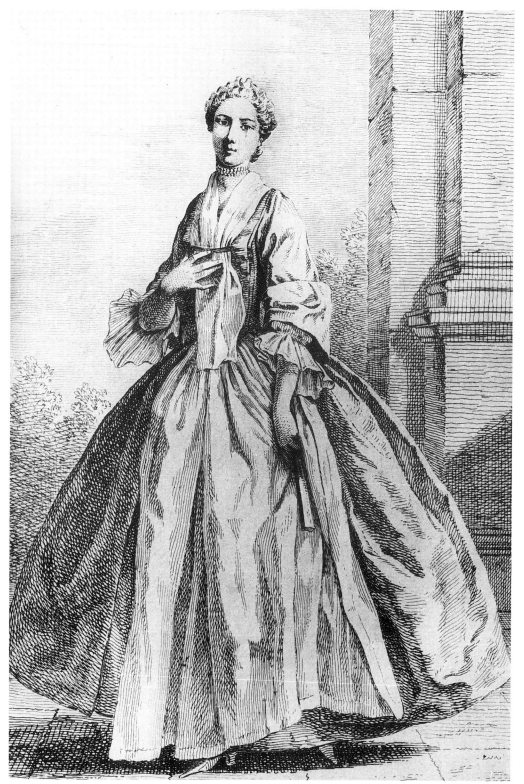

105. Standing figure, *c.* 1745
After Hubert Gravelot

Note Gravelot, the son of a tailor, imbued a series of drawings of English fashions in the mid-1740s with French rococo elegance.

Head A small linen cap is worn over a *tête-de-mouton* hairstyle.

Body It was possible, as Horace Walpole noted of a lady in 1741, for 'her head to be dressed French and her body English'. Here, with the French hairstyle, is a fitted English gown with plain robings and winged cuffs. This may be the dress known as a nightgown (a semi-formal gown by the mid-century), which was often worn with an apron; a plain linen kerchief is held in place by a band across the robings.

106. The months: June 1749
John June (attr.)

Head The hair is curled into the neck at the back; on the head is worn a small lace-edged pinner with vestigial side lappets.

Body The immense sweep of the sack dress over huge square hoops – in 1750 Mrs Delany called them 'tubs of hoops' – dominates this back view; at this stage in its development the sack dress is loose-fitting with unpressed pleats falling from a wide neckline at the back.

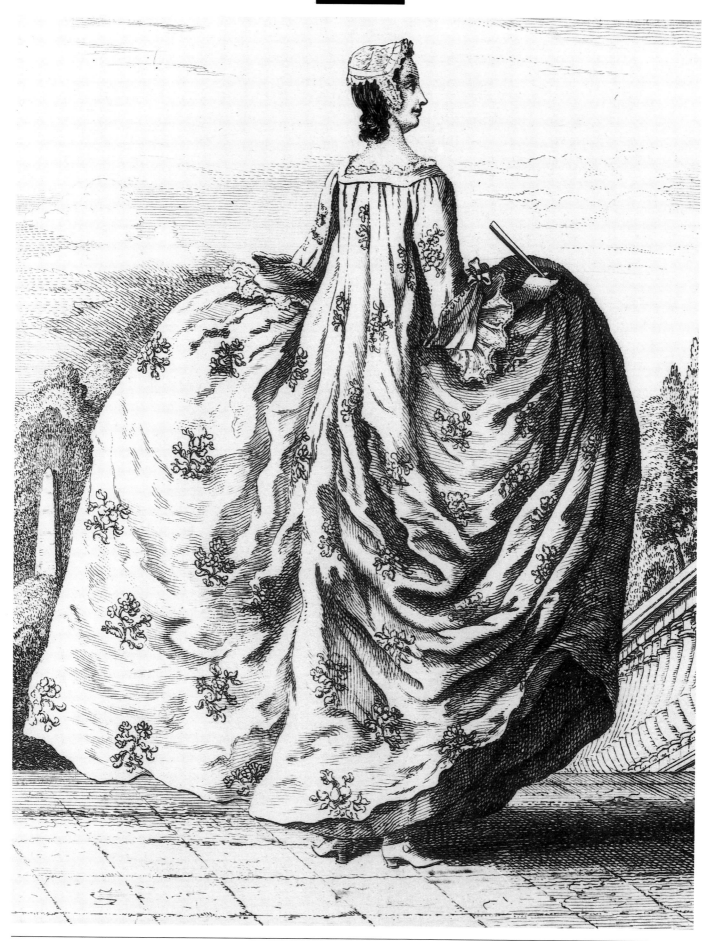

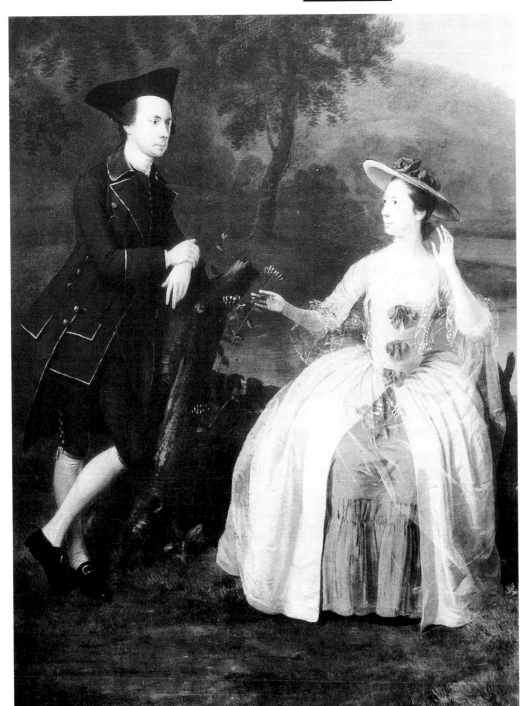

107. **Sir George and Lady Strickland in Boynton Hall Park (detail), 1751**
Arthur Devis

Note A typical conversation piece by this artist shows the landed gentry dressed in suitably rural costume, enjoying their property. In this case it is more than a flourish by the artist, for Strickland was one of the growing band of landowners who devoted himself to the improvement of his lands.

Head For the country the hair is dressed simply. Strickland's hair (his own) has a rolled curl on each side – the contemporary term was a 'buckle' (from the French *boucle*) – and is tied at the back. His wife's hair is combed close to the head, under a straw hat trimmed with green ribbons.

Body The blue frock suit is lightly trimmed with gold braid; the coat is double-breasted, and a much slimmer silhouette is created by the absence of heavy side pleats.

Lady Strickland wears a deliciously impractical gown for sitting on a tree stump, of pale pink silk, with a closed front bodice trimmed with green silk bows, the same colour as her petticoat which has a deep flounce at the hem. The apron is of the finest silk gauze, as are the sleeve ruffles trimmed with silk lace (blonde).

108. Man standing in a landscape, c. 1753–4
Paul Sandby

Head A plain three-cornered hat is worn over a short curled tye wig.

Body The greatcoat with large collar (known as a cape) and wide cuffs is the English contribution to a fashionable man's wardrobe; in Henry Fielding's novel *Joseph Andrews* (1742) it is the only garment that the man-about-town Bellarmine will commit to an English tailor. To achieve the fashionable slim silhouette, it is possible to wear a greatcoat only if the suit beneath it is well-fitting; in this drawing we can see the greatly reduced width of the suit coat, the short waistcoat, and the knee-breeches tailored closely to the thigh.

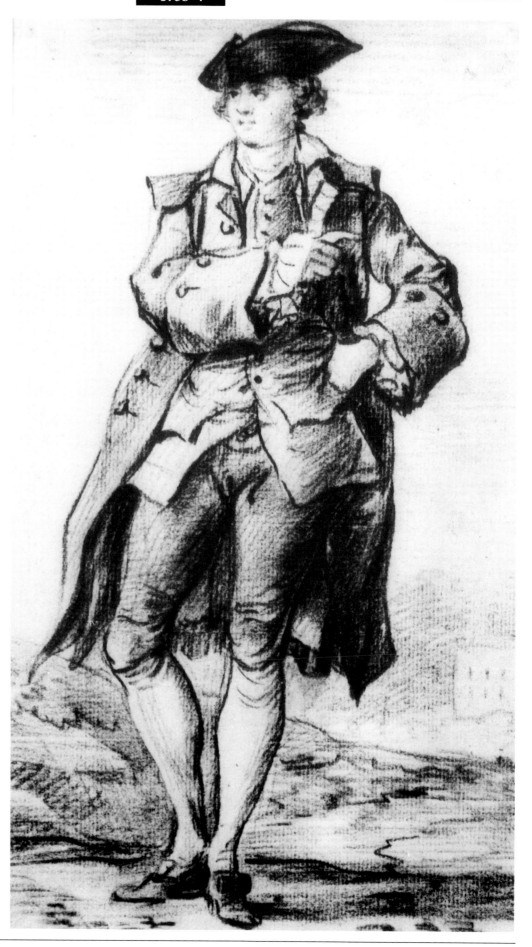

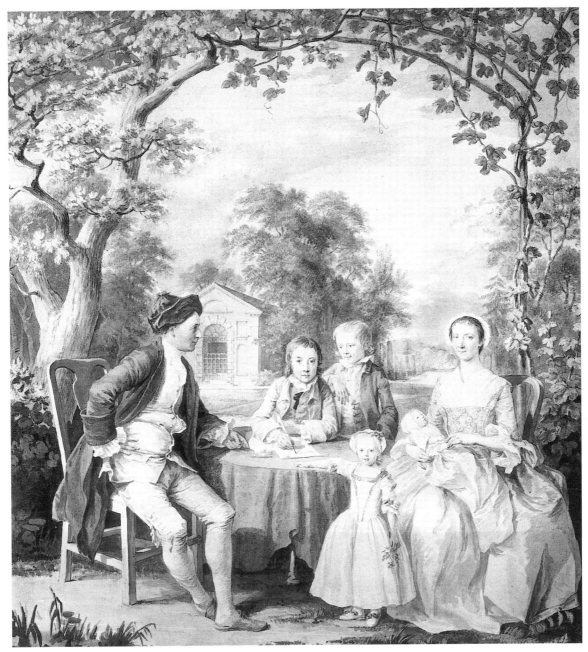

109. **A family group in a garden,** *c.* 1754
British School, watercolour

Head The father wears a turban over his shaved head, and the mother displays a round-eared cap over her plainly styled hair; a similar cap worn by her daughter has a sprig of flowers in it.

Body The informality of the morning gathering is most obviously displayed in the costume of the man, a banyan worn over a short waistcoat, and his breeches unbuttoned at the knee. His wife wears an open gown, the widely spaced robings revealing a broad expanse of stomacher covered in puffed trimming, forming a lattice design; one flounce, narrow at the elbow and wide behind, edges the sleeve. The small sons have plain frock coats, and their shirt collars turn down to form a ruffle, a style characteristic of small English boys at this date, and sometimes tied with a black ribbon.

Accessories The heelless, backless slippers or mules were customary morning wear with the banyan or dressing gown.

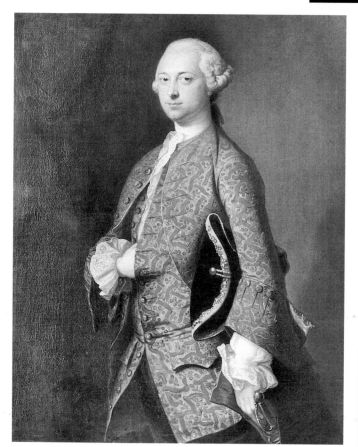

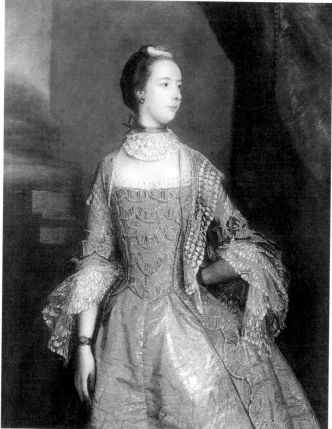

110. **Sir Henry Oxenden,** *c.* **1755**
Thomas Hudson

111. **Susanna Beckford, 1756**
Sir Joshua Reynolds

Note This is probably a portrait painted to commemorate the sitter's marriage in 1755.

Head A bag wig is worn with one large, slightly curving roll of hair at each side.

Body Sir Henry wears a formal suit of blue silk, the stylized floral compartmented pattern being typical of surviving museum pieces; the coat curves away from the top of the chest, and like the waistcoat, it is lined with white satin.

Accessories The hat carried under the arm is the regulation black beaver, but trimmed with silver braid, button and loop.

IX **Miss Eleanor Dixie,** *c.* **1755**
Henry Pickering (attr.)
Colour illustration, between pages 128 and 129

Note William Hogarth in his *Analysis of Beauty* (1753) summed up the rococo by his description that 'the beauty of intricacy lies in contriving winding shapes'; nowhere is this more evident than in this portrait.

Head The hair is beginning to have a slight fullness at the back and sides, and on top the effect is created with a pompon of white feathers and blue ribbon.

Body The dress is an open sack, of turquoise blue and silver watered silk, decorated down the sides to the hem with serpentine robings of the same silk, ruched; the bodice is cut wide to show a stomacher trimmed with the same silk. The sleeve ruffles and the handkerchief hanging on the shoulders are of blonde lace made of silk, and its sheen complements that of the gown.

Accessories There is a necklace of blonde lace and blue silk. The jewellery is simple almost as a deliberate contrast to the splendour of the dress. The sitter wears clip-on earrings called 'snaps' probably of paste; on her arms she wears bracelets of black silk, each with an agate surrounded by paste brilliants.

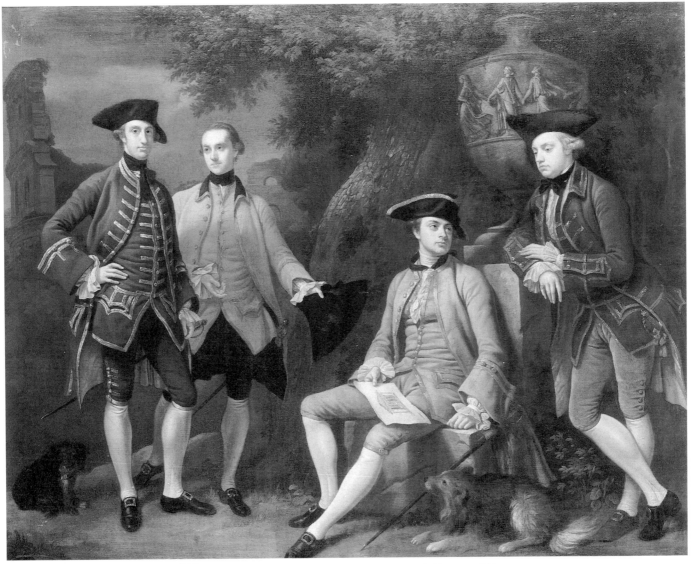

112. **Sir James Grant, Mr Mytton, the Hon. Thomas Robinson and Mr Wynn, 1760–61**
Nathaniel Dance

Note This is one of four versions of this picture, intended presumably so that each sitter could have one.

Head All these gentlemen on the Grand Tour wear their own hair in a virtually identical style with regard to the single side curl, but the two on the right have chosen to tie the back hair *en solitaire*. On the left, Grant and Mytton have adopted the black military stock.

Body The suits are either unified in colour and trimming for more formal wear, or, less formally, are composed of a frock and matching waistcoat with different coloured breeches. Both coats and frock coats are lined and they show a notable front curve which results in the diminishing side pleats being moved towards the back. The coat cuffs are still quite wide compared to those of the frocks, and on the far right Wynn wears a cuff *à la marinière*.

Accessories All wear swords, a custom more usual on the continent than in England, which by this time tended to restrict this practice to more formal occasions. Wynn's sword is decorated with a red ribbon knot.

113. Harriott, Lady Brownlow Bertie, *c.* 1762
Francis Cotes

Note Although this portrait has been identified by one scholar, as that of the second wife of Lord Brownlow Bertie, the compiler believes it to be, on the grounds of the costume and the age of the sitter, the first wife, married in 1762.

Head The hair is plaited and gathered up to a soft knot on the crown, where it is trimmed with a white feather pompon.

Body This is an early example of a new style of open gown, with the bodice buttoned up with a sewn-in false front, and with long tight sleeves to the wrist. These functional sleeves and the unboned bodice made this a popular travelling costume, sometimes called the Brunswick or German habit from its wide use in that part of Europe. Here it is worn as a morning dress; the gown, with a sack-back, has a ruched trimming at the sleeve elbow and robings to the hem, echoing those on the bodice. The fabric is a pink silk brocaded with tiny green flowers and silver leaves; such an up-to-date pattern, which anticipates the popular spot designs of the 1770s and 1780s, is typically to be seen first in an informal gown.

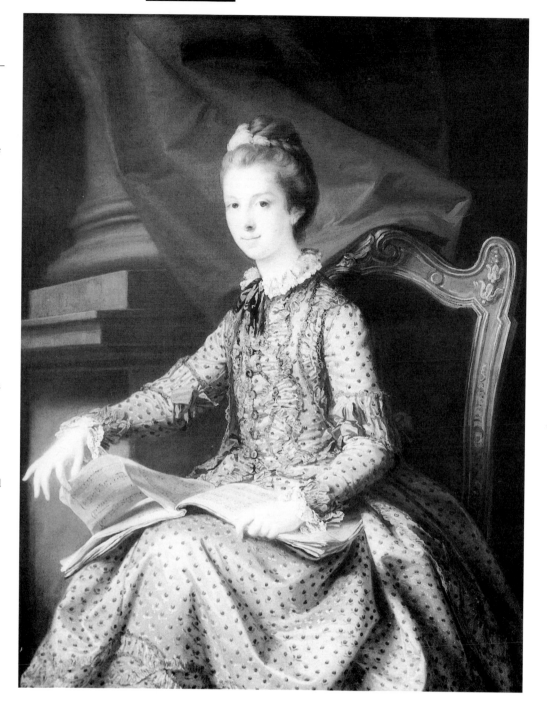

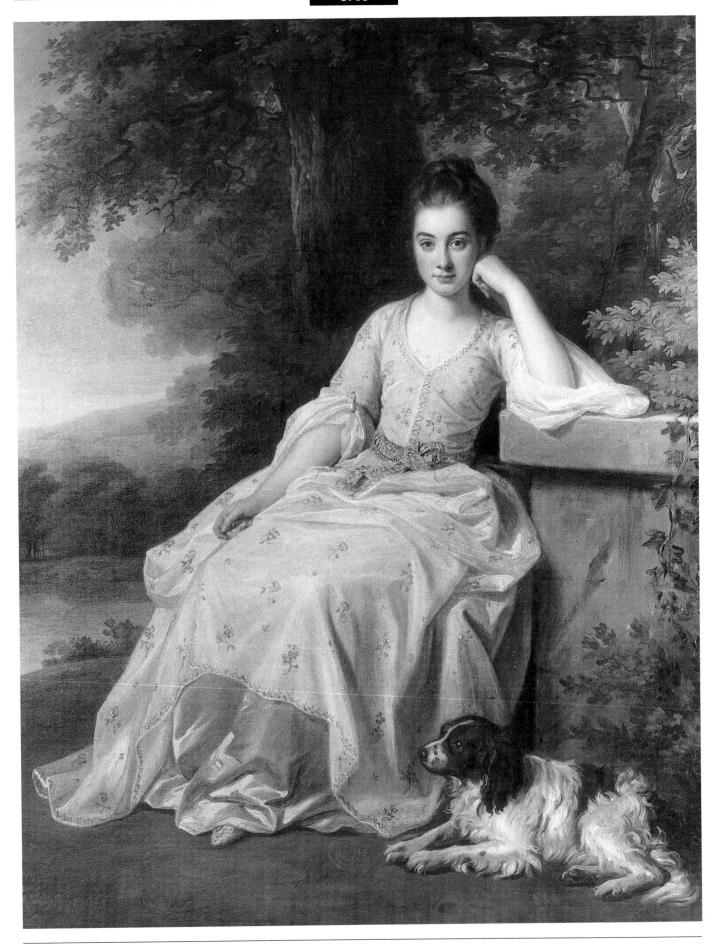

114. A girl with a dog, *c.* 1766
Nathaniel Dance

Head The hair is beginning to rise perceptibly, and is loosely plaited into a knot on top.

Body This dress consists of a petticoat of pink satin, and an overgown of white Indian muslin embroidered with gold, which is front-fastening and tied around the waist with a striped pink silk sash. The costume reflects the growing taste for the oriental in dress in this decade, combining the love of the exotic with a preference for the informal.

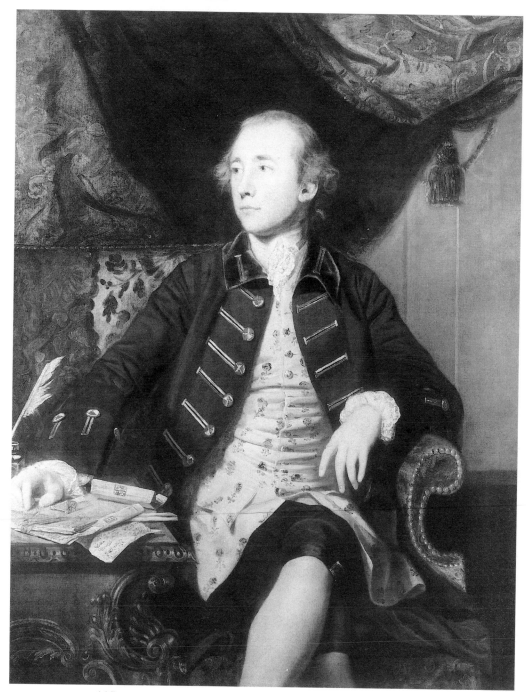

115. Warren Hastings, 1766–8
Sir Joshua Reynolds

Head An informal style which was popular with Englishmen in the Indian climate was to cut the hair short on top but otherwise to follow the fashion for a single roll of hair at the side.

Body He wears a blue frock coat with velvet collar; the buttons and buttonholes are made of gold thread. The waistcoat is probably of cream printed cotton, very possibly purchased in India; such items were part of the wardrobe of fashionable expatriates and some were exported to England to be greeted with the enthusiasm that was accorded to anything oriental.

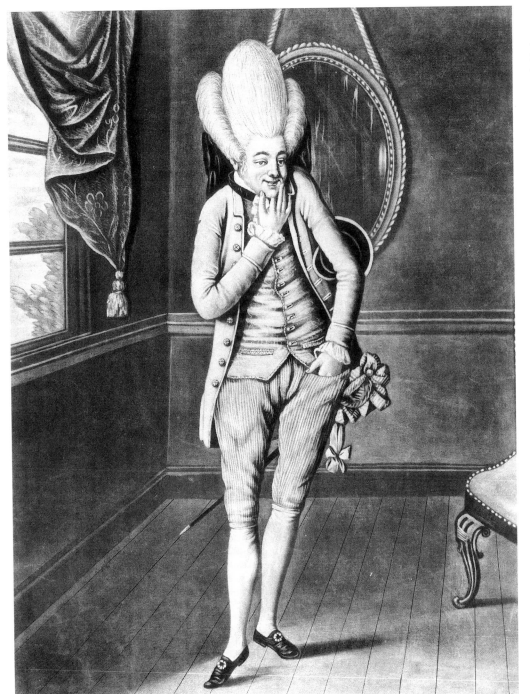

116. 'How d'ye like me?' 1772
Anon. engraving

Note The word 'macaroni' first appears in the 1760s to describe ultra-fashionable foppish young men-about-town. According to the *Town and Country Magazine* (1772) the word was applied by those who had been on the Grand Tour, and especially to Italy, to anything they found 'elegant and uncommon'. Their extremes in fashion provided considerable material for the caricaturists who flourished in the 1770s.

Head The bag wig is of an enormous height with a vast, almost vertical side curl.

Body The frock coat (now *de rigueur* for all but the more formal occasions) is very short and tight-fitting; in pursuit of an unbroken line, the macaronis dispensed with the flapped outside pocket in favour of an inside one. The waistcoat is short, with slit pockets. To accentuate the slim line, the macaronis popularized the use of stripes, most notably for breeches, as here, and for stockings.

Accessories The new small round hat is clutched under the arm. The large striped silk sword knots draw attention to the fact that this macaroni is unlikely to use his weapon. The macaronis were often accused of effeminacy, and this caricature depicts a man with a rather mincing gait emphasized by the flat-heeled dancing pumps with their round, jewelled buckles.

117. Fashionable dresses in the rooms at Weymouth, 1774
Anon. engraving

Note This is a fashion plate from the *Lady's Magazine* which began to appear regularly from 1770. Such fashion plates have little artistic merit but they are often useful guides to an increasingly complex range of women's dress for different occasions.

Head The high-piled hair requires either the straw hat tilted at an angle over the forehead (left-hand figure in foreground) or a large calash or travelling hood (extreme right-hand figure). In the background can be seen two examples of the chignon or flat, heavy loop of hair reaching to the nape of the neck, worn with (on the extreme left) a bicorne riding hat, and an undress ribboned cap (right-hand figure in foreground).

Body The most formal dress is the hooped open robe seen in the foreground, with double sleeve flounces and lace ruffles; a starched or wired 'Medici' collar indicates the fashionable influence of the styles of the late 16th century.

Her companion wears a morning informal dress, an open gown with the skirt fastened up at the sides, an apron and a hooded pelerine. In the background is a riding jacket and skirt.

Sleeve ruffles are worn only for formal dress; the most usual sleeve is tight to the elbow, finishing in a small winged cuff, or a round cuff, or with an over-cuff of pleated linen.

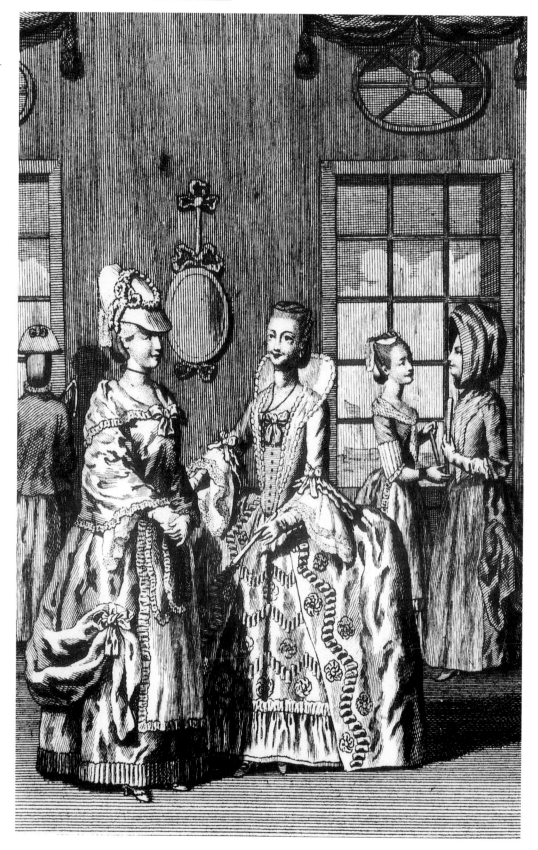

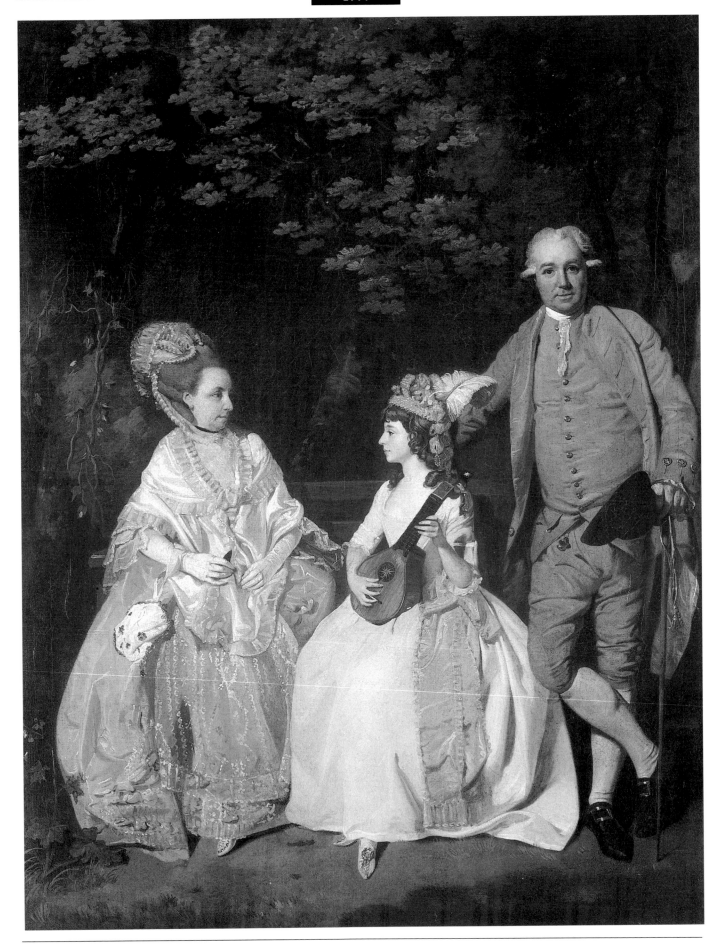

118. Family group, *c.* 1777
Francis Wheatley

Head From this time the high-piled hair of fashionable women begins to slope diagonally backwards from the forehead; it forms a striking contrast to the fringe and naturally curling hairstyle of the daughter. The mother wears a French nightcap or *dormeuse* of silk gauze, tying under the chin with lappets. The girl is depicted in a curiously elaborate confection of feathers, beads and lace, which one sees in a number of portraits in this decade.

Body The suit worn by the rather portly middle-aged man has roomy breeches worn more for comfort than for fashion; the coat is fairly tight-fitting and is no longer intended to fasten all the way down the front.

The seated woman wears a white silk open robe with an embroidered gauze apron; the front of the bodice is hidden by a white pelerine. The girl wears a lightly boned back-fastening bodice, the sleeves reaching to just below the elbow with a small round cuff, and a petticoat of light pink silk; around her waist is a deep pink sash edged in silver braid.

Accessories Knotting is a fashionable pastime throughout the eighteenth century; it consisted of knotting a silk or linen thread into a decorative braid for furnishings or to trim items of clothing such as waistcoats. Knotting bags, like the one depicted here, are often made of embroidered silk.

The man's waistcoat, cut away from the waist, reveals a bunch of seals which are both functional and decorative items of male jewellery.

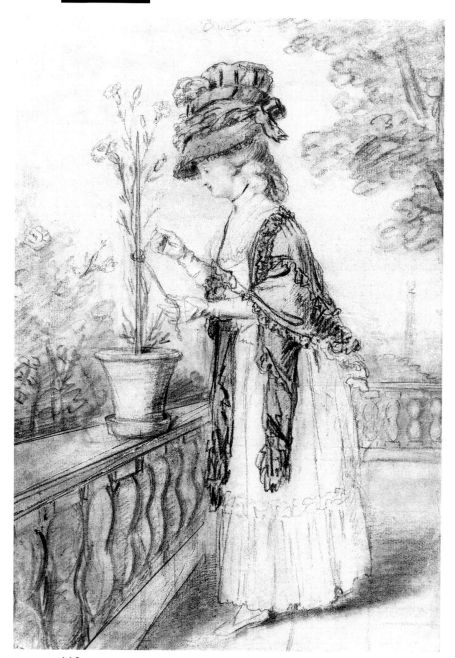

119. Lady on a terrace, attending to a carnation plant, *c.* 1778
John Raphael Smith

Note This artist had an early informed interest in costume, for he was apprenticed to a linen draper, and owned a shop in the Strand selling haberdashery items, while at the same time producing drawings and mezzotints of fashionable people and situations.

Head The hair is soft and rather squashy at the side with large roll curls. A large round silk hat is worn; it has a soft crown trimmed with ribbons and a lace-edged brim.

Body This is an informal costume of jacket and skirt, probably of linen or muslin; the jacket or bodice slopes away from a central rosette, and the ensuing triangular gap is filled by a false waistcoat, sometimes called a 'zone'.

Accessories She wears a hooded black silk pelerine, white mittens with turned-over flaps, and low-heeled comfortable shoes.

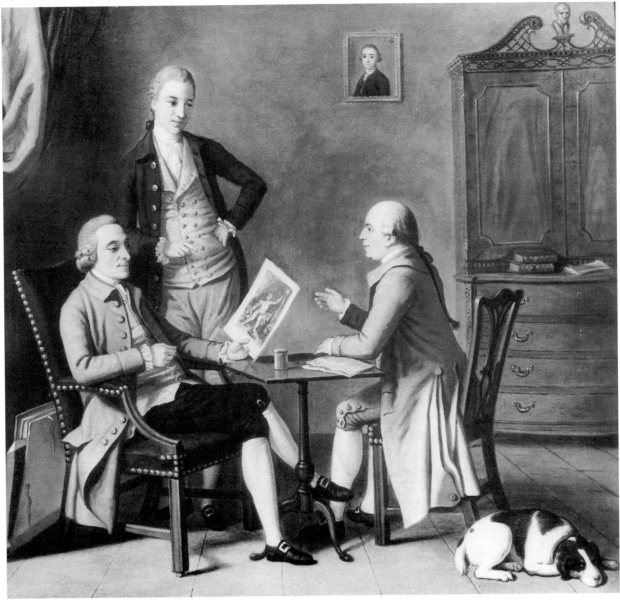

120. **The connoisseurs,** *c.* 1780–1
David Allan

Note The sitters, almost certainly members or connections of the Scottish Hope family, are examining an engraving after Raphael.

Head On the left, the older man, Charles Hope Vere, wears an old-fashioned short bob wig with two rows of rigid curls; sitting opposite him is a man, provisionally identified as Archibald Hope, with his own hair rolled into a small side curl, and the back hair in a long plait. The standing, young man is more up-to-date with his own hair frizzed and knotted at the back.

Body Untrimmed English frocks in sober colours are the rule, with close-fitting sleeves and small round cuffs. Charles Hope Vere wears a grey cloth frock with flapped pocket; Archibald Hope's has a buttoned side vent and large collar, indicating perhaps that this is more a riding or travelling style; the young man has a brown frock with metal buttons.

Short waistcoats are in vogue, and the most fashionable of all is worn by the youngest man; it is double-breasted and cut straight across the waist.

121. A lady sketching, 1785
British School, watercolour

Head Masculine influence, a recurrent feature of English women's riding and walking dress throughout the century, extends to the adoption of the round hat with ribbon hatband. For outdoors, the hair is often left unfrizzed, to fall down the back in waves.

Body The riding jacket and skirt have become a costume for any outdoors activity. The jacket is cut tight at the waist and flares out in a pleated frill at the back, sloping away at the sides like the fashionable man's coat; other masculine features include the high collar and revers, the large buttons and the cuffs *à la marinière*.

X The Morning Walk, *c.* 1785
Thomas Gainsborough
Colour illustration, between pages 128 and 129

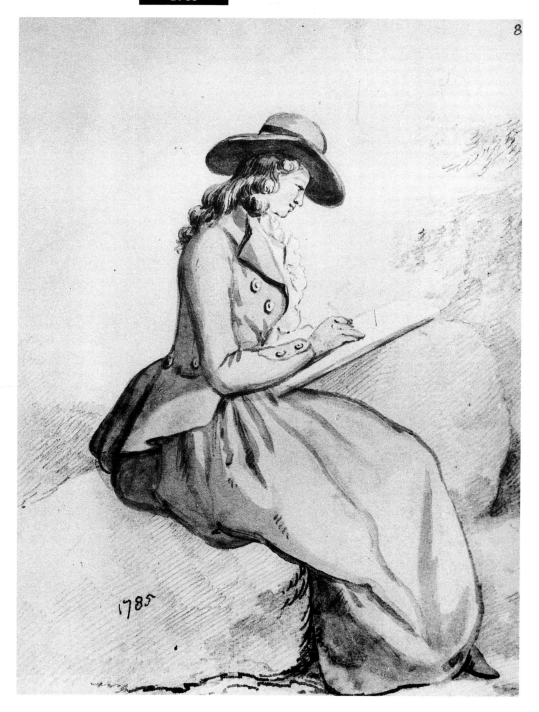

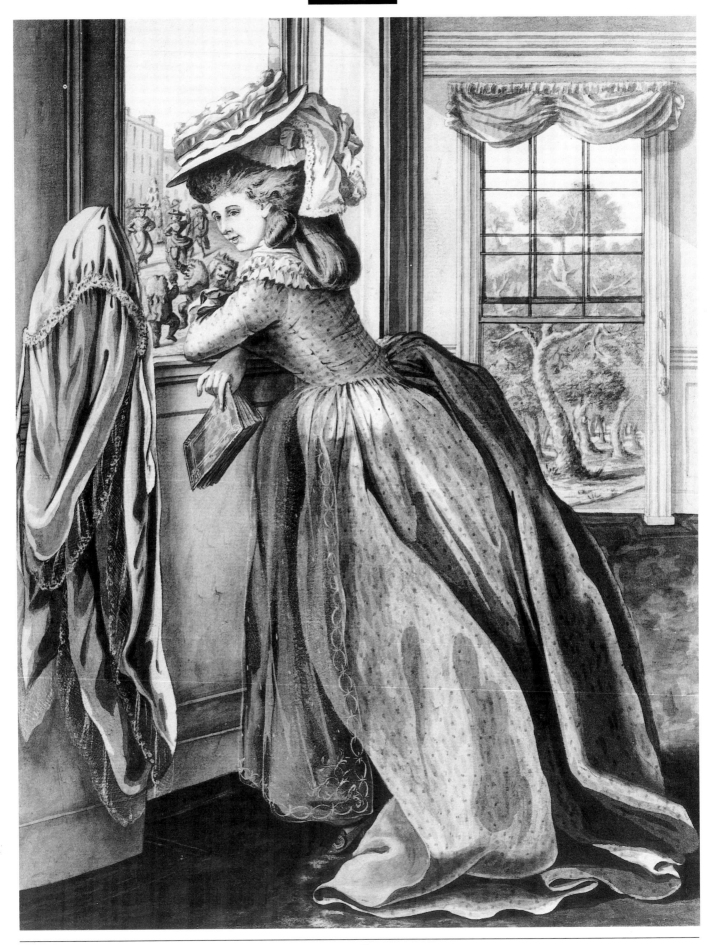

122. The Months: May, *c.* 1785
Robert Dighton

Note This continues the tradition (see 106) of using the months of the year to represent the changing seasonal fashions.

Head The hair is frizzed out at the sides, with a thick loop at the neck; false hair and pomatum must be added to create the fashionable bulk. On the head is a *dormeuse* nightcap, and then a hat with small brim and wide crown trimmed with ribbon.

Body This is a good view of the *robe à l'anglaise* with its *fourreau* back; the dress is an open robe, worn over hip pads, which give the fashionable side bounce and which by now have virtually replaced side hoops. The design of the silk pattern, of tiny dots and stripes, is typical of this period. Over the petticoat is worn a fine embroidered silk gauze apron.

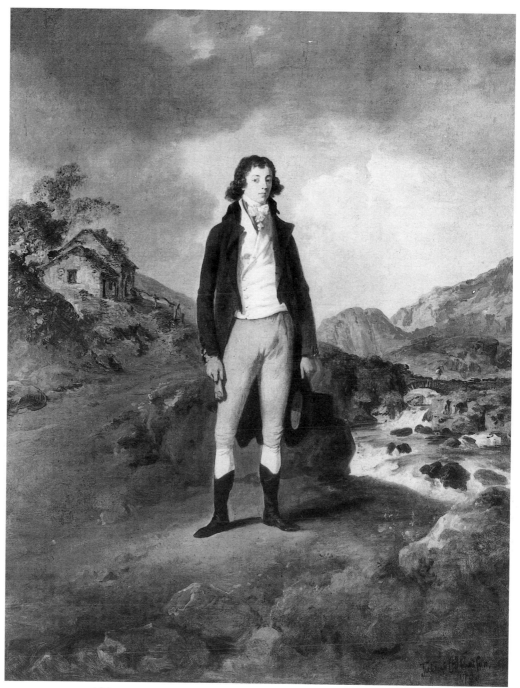

123. Portrait of a young man, 1790
Julius Caesar Ibbetson

Note The vogue for the picturesque, in the form of wild scenery, is thought a suitable background to the casual, 'natural' clothing of this fashionable young man.

Head The hair has a boyish fringe and curls over the coat collar.

Body The dark grey frock, with a high velvet collar, is cut away at the waist, one of the earliest examples of this style. The waistcoat has wide, sloping revers, and is worn over an under-waistcoat, a glimpse of which can be seen at the neck. The shirt collar is high, and the cravat tied in an elaborate puffed knot.

Accessories The round hat with a tall crown is an early example of the top hat of the nineteenth century. The short boots with a dip in the front are called hussar buskins.

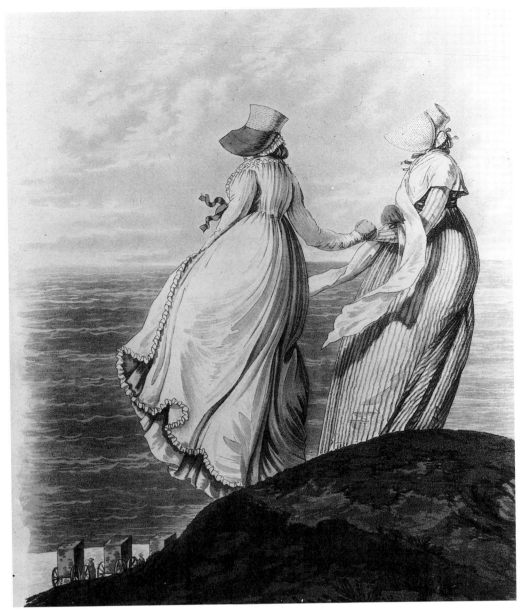

124. Morning dresses
Heideloff's *Gallery of Fashion*, 1797

Note Niklaus von Heideloff, a German engraver who fled from Paris to London during the French Revolution, published his *Gallery of Fashion*, monthly, from 1794 to 1803. Unlike previous English fashion plates, Heideloff's were of high artistic quality; they show, in contrast to the often deliberately provocative extremes of the neo-classical in French dress, a modest and practical English compromise between fashion and comfort.

Head The ladies wear bonnets over lawn caps; on the left is a 'Menton poke straw bonnet with a green silk calash', and on the right a 'Quaker Dunstable hat, tied behind and under the chin with French grey riband'.

Body The newly fashionable slender look still retains some soft fullness at the back; these are informal 'loose gowns' for walking. On the left we have a dress of 'fine India calico' trimmed with ribbon, and on the right a green and white striped gingham; 'Indian' fabrics were very fashionable.

Accessories Although sea-bathing was in fashion, the skin had to be kept white and untouched by the sun, which explains both the face-shading bonnets, and the gloves.

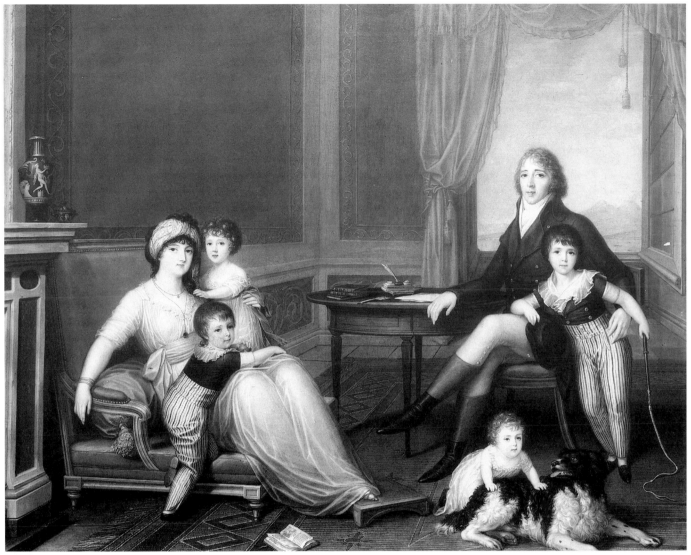

125. **The Lambton family, 1797**

Augusto Nicodemo

Note The interior of this house in Naples shows the prevailing neo-classical taste which also influences women's dress.

Head Anne Lambton's clustering curls and embroidered silk turban show a typical combination of the classical and the oriental. Her husband's lightly powdered hair is cut quite long at the back, and falls over his forehead in a fringe.

Body The dress of mother and small daughters is virtually indistinguishable. Anne Lambton wears a classically inspired white muslin chemise dress, tied around the waist with a yellow silk sash. William Lambton wears a dark blue double-breasted coat, a white waistcoat, and breeches of buff-coloured nankeen which fit the legs without a wrinkle. The two older boys are in skeleton suits consisting of blue cotton jackets onto which button high-waisted striped cotton trousers.

Accessories William Lambton wears French top boots with a turned-over top cut straight round. His wife has pointed white silk shoes crossed with ribbon in imitation of classical sandals.

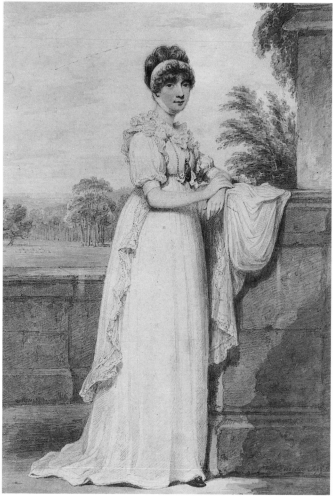

126. **Princess Sophia, 1802**
Henry Edridge

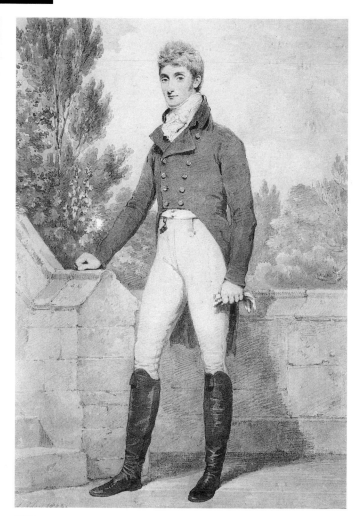

127. **Thomas, Earl of Haddington, 1802**
Henry Edridge

Note For day wear, low necks were often filled in by a handkerchief, chemisette or tucker, and thin fabrics augmented by a variety of shawls, mantles, cloaks, tunics, 'vests' and pelisses.

Head The short hair 'à la Titus' is encircled by a bandeau extending under the chin.

Body The apron-fronted dress is of white muslin, the skirt ties passing right round the body and forming a bow under the bust, the neckline edged with the frill of a tucker or chemisette. It has short full sleeves, and a skirt with a short train and tucked hem, a fashionable feature of this year. She wears an overtunic or mantle with a frilled edge (the sleeves may belong to this rather than to the dress).

Accessories The pointed toes have ribbon ties and very low heels. She wears a necklace and cameo brooch, in the classical style.

Note Fashionable morning and walking dress has adopted elements of military and country wear, in the form of the riding coat, with its curved fronts, and long boots. Breeches were being replaced by pantaloons, which were tighter fitting and extended to the mid-calf or below. They were usually worn with hessian boots made of patent leather, as developed in the 1790s.

Head The hair is 'à la Titus'.

Body He wears a fine white linen shirt and cravat, double-breasted riding coat, a short waistcoat, and light-coloured breeches or pantaloons.

Accessories He has V-fronted, tasselled hessian boots, and short gloves of cotton or leather. Seals hang at his waist.

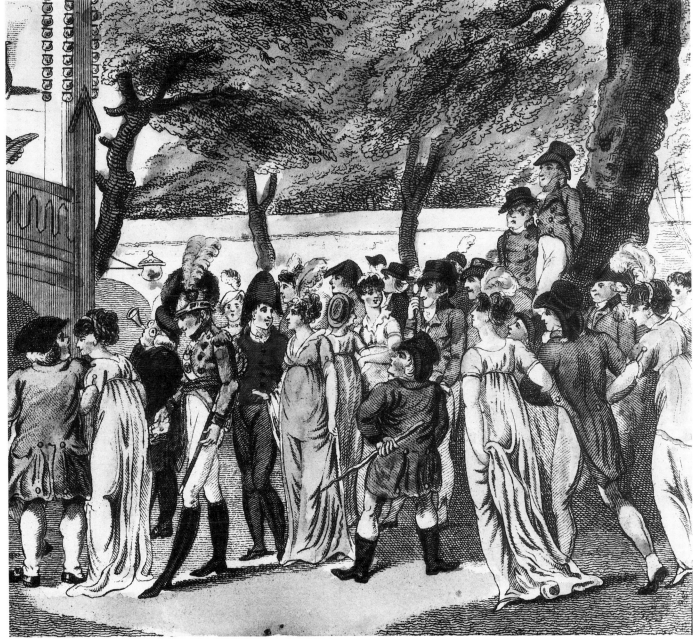

128. **Vauxhall Gardens (detail), 1805**
Anon. engraving

Note Vauxhall Pleasure Gardens were frequented by all ranks of society.

Head The women wear their hair trimmed with jewelled bandeaux, ornamental combs and feathers.

Body The outfits include several formal afternoon or evening dresses, similar in style to day dresses, but with lower necklines and longer trains. Frilled V-necks are popular, with short puffed sleeves draped or caught up and buttoned on the outer arm.

The men's outfits range from the stylish full evening dress of the man in the centre, with his crescent-shaped opera hat or 'chapeau bras', dark evening coat and pantaloons and lace-up pumps, to the old man on the left who still wears the three-cornered hat, curled wig, loose frock coat and breeches with stockings and buckled shoes, which were last fashionable in the mid-18th century.

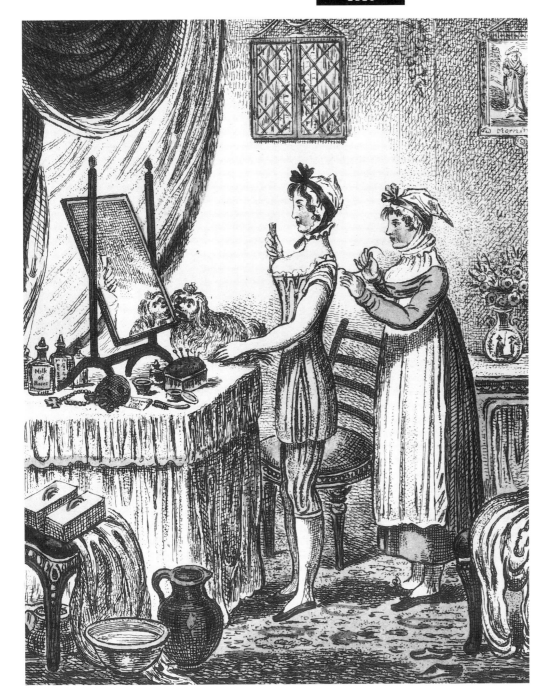

129. 'Progress of the Toilet: the Stays', 1810
James Gillray

Note Despite the ideal of body-revealing draperies, the fashionable, willowy silhouette of 1810–20 was achieved by hip-length boned stays (Gillray exaggerates the length). To maintain the narrow line, drawers were sometimes preferred to layers of petticoats, but did not become general wear until the 1840s.

Head The fashionable lady being dressed has short hair under a ribbon-trimmed morning cap of fine muslin or lace. The maid wears a cornette.

Body The lady has a short-sleeved chemise with frilled neck, boned stays (into which she inserts a busk), and knee-length drawers. The maid's dress has a fashionably high waistline and long, tight sleeves, but the coloured cotton fabric and ankle-length skirt, and the addition of an apron, are governed by practicality. Her chemisette is normal daytime wear for all classes.

Accessories The lady's silk stockings with decorative clocks, and elegant low-cut shoes contrast with the maid's practical lace-ups.

130. Sir David Wilkie, 1816
Andrew Geddes

Note The dressing-gown was a long, loose garment worn indoors over the shirt, waistcoat and legwear, as an informal alternative to the coat. Although straight-fronted, with an easy shawl collar, this gown has a gore in the side to give a flare to the skirt and emphasize the waist, so following a general trend in menswear for a closer fit.

Head He has short, tousled hair.

Body He is dressed in a frilled white shirt and cravat, a dressing-gown of silk or wool damask patterned with leaves and flowers, and trousers with the legs buttoning at the outer ankle.

Accessories He has light stockings, and slippers in the form of flat, heelless mules with a pointed vamp, in the Turkish style.

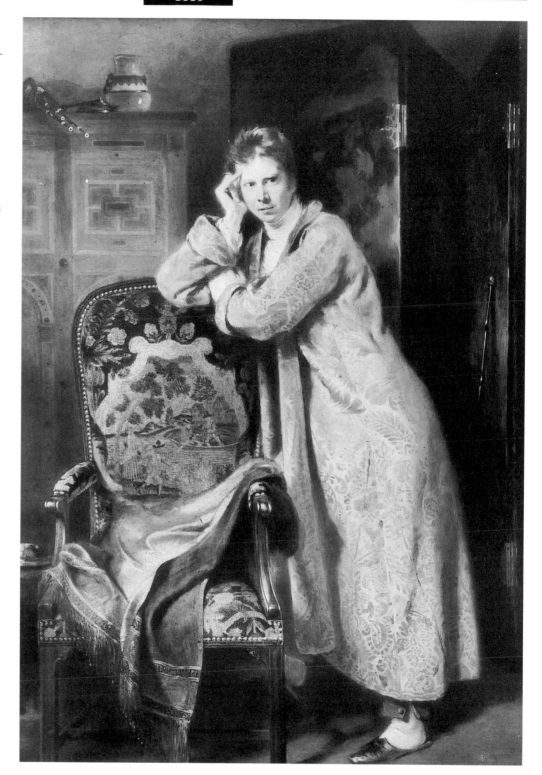

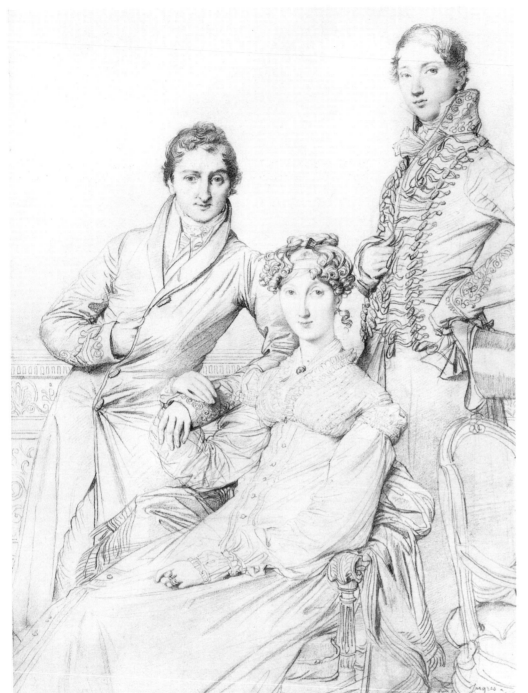

131. **Mr and Mrs Woodhead and the Rev. Henry Comber as a youth, 1816**
Jean-Auguste-Dominique Ingres

Head Mrs Woodhead's hair is coiled and held by a comb and bandeau.

Body She wears a spencer, probably of cotton, decorated with bands of ruching caught down with narrow cords, over a dress featuring the very high waist of 1815–20.

Both men wear versions of the greatcoat, a form of overcoat fashionable about town and typically long and loose, with straight fronts and buttons to the waist. Woodhead's (left) has a shawl collar, and Comber's a high 'Prussian' collar. When such coats were decorated with braid and loop or frog fastenings, like Comber's, they were called 'Polish', 'Hungarian', or 'Russian' coats, and were sometimes fur-lined. Around this date they began to be cut with a close fit and were worn as informal coats with trousers, early versions of the straight-fronted frock coat.

Accessories Mrs Woodhead's neckline is filled in with a handkerchief fastened with a brooch. The dress buttons are almost certainly ornamental. She has a fashionable fringed shawl.

XI **The Cloakroom, Clifton Assembly Rooms, 1817**
Rolinda Sharples
Colour illustration, between pages 128 and 129

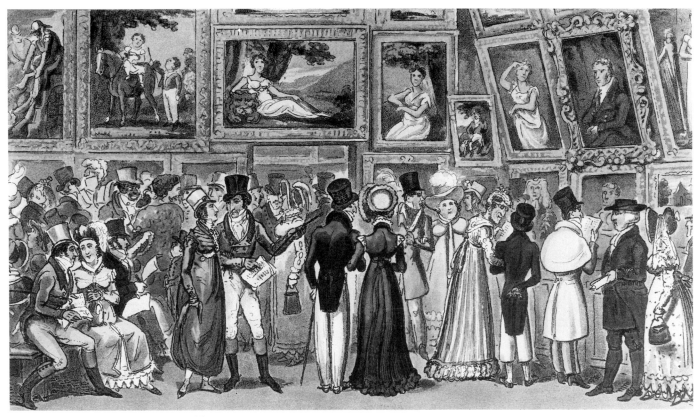

132. **Tom and Jerry at the Royal Academy (detail), 1821**
Robert Isaac and George Cruikshank

Note Fashionable day dress is shown in this scene.

Head Women's headwear includes (from the left) a feathered turban, a high-crowned hat, and a range of wide-brimmed bonnets trimmed with ostrich plumes and a veil.

Body Women's pelisses are very high-waisted, with mancherons and braid trimming. Hem lengths vary, but puffs and vandyking are featured. On the left is a riding habit, trimmed with military-style braid.

The men wear morning coats, or (at the back) a frock coat, while the parson on the right wears clerical dress. Greatcoats feature cape collars (back view right). Breeches still compete with straight trousers of varying lengths, including (centre) voluminous 'Cossacks', pleated to the waist and gathered to the ankle, a style inspired by the Czar's visit to London in 1814.

Accessories Women carry reticules of fabric or leather.

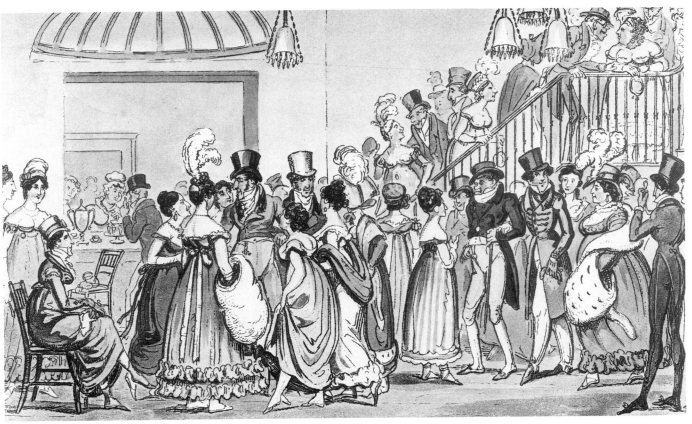

133. Tom and Jerry in the Saloon at Covent Garden (detail), 1821
Robert Isaac and George Cruikshank

Note The men generally wear day dress, but many of the women are in full evening dress.

Head Evening headdresses for women include curled hair in a knot, with combs and feathers, or feathered turbans.

Body Evening dresses have low décolletage with puffed sleeves and padded hems. Day dress necklines are modestly filled in with a chemisette, while the woman in the riding habit (left) demonstrates the fashionable obsession with informality, and the popularity of riding dress for all occasions.

The men generally wear morning coats and knee breeches or pantaloons. An exception (right) is the frock coat with military-style frogging, and trousers with instep straps to keep them taut (popular from 1817).

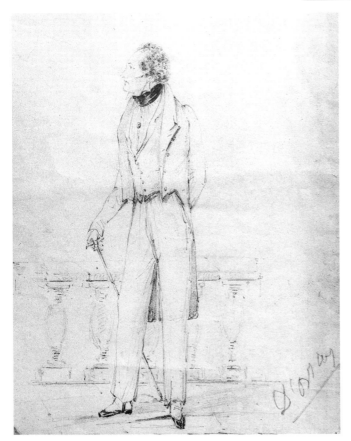

134. Lord Byron, 1823
Count Alfred D'Orsay

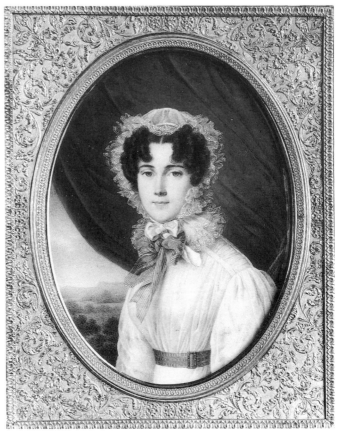

135. Portrait of a woman, 1824–7
'Mansion' (André Léon Larue)

Note Byron is here newly recovered from an illness, and his fashionable day clothes hang rather loose upon him. In this decade the clothes of both sexes feature fuller shoulders and a narrower waistline.

Head His hair is short and tousled.

Body His shirt is finely gathered to a high, pointed collar, and he wears a black silk stock. He wears a morning coat with a roll collar cut high at the back and M-notch lapels. The cut-away fronts are now squared off, and the tails broad and square; the shoulders are gathered and the sleeves long and tight. The waistcoat is cut in the latest fashion with a slightly pointed waist. The trousers have instep straps.

Accessories He is probably wearing light-coloured gaiters over square-toed boots. There is a decorative, perhaps jewelled, pin fastening the shirt front. He carries a cane with a plain short handle.

Note Between 1822 and 1827 the waistline drops to its natural level, sleeves widen, and with 'Marie Stuart' caps and ruffs, the look is self-consciously 'Elizabethan'.

Head Fashionably parted hair with side curls and a knot on the crown is worn under a 'Marie Stuart' morning cap of fine muslin, the double frill edged with lace, and silk ribbon ties under the chin.

Body A matching neck ruff is attached to a chemisette, and she has a bow of striped silk gauze ribbon. Her day dress is of fine lawn or muslin, the fan-shaped gathers emphasizing shoulders and waist. The straight edge of the cotton lining is visible, level with the shoulder. The sleeves are gathered at the shoulder over short puffed undersleeves. The flared skirt is gathered to the bodice at the sides and back (probably over a small bustle pad).

Accessories She wears a belt of watered silk with a metal and paste buckle.

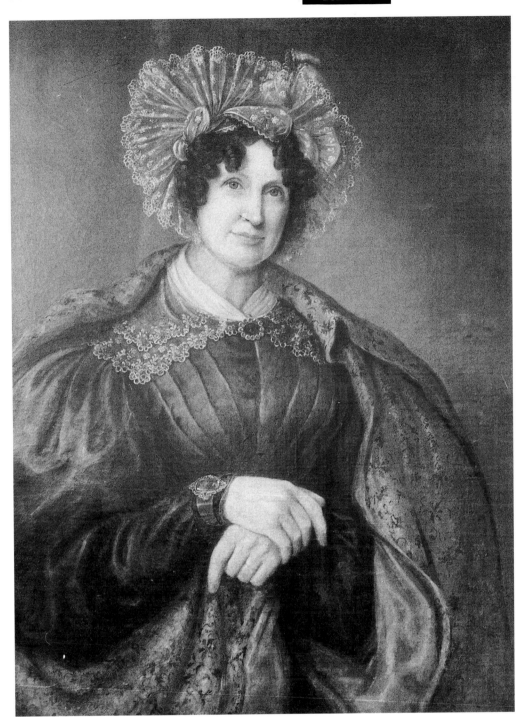

136. Mrs Ellen Sharples, 1829–31
Rolinda Sharples

Note The artist's mother wears fashionable day dress. Still wider gigot sleeves are emphasized by wide caps, pelerines and capes. Within a year or two, bodice pleats will converge well above the waist, adding another almost horizontal line.

Head The hair in side curls and a knot is hidden by a cap of pleated, stiffened blonde lace.

Body Her neckline is filled by a kerchief and she wears a double pelerine of blonde lace. The silk dress has a bodice with flat pleats converging at the waist and padded gigot sleeves. The cloak, apparently of figured or brocaded silk, has a plain lining and an attached cape.

Accessories She wears a brooch at the neck, and on her right wrist a bracelet set with a cameo, mosaic or semi-precious stone.

137. Benjamin Disraeli, 1833
After Daniel Maclise

Note Young Disraeli's style of morning dress reflects his dandified tastes. In this decade, lavish tastes found expression in colourful patterned waistcoats and a variety of jewellery, including studs, pins, rings etc.

Head The hair is fashionably mid-length with a side parting.

Body The shirt has a frilled front and cuffs, and the wide cravat is tied in the 'waterfall' style, with a decorative pin (Disraeli favoured white satin cravats). His shawl-collared waistcoat is very tight. Fitted, and possibly padded, the morning coat has a roll collar and lapels cut high at the back, M-notch lapels, and very long sleeves, and it is worn open to reveal cravat and waistcoat. His trousers have instep straps.

Accessories His footwear consists of square-toed pumps with ribbon bows. He has a watch and chain tucked into the waistcoat watch pocket.

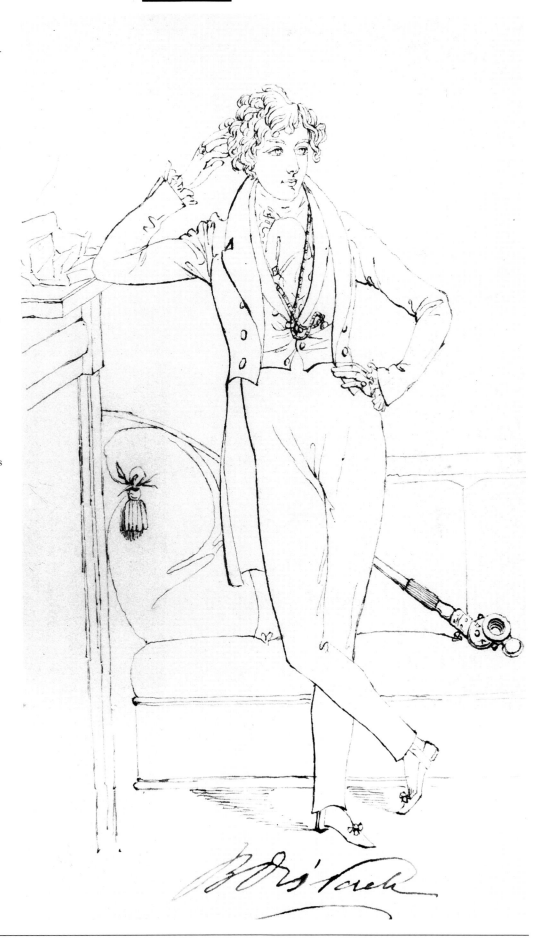

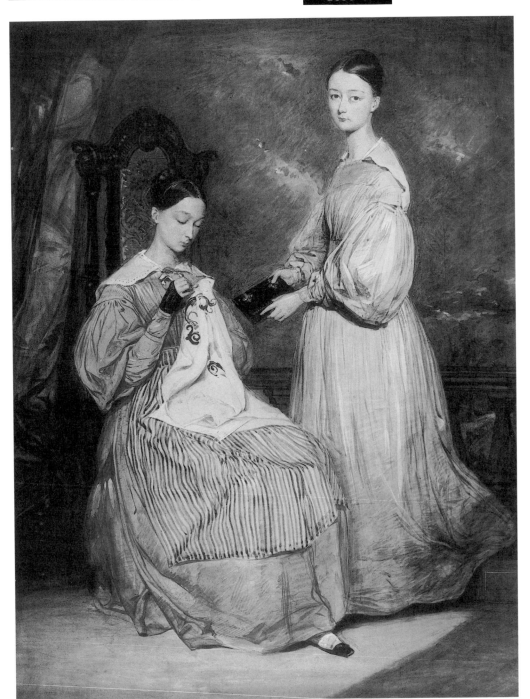

138. Florence and Parthenope Nightingale, 1836–7
William White

Note These are middle-class girls in informal morning dress. From 1836 shoulder lines dropped, sleeves began to deflate, and hemlines fell from the ankle to the instep. Mittens were fashionable for day and evening in the 1830s and 1840s.

Head Both women have centrally parted hair smoothed into a plaited knot on the crown.

Body They are wearing white muslin pelerines and day dresses with simple draped bodice and belted waist. The smooth, dropped shoulder line leads to versions of the full gigot sleeves; (right) the 'Imbecile', full to the cuff, and (left) the 'Donna Maria', full to the elbow, and then tight to the wrist. Their skirts are full and gathered.

Accessories The sister on the left has square-toed shoes, short mittens of black net or lace, and a linen or cotton apron.

139. Lady Elizabeth Villiers, 1841–3
After Alfred Edward Chalon

Note She is wearing fashionable day dress. Although the fullness is still centred on the back, skirts are becoming wider. From 1841 they contain more material which is gauged to the waist, a technique whereby the fabric is finely gathered and attached by alternate pleats; this produces a characteristic dome-shaped skirt. Here, the width is emphasized by the horizontal bands of trimming.

Head Her long hair is arranged in a knot and ringlets.

Body The dress of watered silk is trimmed with bands of velvet and black lace flounces, giving the effect of a bertha on the bodice. The long, tight sleeves have a band of trimmings as the only remnant of the bouffants of the late 1830s. The skirt is full and gathered.

Accessories She carries the ubiquitous lace-edged handkerchief.

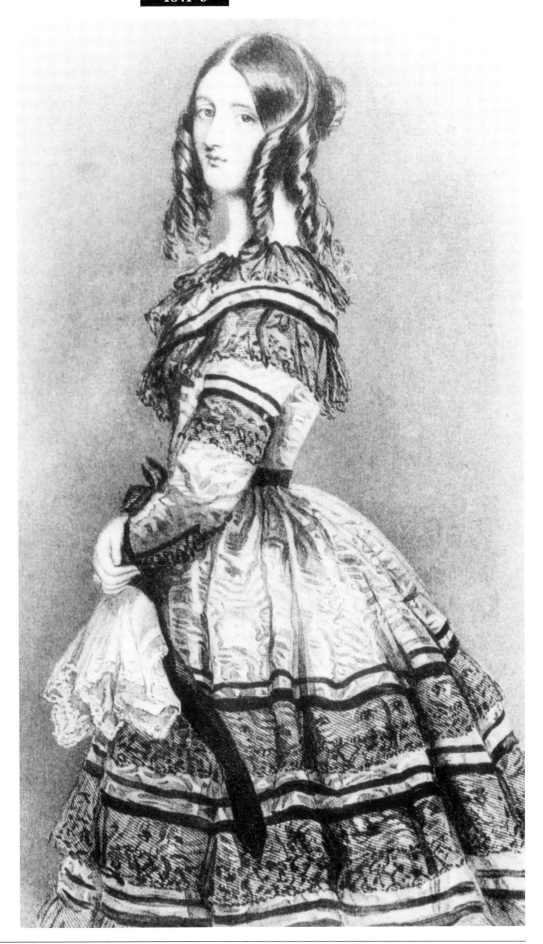

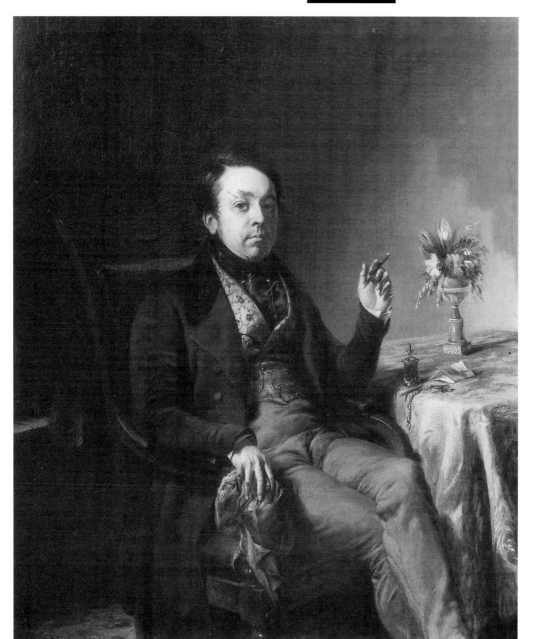

140. Unknown gentleman, 1842
William Huggins

Note Fashionable day clothes are worn here. Gathered sleeves and chest padding are reduced, waists lengthen, and waistcoats are cut with a pointed front, all features which echo changes in women's fashions, and which produce a more streamlined silhouette. His trousers feature a fall front, although the fly fastening, first used around 1823, became general in the 1840s.

Head He has smoothed hair with a side parting (many wore it longer and curled under at the back).

Body He has a high shirt collar with a large silk cravat or 'scarf', covering the shirt front. The double-breasted frock coat has a velvet collar, narrow sleeves and cuffs. The waistcoat, of embroidered or brocaded silk, has a wide roll collar and lapels, and pointed waist. The narrow trousers probably have instep straps.

Accessories His jewellery consists of a chained cravat pin, watch chain and ring.

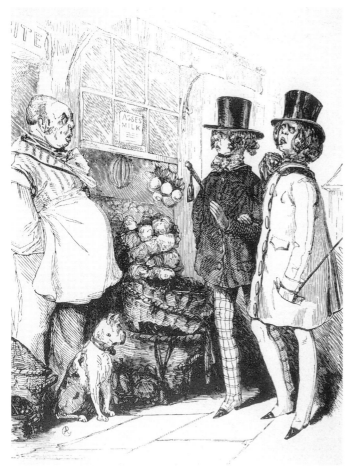

141. Two dandies
Illustration from *Punch*, 1843

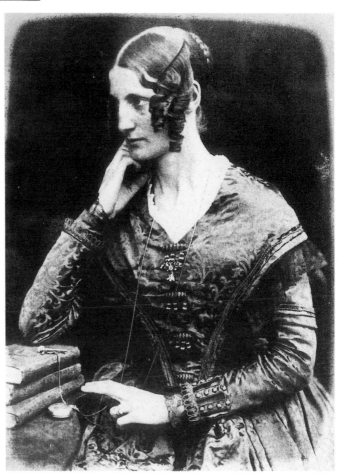

142. Mrs Bell, 1843–8
David Octavius Hill and Robert Adamson

Note As the male silhouette becomes more streamlined, flamboyance is expressed in brightly patterned neckwear, waistcoats and trousers. Paletots, short informal coats, had many versions; these may be (left) the short pea- or monkey-jacket, and (right) the pilot coat, noted for its large buttons and slanted pockets.

Head They have long hair and flat-brimmed top hats.

Body They wear high shirt collars with (left) a brightly patterned silk cravat tied in a bow, and (right) a scarf cravat. Their paletots have fashionable turn-down collars, and horizontal slit or flapped pockets. By contrast, the shopkeeper is unfashionable with his short hair, frilled shirt front and baggy trousers.

Accessories Footwear consists of narrow, square-toed shoes. They wear short gloves and carry thin canes, probably of ebony or bamboo, with gold knobs and tassels.

Note She has centrally parted hair with plaited knot, comb, and ringlets.

Body Her day dress is of silk, figured or damasked with stylized scrolling leaves recalling medieval designs, and has trimmings of tucks, velvet ribbon and black lace; the neck is edged with a frill of muslin or lace. The bodice has a cap-like front panel, emphasizing the sloping shoulders, low-set sleeves, and long pointed waist. A trimming of ornamental, thread-covered toggles and beads runs down the centre front (a precursor of the front-buttoning jacket bodice of the 1850s). The long tight sleeves have braid trimming at the cuffs.

Accessories Her neck chain has a watch, and key or seal. She wears a brooch of delicate intertwined flowers and stems, with pendant flower, in the Romantic style.

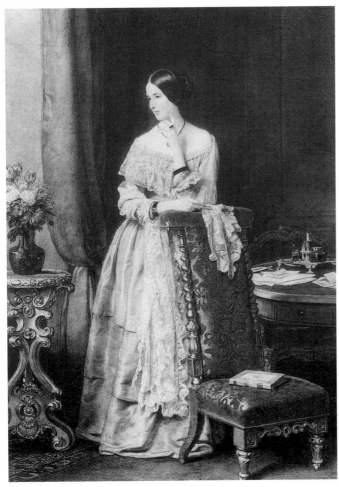

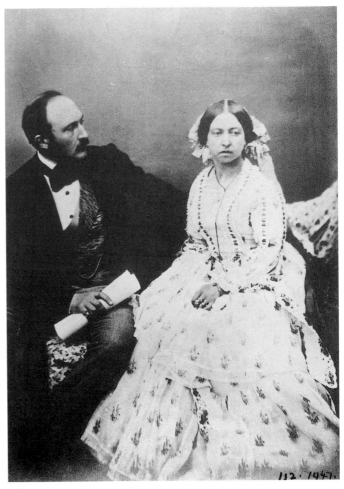

143. **Angela Georgina, Baroness Burdett-Coutts, 1847–50**
Sir William Charles Ross

144. **Queen Victoria and Prince Albert, 1854**
Roger Fenton

Note The evening dresses of this decade were restrained in style, characterized by the contrast between plain silk and rich lace; this is probably expensive hand-made bobbin lace (but the cheaper machined laces were stylish and popular). The fashion plate ideal would have a wider skirt, and flowers in the hair.

Head Her hair is looped back in a plaited knot.

Body The silk dress has a décolletage edged with a tucker and a flounced lace bertha, sleeves with lace ruffles, and a flounced skirt.

Accessories She wears a lace shawl, neck ribbon with pendant, and bracelets including two of black velvet ribbon with a decorative clasp or locket.

Note The royal couple are in fashionable day dress.

Head The Queen's hair is draped over her ears into a knot at the back of the head. Her elaborate cap of frilled muslin, lace and ribbons, with hanging streamers, is worn on the back of the head like a fashionable bonnet.

Body The dress, of spotted muslin warp-printed with bouquets, and arranged in flounces, is trimmed with lace and threaded ribbons; it helps to create the characteristic blurred silhouette seen in women's dress in the 1850s. It has the fashionable pointed waist and pagoda sleeves.

The Prince wears a bow-tied cravat, and shirt with decorative studs. Patterned waistcoats were popular even, as here, with a dark formal frock coat.

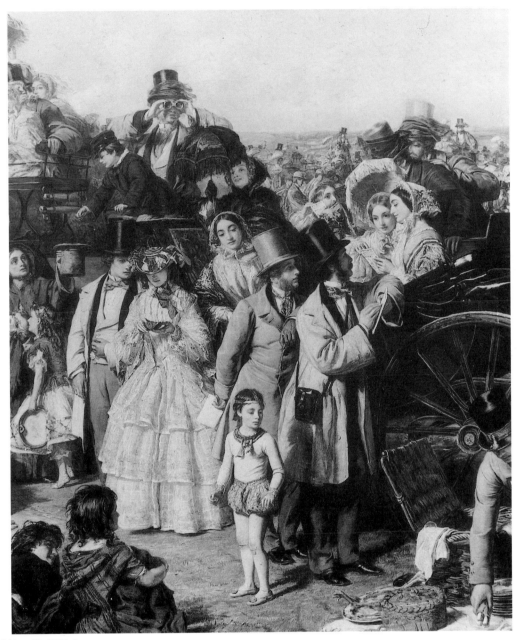

145. 'Derby Day' (detail), 1856–8
William Powell Frith

Head The fashionable men wear top hats with the straight sides and almost flat brim typical of this decade.

In the carriage on the right, the fashionable women wear their hair turned under at the ears, into a low-set knot. Their silk bonnets have the sloping crown which grows progressively smaller and slides further down the head, throughout the 1850s. The one on the far right has trimmings of artificial flowers with bobbin lace on the edge and inside the brim and round the *bavolet*. Women's hats went out of fashion after the mid-1830s, but by the late 1840s a large round straw hat with turn-down brim was appearing for seaside and country wear. By 1857 more stylish versions, such as the mousquetaire – a low-crowned, wide-brimmed hat with a feather plume – were worn by fashionable young women. On the centre left, the young woman examining her purse wears her hair in a knot and ringlets under a mousquetaire hat of striped straw trimmed with ruched silk ribbons and feathers and tied under the chin with wide silk ties.

Body The fashionable man on the centre left, like the others in the foreground, wears a dark coat with a lighter-coloured greatcoat. His shawl-collared waistcoat is now cut without the pointed waist of the 1840s, and with the shorter length introduced by 1855.

His female companion wears a frilled cotton collar, and a dress of muslin woven with a check, the flounces printed with flowers *à disposition*. The softly pleated bodice has a pointed waist trimmed with a sash; her pagoda sleeves have separate gathered undersleeves of broderie anglaise. The woman on the far right has a broderie anglaise collar, and silk day dress with flounced sleeves and fringe trimming.

Accessories Fringe trimming on dresses and accessories was popular from the mid-1840s; a fringed parasol is carried by one of the women in the carriage.

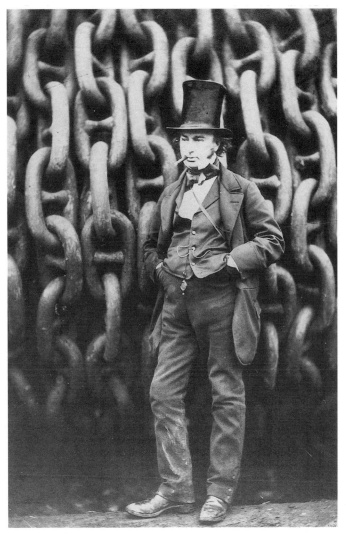

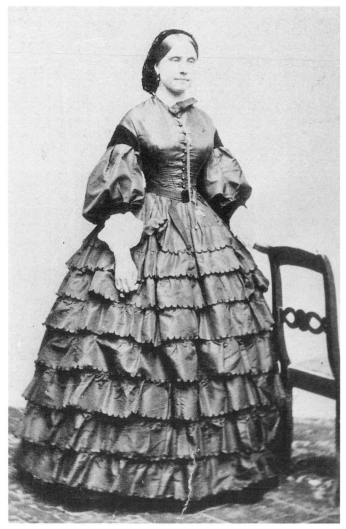

146. **Isambard Kingdom Brunel, 1857**
Robert Howlett

147. **Unknown woman, 1862**
Anon. photograph

Note Although jacket and trousers are of the same tone, this is not a matching suit. The heavy wool fabrics of the mid-century sag and crease, producing a look totally different from the fashion-plate ideal.

Head His top-hat is fashionably straight.

Body He wears a pointed standing collar with a bow-tie. His morning coat, the popular coat of the decade, is distinctive in its slightly cutaway front skirts, combined with waist seam, stitched edges, and flapped pockets. An extra buttonhole in the left lapel (for a flower) was introduced in the 1840s. He has a fashionably short waistcoat with lapels, and trousers with fly front, high-set slant pockets and buttons at the outer side seams.

Accessories The wide, square-toed boots have the high toe spring typical of this decade, and stacked heels. He has a watch and chain.

Note Velvet was a popular trimming on plain silk, and was often echoed in hair nets of chenille. Creases betray the tight fit of the boned bodice. The pointed waist is now shorter, and was often replaced by the princess line, cut without a waist seam.

Head The woman's hair is in a low chignon, worn inside a net.

Body She wears a narrow white collar with tie, and a silk day dress with velvet-trimmed bishop sleeves and cotton undersleeves. The skirt is trimmed with pinked flounces and worn over a crinoline.

Accessories These include earrings, a neck chain with attached watch or scent bottle tucked into the belt, and keys or seals hanging below.

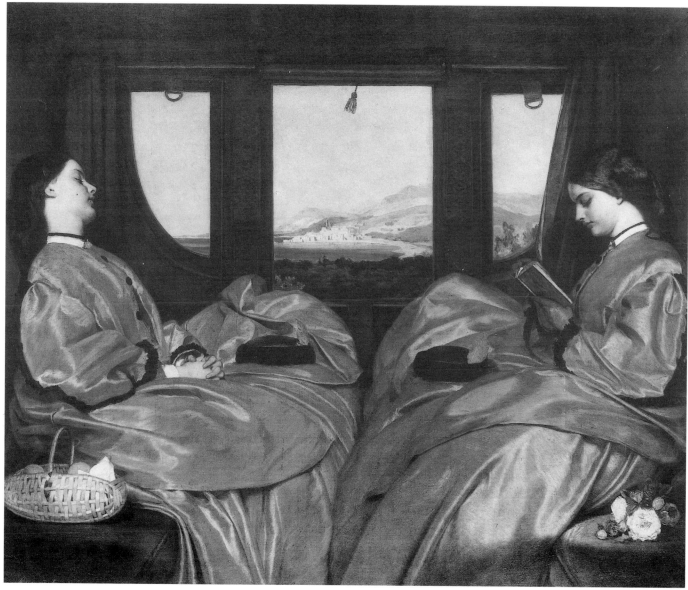

148. 'The Travelling Companions', 1862
Augustus Egg

Note These are fashionable middle-class sisters travelling through Europe, their balloon-like crinolines filling the railway carriage. When sitting, the hoops telescoped at the back, and rose slightly at the sides.

Head They wear their hair in a very large, low chignon; such chignons were often supplemented by false hair.

Body They wear narrow collars. Their day dresses are worn under matching three-quarter-length coats which are loose or slightly waisted, buttoning at the front and with full, braid-trimmed sleeves; these coats may be *paletots* in contemporary terminology.

Accessories Ribbons with pendants are worn at the neck. On their knees are round hats of felt or velvet with turned-up brims, trimmed with a feather; this was a popular style for young women and was often called a 'pork-pie' hat.

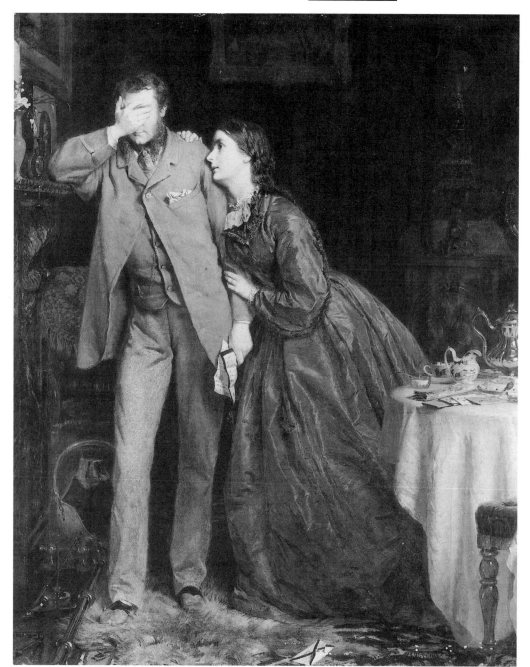

149. 'Woman's Mission: Companion of Manhood', 1863
George Elgar Hicks

Note Both wear informal morning dress.

Head The husband has fashionably short, side-parted hair, with long drooping 'Dundreary' side whiskers (as popularized by a character in the play *Our American Cousin* in 1861).

The wife wears her hair loose at the back, although a chignon, and perhaps a morning cap, were more usual, even before breakfast.

Body The husband wears an informal three-piece lounge suit; the jacket, edged with braid (this was a general feature from the 1850s) has the narrow cuffs and high-set button typical of the 1860s.

His wife's day dress is fashionably plain, with bishop sleeves; she appears to wear a crinoline.

Accessories The husband's Turkish-style slippers are informal indoor wear.

XII The Dancing Platform at Cremorne Gardens, 1864
Phoebus Levin
Colour illustration, between pages 128 and 129

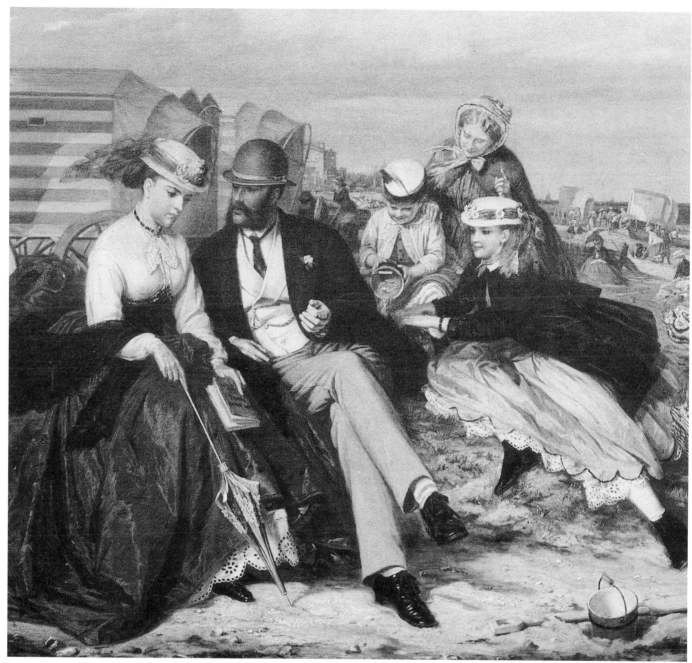

150. **On the Beach: a Family on Margate Sands (detail), 1867**
Charles Wynne Nicholls

Note The bowler hat and lounge jacket, although informal, could be extremely stylish.

For women, an innovation of this decade was the wearing of contrasting blouse and skirt for country, at home, or at the seaside. The skirt often had a matching cape or jacket, forerunner of the tailor-made suit.

Head The man has short hair, moustache and 'mutton-chop' whiskers. He wears an early form of the bowler hat, a hard felt hat with distinctive bowl-shaped crown and curly brim, introduced for informal wear.

Over her high chignon, the young woman wears a straw hat with net and feather trimming, and a net veil.

Body He has a narrow turn-down collar and neck-tie. His dark cloth or velvet lounge jacket has a flower in the buttonhole. He wears a fashionably short, plain, shawl-collared waistcoat and narrow trousers.

She wears a muslin chemisette trimmed with lace and threaded ribbon; beneath it are visible the low neckline and short ribbon-threaded sleeves of her chemise, and across the bust, the top of her stays. She wears a Swiss belt and a silk skirt with braided hem (a protection against wear). The cotton petticoat with broderie anglaise hem is probably worn over a crinoline.

Accessories For the man, one might note the striped hose (striped stockings were also fashionable for women in this decade).

The woman's accessories include lace-up boots, short gloves with decorative points, a black lace shawl, and a silk and lace parasol.

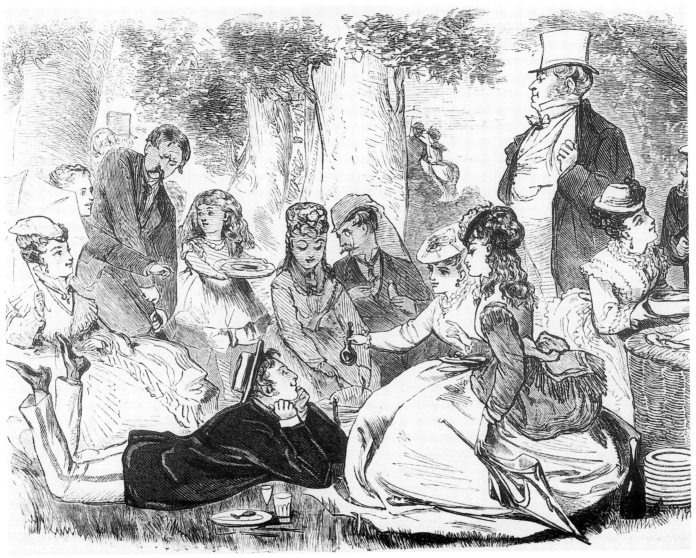

151. **An August Picnic**
Illustration from *The Girl of the Period,* 1869

Head The older man wears formal day dress, including a top
hat, but more casual styles are favoured by the younger men.
The one in the foreground has a straw sailor hat, later called a
boater; the man in the centre has a protective veil, fashionable
for men as well as for women.

The young women wear a variety of small hats, now tilted
forward to accommodate the still rising and ever larger chignon.
The girl in the right foreground shows the fashion for loose back
hair, introduced from America in 1868.

Body The older man's formal standing collar and frock coat
contrast with the casual lounge jackets of the younger men; the
one in the foreground may be velvet, and is worn with
fashionable braided trousers and elastic-sided boots.

The full crinoline disappeared in 1868, and the girl in the
foreground has the looped polonaise overskirt and bustle
fashionable from that date.

152. The Marchioness of Huntley, 1870
Sir John Everett Millais

Note The Marchioness avoids fashion extremes to achieve romantic simplicity. Her square neckline and high round waistline are typical of 1868–74, although her epaulettes are no longer high fashion by 1870. The skirt, with its flat front, gored sides and long train, shows the transitional stage between crinoline and bustle. Here it is worn without either, but the trimmings suggest the more fashionable alternative of an apron-fronted overskirt, which high fashion would have worn draped and puffed over a bustle and half-crinoline.

Head Her hair is in a high but plain chignon trimmed with ribbons.

Body Her summer day dress of muslin is trimmed with threaded silk ribbons and lace.

Accessories She wears drop earrings, a neck ribbon with a pearl drop pendant, and a bracelet. Her gloves are probably of soft leather.

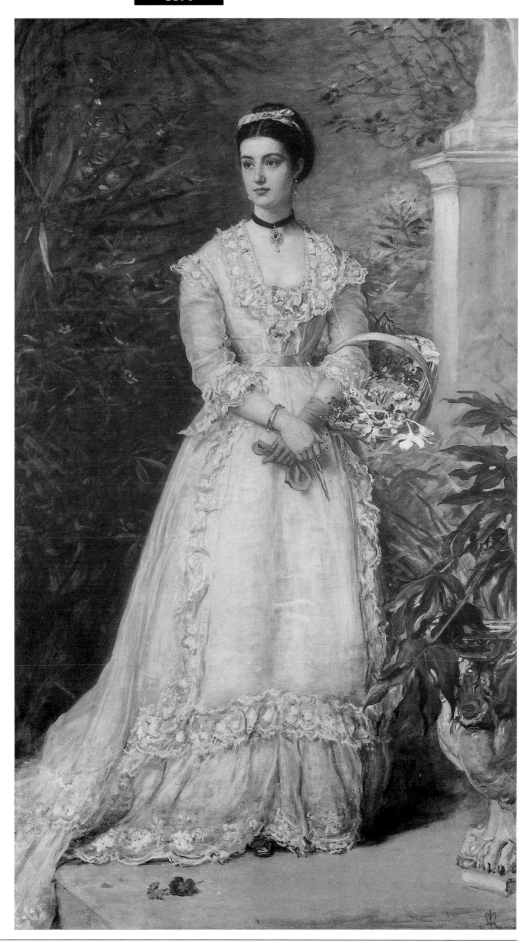

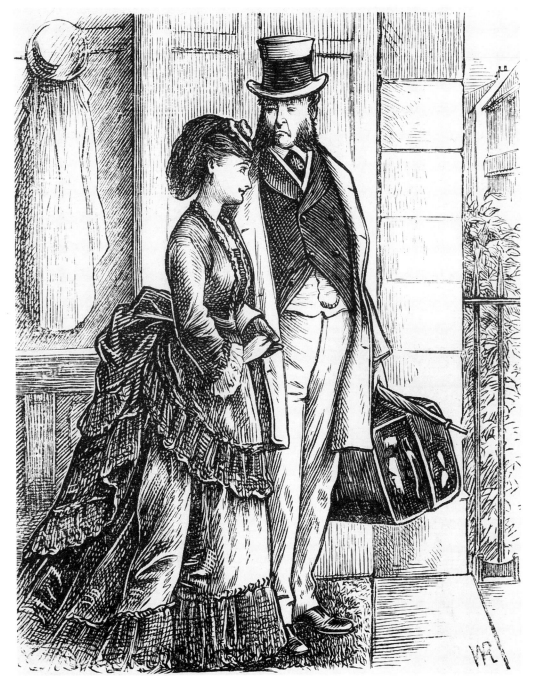

153. **Travelling scene**
Illustration from *Punch*, 1874

Note A middle-class couple dressed for travelling.

Head The fashionable wife wears her hair in a full chignon, with an exaggeratedly small, forward-tilted hat. Her husband has full side whiskers and the curved and curly top hat of the first half of the 1870s.

Body He wears a greatcoat or paletot over his cut-away morning coat and waistcoat.

She wears fashionable day dress, the square-necked jacket bodice with slightly pagoda-shaped sleeves, and ruffles, the skirts draped to give an apron-front and puffed back. Her matching underskirt has a flounced hem, and a train supported by a bustle.

154. Woman in day dress, 1876
James Tissot

Note By 1876 the overall silhouette was sheath-like, the bustle giving way to a waterfall of drapery extending as a train. Trimmings of flounces, pleats and ruching became more elaborate as the decade progressed.

Head The curly-brimmed hat is decorated with feathers, probably ostrich.

Body The dress of striped muslin trimmed with silk bows, has a short polonaise bodice, the frilled edge forming the fashionable high collar and frilled cuffs. There is a separate overskirt with frilled edge dipping down at the back, and a flounced underskirt.

Accessories A large plain parasol was a fashionable alternative to those with lace edgings or trimmings of ribbon bows or ruchings.

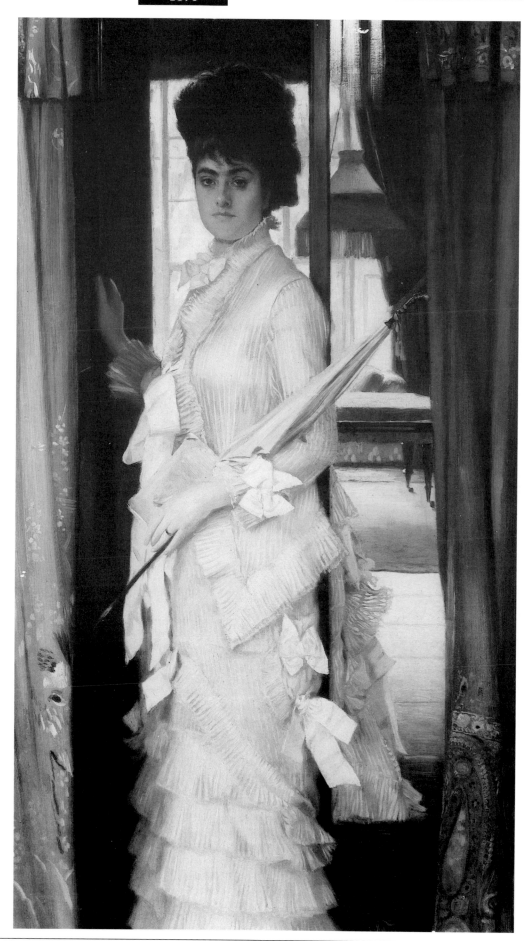

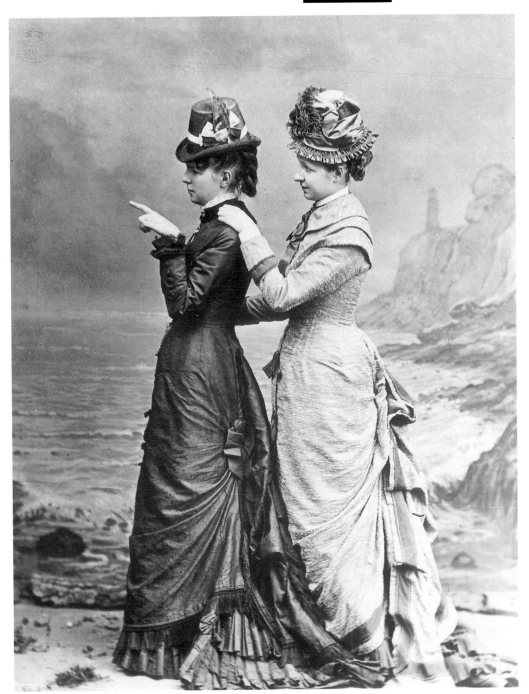

155. Two women in day dress, 1878
Elliot and Fry

Note Skirts were now so sheath-like that long stays were essential, and combinations were introduced to dispense with the bulk of separate chemise and drawers. Petticoats were few and narrow, with extra flounces at the back to support the fall of drapery which replaced the bustle from 1876–80.

Head They wear their hair in chignons under (left) a hard felt Tyrolean hat trimmed with ribbons and a bird's wing, and (right) a soft-crowned toque trimmed with feathers.

Body Each wears a dress in the form of a princess-style polonaise, with narrow cuffed sleeves, a centre-front opening decorated with bows, and a tie-back skirt with back draperies and train. The pleated flounces at the hem may belong to a separate underskirt, but more probably are attached directly to the lining of the main skirt.

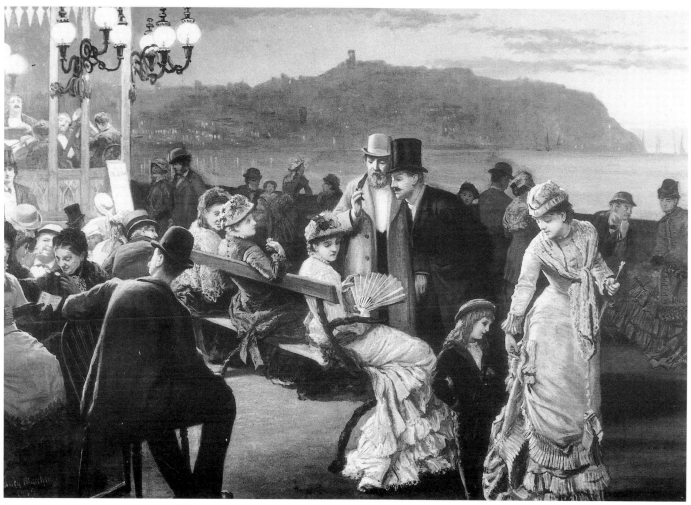

156. Scarborough Spa at Night, 1879
Francis Sydney Muschamp

Head The women wear small hats or toques trimmed with flowers and feathers, or high-crowned hats with birds' wings.

The men favour the tall straight-sided, small-brimmed top hats of the late 1870s, or bowler hats, both high- and low-crowned.

Body The princess polonaise is the most popular dress, decorated with bows and pleated frills. The woman on the right loops up her train for walking. On a warm summer night, lace shawls are the most popular outerwear, tied fichu-style (right).

The men wear high-buttoning frock coats or overcoats. The little boy has the long hair more usually associated with aesthetic dress, and a sailor hat and suit with knickerbockers.

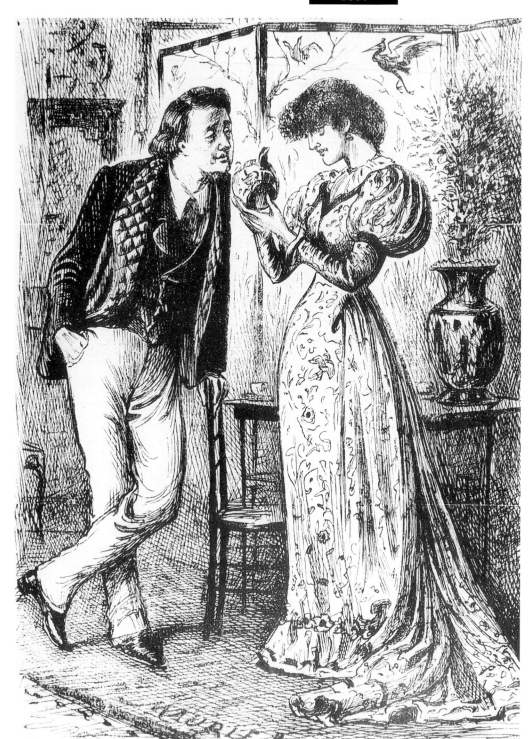

157. Couple in aesthetic dress
Illustration from *Punch*, 1880

Note In artistic circles in the late 1870s the extremes of high fashion were rejected in favour of 'aesthetic' dress. For women this meant romantically loose or frizzed hair, loose dresses worn without stays or stiffened petticoats, and large puffed sleeves in the 'Renaissance' style. Aesthetic women either wore soft oriental silks in the muted 'greenery-yallery' colours which they obtained from Liberty's, or exotically embroidered or brocaded silks which were thought to be 'Renaissance' in design.

Head The man's long hair and clean-shaven face brand him as an aesthete; a similar message is conveyed by the women's loose frizzed hair, in the style popularized by the Pre-Raphaelite artists.

Body The man's turn-down collar, soft tie, and lounge jacket (probably of velvet with a quilted silk collar), are fashionable informal dress, although velvet jackets were particularly associated with aestheticism.

The woman's dress, probably of brocaded silk, has the low neck, puffed 'Renaissance' sleeves, lack of waist seam, and loose flowing skirt typical of aesthetic gowns.

158. Marion Hood, 1884
Elliot and Fry

Note This is fashionable, formal day dress, the draperies of which were at their most exuberant in the mid-1880s, just before they disappeared almost entirely.

Head She wears her hair with a fringe (fashionable since 1882), and a loose version of the low-set chignon.

Body The velvet bodice has a standing collar, fashionably short sleeves and a pointed front waist, with a lace neck frill, sleeve ruffles, and plastron. The silk skirt, with train, is made up from panels of draped and ruched silk, intermingled with swags and frills of lace, attached to a plain lining which is tied with tapes inside the back, and worn over a bustle.

Accessories She wears a necklace, possibly of amber, and kid or suede gloves. Her shoes are of fancy leather, with pointed toes, decorative rosettes and heels of probably one-and-a-half to two inches in height.

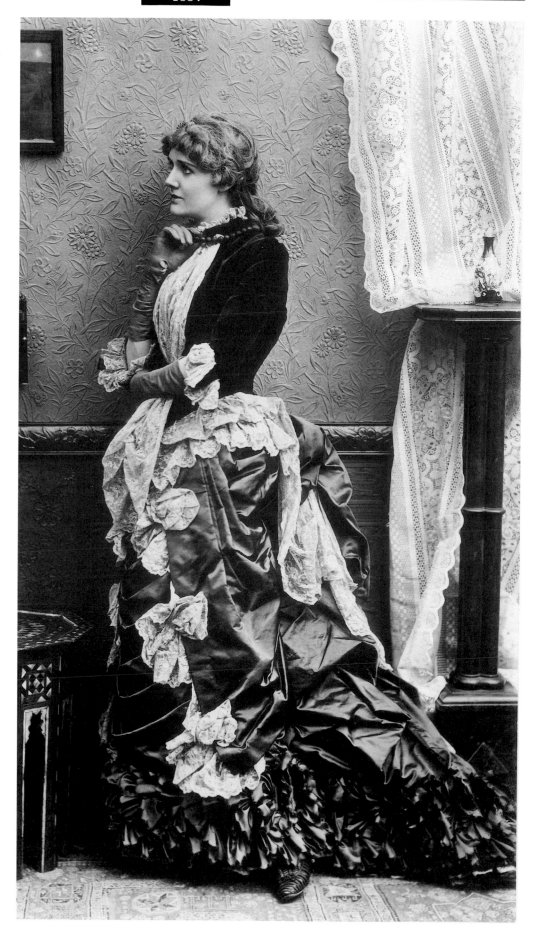

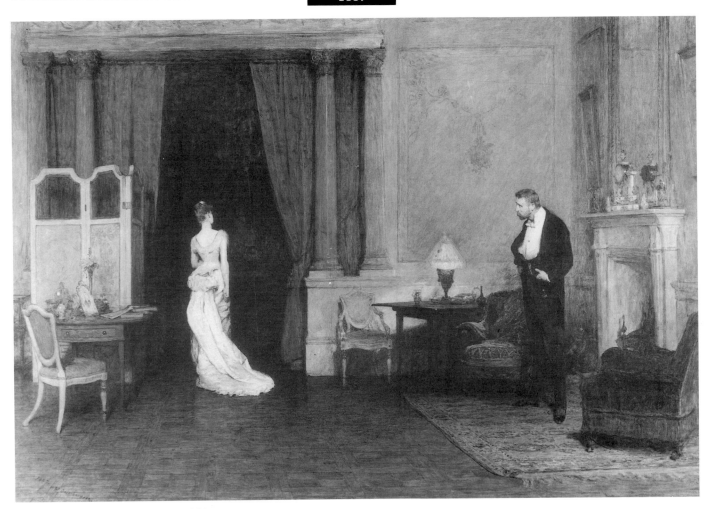

159. 'The First Cloud', 1887
Sir William Quiller Orchardson

Note This upper-class couple are in full evening dress.

Head The woman wears her hair swept into a knot, with flower or feather trimming.

Body Her silk gown has the extreme décolletage and vestigial sleeves typical of the late 1880s. Her draped tie-back skirt is worn over a bustle, narrower and more angular than that of the 1870s; worn over a train, it gives a greater sense of movement. The man has the fashionable standing collar, white bow tie, starched shirt front and cutaway dress coat (although by the mid-1880s lapels were generally superseded by the roll collar for evening).

160. Sir Arthur Sullivan, 1888
Sir John Everett Millais

Note Sir Arthur wears fashionable formal day dress. Coats were buttoned very high in this decade. Collars, shirt fronts, and cuffs were heavily starched in the latter half of the century.

Head He has short hair, probably sleeked with macassar oil, and centrally parted. Moustaches were usual, with or without short side whiskers.

Body He wears a winged collar and unusually wide tie; the shirt cuffs are as heavily stiffened as the collar. He wears a double-breasted frock coat with cuffs, and trousers in a contrasting colour.

Accessories A monocle hangs from a cord round his neck, a popular accessory since the middle of the century, and particularly associated with ultra-fashionable 'swells'.

XIII St. Martin-in-the-Fields, 1888
William Logsdail
Colour illustration, between pages 128 and 129

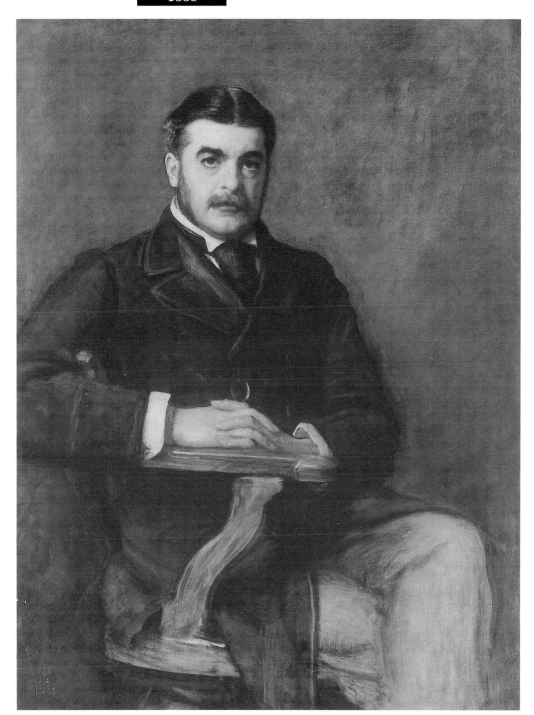

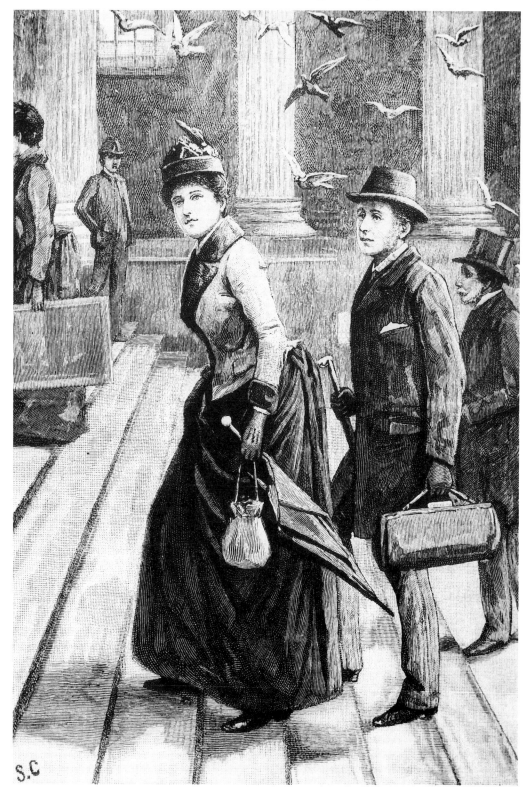

S.C

161. City scene
Illustration from *The Family Friend*, 1890

Note A middle-class couple in simple, conservative, outdoor dress.

Head The woman has a fashionable frizzed fringe and high-set knot of hair, under a toque trimmed with ribbons and a bird's wing. The man wears a semi-formal felt hat.

Body The woman's fitted jacket is a less dressy alternative to the popular mantle, and is probably made of cloth trimmed with darker fabric or fur. Her day dress has a simple draped skirt worn over a bustle.

The man wears a Chesterfield overcoat, distinguished by its straight lines and outside pockets.

Accessories Her reticule or dress bag is probably home-made, for during the 1880s soft drawstring bags were being superseded by commercially-made leather handbags, more stylish versions of the man's travelling bag.

162. Middle-class couple, holidaying in the country
Illustration from *The English Illustrated Magazine*, 1894

Note Their dress is smart but informal.

Head The woman wears her hair frizzed and probably padded, in a heavy knot or coil. Her wide-brimmed hat is trimmed with either ribbon bows or birds wings. Her husband wears the soft, peaked cap which was originally sportswear, but became popular in the 1890s for general leisure activities.

Body The woman wears a contrasting jacket and skirt, with a blouse. Fashionable features are the high standing collar, gigot sleeves, and applied trimmings of braid or ribbon. The cut of the skirt is typical of 1890–7, when gores and darts gave a snug fit on the hips, while deep pleats, cut on the cross, gave a flowing line at the back.

The man's lounge suit displays the large checks often used for informal wear in this decade.

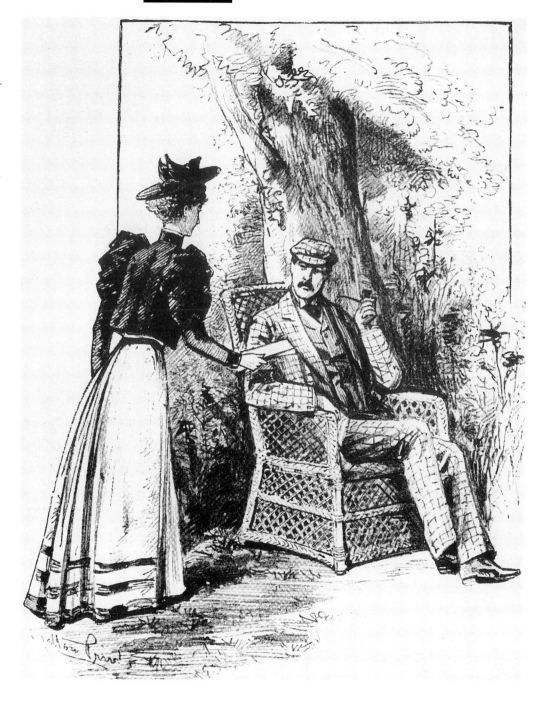

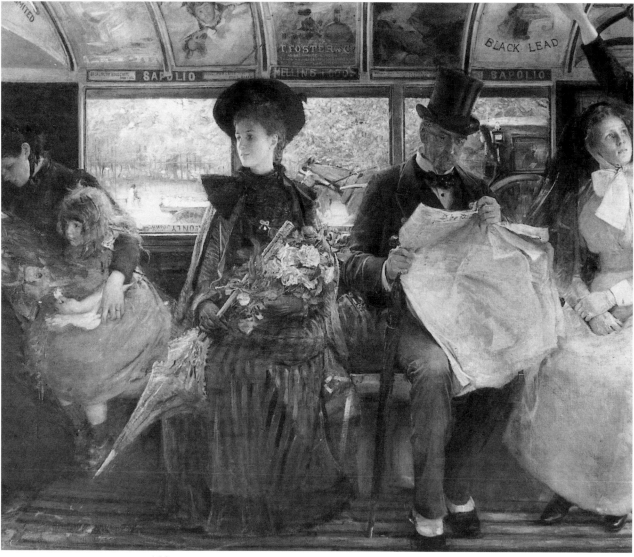

163. 'The Bayswater Omnibus' (detail), 1895
Thomas Matthew Joy

Note The fashionable woman is dressed for city travelling, and the businessman wears correct dress for formal day and city wear.

Head She wears a wide-brimmed 'picture' hat. He has very short hair and a heavy moustache; he wears a curly-brimmed top hat.

Body She wears a high-collared day dress of striped fabric, probably silk, and a cape or cloak with wide frilled collar. His dress consists of a high starched wing collar, with a spotted bow tie; a frock coat with braided edges; a high-buttoning waistcoat; and narrow trousers.

Accessories She wears short day gloves, probably of suede, and holds a long parasol, with fashionable frilled edge. Her bow-shaped brooch is probably of paste stones, with a pendant pearl. He wears pointed boots and spats (popular with frock coats from 1893), and has a metal-framed business bag. The long furled umbrella is, in the 1890s, a fashionable alternative to the cane. For men, a signet ring is now the only fashionably acceptable form of jewellery apart from the tie-pin. Gloves of fawn kid or grey suede were popular with frock or morning coats, but he may have removed them while reading his newspaper.

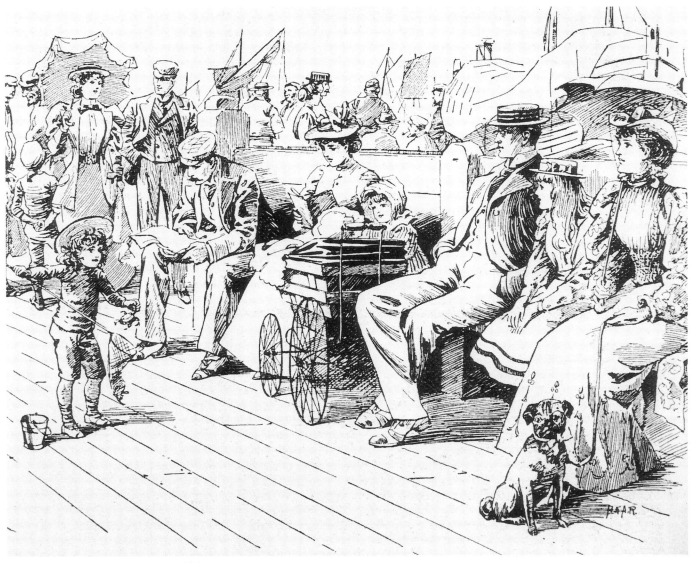

164. 'In the holidays'
Illustration from *The Windsor Magazine*, 1897

Note Middle-class families in fashionable but informal seaside wear.

Head Straw sailor hats are popular for men, women and children; alternative styles are soft-peaked caps for men, more dressy wide-brimmed hats for women, and cotton sunbonnets for little girls (copies of those worn by countrywomen).

Body and Accessories For women, a tailored jacket, blouse and skirt (left) are an alternative to day dress (right), but both feature high collars, gigot sleeves, narrow waists and flared skirts. The older girl wears a calf-length version of adult dress, but the younger ones complement their sunbonnets with loose, yoked dresses or overalls, based on the countryman's smock. Their brothers wear jerseys and open-legged knickerbockers. Men favour informal suits and two-tone brogue shoes.

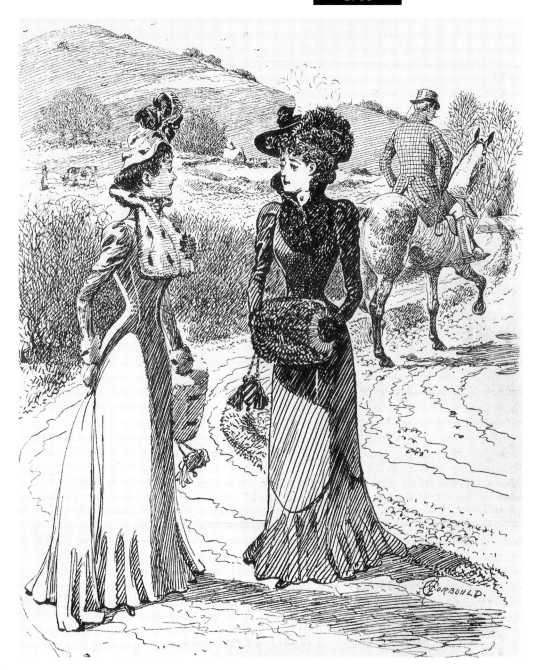

165. Fashionable walking dress
Illustration from *Punch*, 1900

Note The emphasis is on height, achieved by the padded hair and plumed hats, puffed shoulders, narrow, fitting costumes, and high-heeled boots and shoes. Nevertheless, padded busts and hips, and heavily boned long-fronted stays, create an S-shaped silhouette, completed by the flowing skirts.

Head The women's hair is rolled and padded with a knot on top. Their wavy-brimmed hats are trimmed with feathers and fur.

Body They wear long fitted pelisses of cloth or velvet, trimmed with fur, and with high wired collars, wide lapels, narrow sleeves with small shoulder puffs, and skirts with short trains, cut to flare out from below the knee.

Accessories They carry muffs to match the fur on their costume; attached to these muffs are metal-framed purses, decorated with tassels, and, on the left, a posy of artificial flowers.

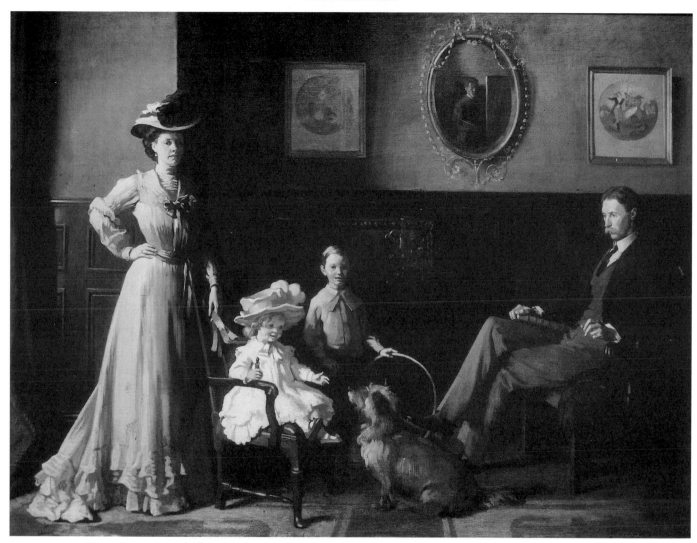

166. **The Family of George Campbell Swinton at Pont Street, London, 1901**

William Orpen

Note The sitters are Elizabeth Ebsworth, Mrs Swinton; Mary Swinton (later Lady William Percy); Alan Henry Campbell Swinton and George Campbell Swinton. Orpen's portrait appears as a mirror-reflection on the wall. The fashionable cut of Mrs Swinton's dress, the elaborate nature of the children's clothes and the quiet but well-tailored elegance of their father suggest that this is a well-to-do family. Mrs Swinton's confident pose with her hand on one hip (which incidentally draws attention to the narrowness of her waist) was a favourite stance at this period.

Head Although they are indoors both Mrs Swinton and her infant daughter wear hats. Mrs Swinton's has a wide, curved brim trimmed with ostrich feathers; the little girl's has a deep crown and wide brim. Mr Swinton's hair is parted at the centre and he has a long moustache.

Body Mrs Swinton's day dress has a V-shaped opening with turned-back collar filled in with a high-necked dress front. Her flounced skirt is cut with additional fullness at the back to form a short train. Mr Swinton wears a dark frock coat with lighter-coloured waistcoat and trousers; his shirt has a stiff, double collar. Mary Swinton is dressed in a flounced coat and dress, her brother in a shirt with a wide collar and knee breeches.

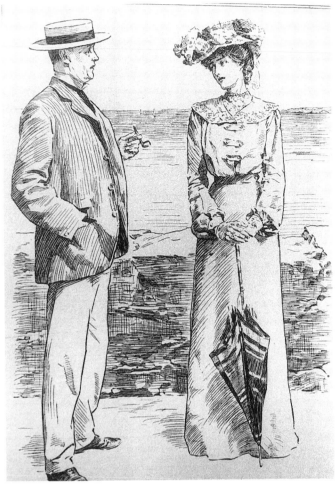

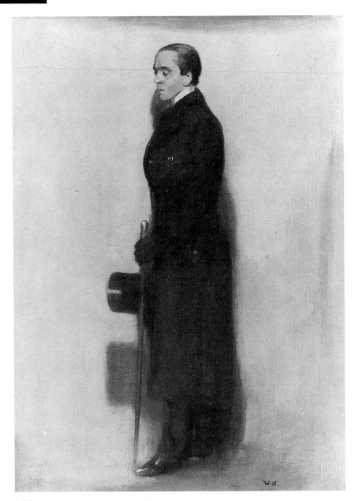

167. **Seaside wear**
Illustration, *Punch*, 1902

Note The man and woman in this *Punch* cartoon wear informal day clothes at a seaside resort. The man has a relaxed air with his pipe in one hand and the other in his pocket. The woman's stance, with hands folded and leaning slightly on her parasol is characteristic of this period.

Head The man's hair is cut very short and he is clean-shaven. The woman's long hair is knotted at the nape of her neck. Both wear straw hats – the man a boater and the woman a large hat trimmed with artificial flowers.

Body The man has on an easy-fitting lounge jacket with narrow lapels and single-breasted fastening, and light-coloured trousers. His shirt collar is stiffened in the wing or butterfly style with a long, knotted tie. The woman wears a blouse and long, tailored skirt. The blouse has a wide collar trimmed with braid and the opening is filled in, high to the neck; although it appears easy-fitting the blouse would have been worn over a rigidly boned corset.

Accessories Gloves are worn by the woman and she carries a parasol or umbrella with a long handle and striped cover.

168. **Sir Max Beerbohm, 1905**
William Nicholson

Note Max Beerbohm (1872–1956), the author and cartoonist, was a noted dandy and one of the few men to praise the costume of his time. He commended 'its sombre delicacy, its congruities of black and white and grey' and the way it produced 'a supreme effect through means the least extravagant'.

Head His hair is short and very neat, being smoothed flat over the crown.

Body He wears a long, fitted, Chesterfield overcoat in dark cloth. His shirt collar is high and stiff.

Accessories He carries a top hat and walking stick and wears gloves.

169. Three gowns by Paul Poiret

Paul Iribe, *Les Robes de Paul Poiret*, 1908

Note Paul Poiret (1879–1944) was one of the most influential French fashion designers in the first two decades of the twentieth century. His work was stylishly publicized in 1908 by the illustrations of Paul Iribe in a *de luxe* booklet called *Les Robes de Paul Poiret*. His designs were notable for their elegance and economy of line.

Head The women's hair arrangements are stylized in this illustration but suggest the neo-classical inspiration with their loose curls and Grecian-type fillets.

Body The dresses are extremely simple and severe in shape with the raised waistline and straight, tubular skirt reminiscent of the neo-classical taste of the early-nineteenth-century period. The natural curves of the female figure have been almost entirely eliminated and there is a marked absence of ornament – the decoration of these gowns is handled with restraint and an almost geometrical precision. Poiret's colour range was bold and brilliant, rejecting the soft, pretty pastel shades popular at the turn of the century.

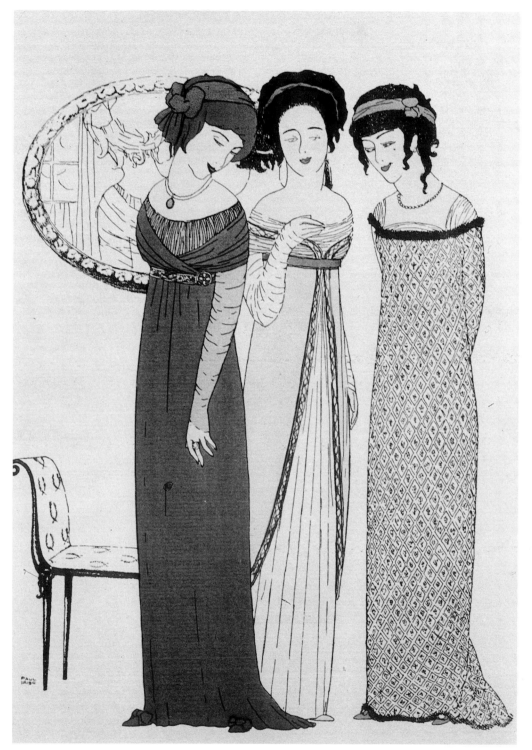

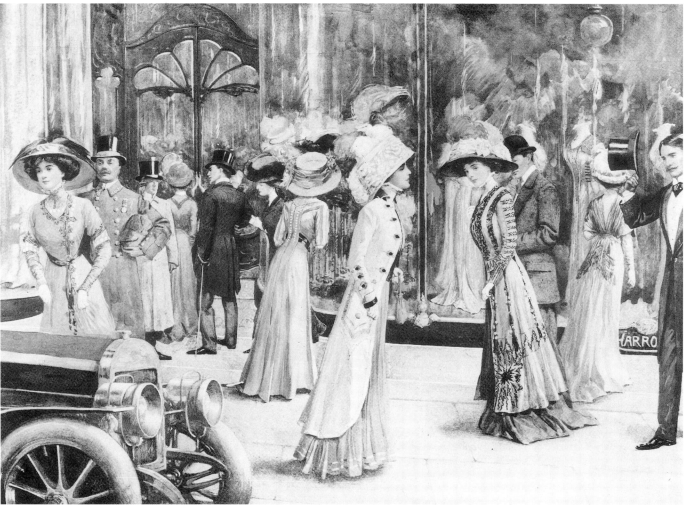

170. **Day dresses at Harrods, 1909**
Anon. illustration

Note The early years of the century saw the heyday of the great London department stores and Harrods, among others, produced regular, lavishly illustrated catalogues of goods for sale.

Head Most of the men wear top hats (the correct accessory to a frock coat or morning coat) but one can be seen in a bowler (worn with a lounge suit). The women's hats are all large, with deep crowns and wide brims, heavily trimmed.

Body Although one man (centre left) wears a morning coat and one (far right) is in a frock coat, a third (right) can be seen in the less formal lounge suit which was becoming increasingly popular for day wear in town. Some of the women wear long coats over their day dresses. The fashionable line continues to narrow as the waistline rises and the skirt contracts. However, there is still a liking for applied ornament and clothes are trimmed with embroidery, braid and decorative buttons.

Accessories The lady in the centre carries a small drawstring 'Dorothy' bag.

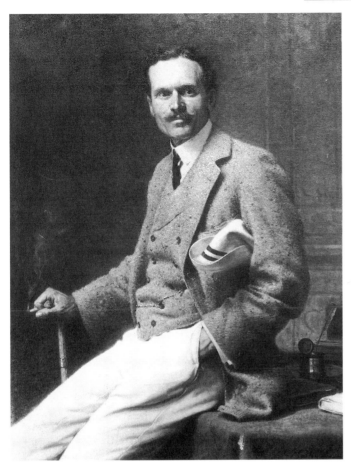

171. Horace Annesley Vachell, *c.* 1910
Gaston Linden

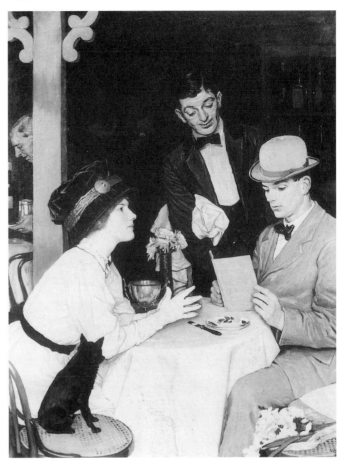

172. Bank Holiday, 1912
William Strang

Note Horace Annesley Vachell (1861–1955) was the author of over 50 novels and fourteen plays. He is dressed here in informal summer clothes.

Head His hair is cut short with no side-whiskers and he wears a moustache.

Body Vachell's suit consists of a matching lounge jacket and double-breasted waistcoat in a light, textured tweed, worn with white trousers. His shirt has a starched turned-down collar and he wears a narrow, dark, knotted tie.

Accessories Under one arm he holds a soft, light Panama straw hat with striped silk hat band (a style which was replacing the boater for summer wear); the other hand, holding a cigarette, rests on a walking stick. A watch chain is worn across his waistcoat.

Note A young, lower-middle-class couple are shown taking a meal out on a public holiday. They are both neatly and respectably dressed but their clothes are neither highly fashionable nor expensively tailored (as can be seen in the cut of the man's suit).

Head The young woman wears a deep-crowned velvet hat under which her hair is brushed low over her forehead and ears. The young man's hair is very short beneath his bowler hat with ribbon-bound brim and he is clean shaven. The bowler was usual with a lounge suit but it was also commonly worn by the less well-off at this time as a best hat (rather than the formal top hat).

Body Her light pink dress has a small turned-down collar and a black belt set higher than the natural level of the waist (but not as high as on the most fashionable dresses at this date). He wears a brown lounge suit with a black spotted bow tie and a low, turned-down shirt collar. The waiter is dressed in a black tail coat, black waistcoat and bow tie; he carries a white napkin, a traditional accessory which can be traced back to the medieval period. The black suit with tail coat (for both day and evening wear) had become usual for waiters by the last quarter of the nineteenth century.

Accessories She wears long white gloves.

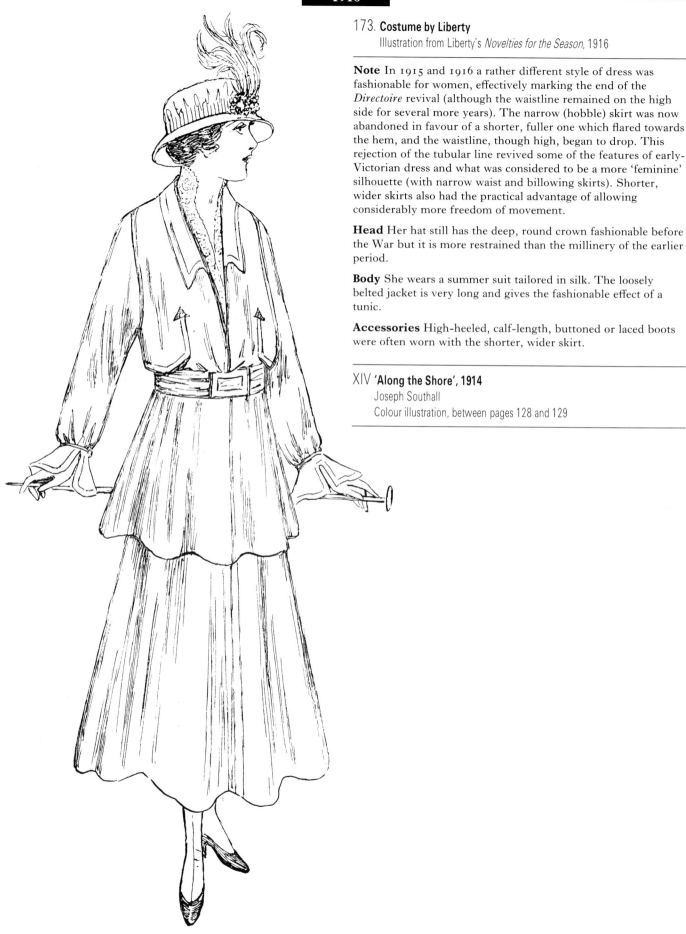

173. Costume by Liberty

Illustration from Liberty's *Novelties for the Season*, 1916

Note In 1915 and 1916 a rather different style of dress was fashionable for women, effectively marking the end of the *Directoire* revival (although the waistline remained on the high side for several more years). The narrow (hobble) skirt was now abandoned in favour of a shorter, fuller one which flared towards the hem, and the waistline, though high, began to drop. This rejection of the tubular line revived some of the features of early-Victorian dress and what was considered to be a more 'feminine' silhouette (with narrow waist and billowing skirts). Shorter, wider skirts also had the practical advantage of allowing considerably more freedom of movement.

Head Her hat still has the deep, round crown fashionable before the War but it is more restrained than the millinery of the earlier period.

Body She wears a summer suit tailored in silk. The loosely belted jacket is very long and gives the fashionable effect of a tunic.

Accessories High-heeled, calf-length, buttoned or laced boots were often worn with the shorter, wider skirt.

XIV 'Along the Shore', 1914

Joseph Southall
Colour illustration, between pages 128 and 129

174. Edward, Prince of Wales, 1922
William Orpen

Note Orpen's portrait depicts the Prince of Wales (later King Edward VIII and Duke of Windsor) as Captain of the Royal and Ancient Golf Club of St Andrew's, Fife. Although the clothes he is wearing were intended for golf (tweed cap, knickerbockers and knitted sweater) they became popular for informal day wear for men in the 1920s and were a fashion particularly associated with the Prince of Wales.

Head The Prince's flat tweed cap has a full, pancake crown.

Body He is casually but stylishly dressed in a soft-collared shirt and tie with a geometrically patterned, knitted pullover, loose, checked tweed knickerbockers or 'plus fours', checked stockings and heavy brogues.

XV **La Caline**
André Marty (attr.)
Colour illustration, between pages 128 and 129

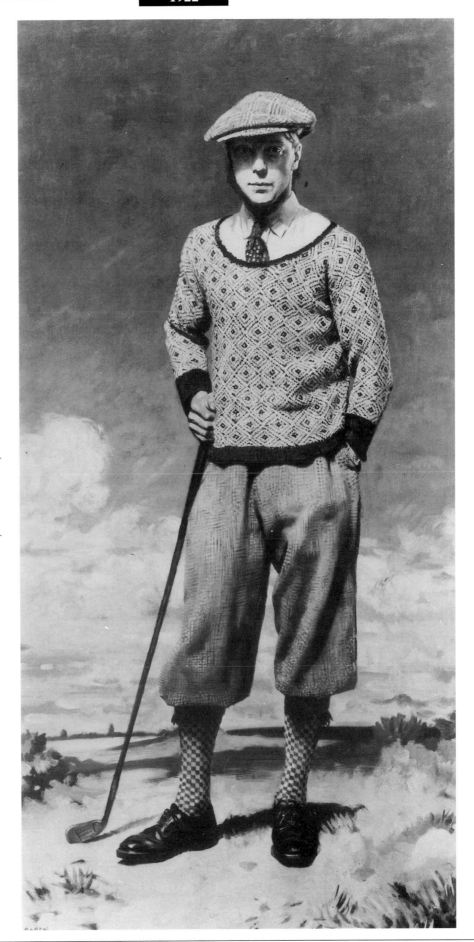

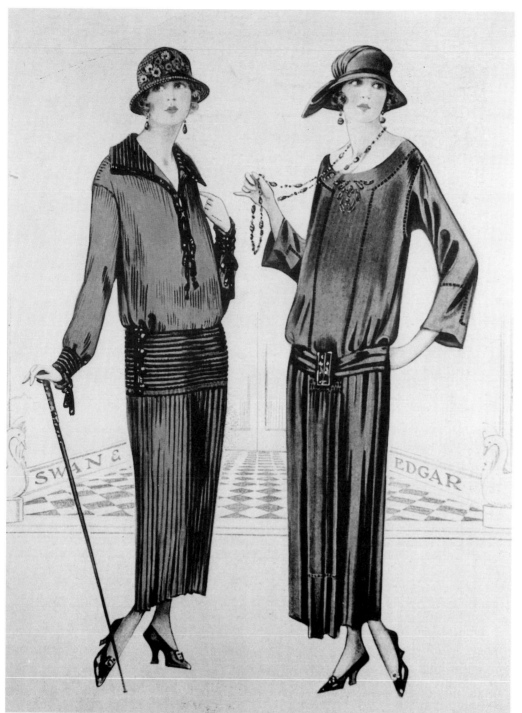

Fashions by Swan & Edgar, 1924
Anon. illustration

Note Skirt lengths fluctuated during the first half of the 1920s but were generally well below the knee for daytime wear and ankle-length for formal afternoon and evening occasions.

Head The hat on the left is described as 'practical' and is of wool-embroidered straw; the hat on the right is in 'superior quality marocain'. Both are the deep-crowned 'cloche' style with a narrow brim.

Body On the left is a knitted wool jumper suit with accordion-pleated skirt, suitable for spring, summer and sports wear. The afternoon frock on the right is made in silk and wool marocain. The garments are unshaped and the waistline is dropped to the level of the hips.

Accessories The costumes are worn with high-heeled court shoes trimmed with decorative buckles; both women wear pendant earrings (which have now become fashionable with short hair) and one has a long string of coloured beads.

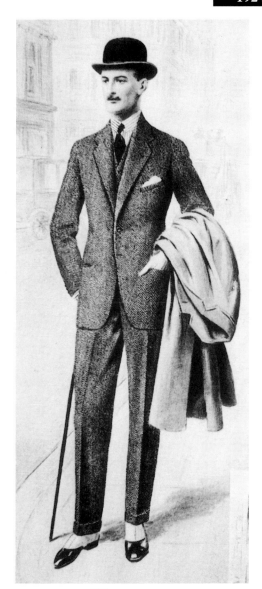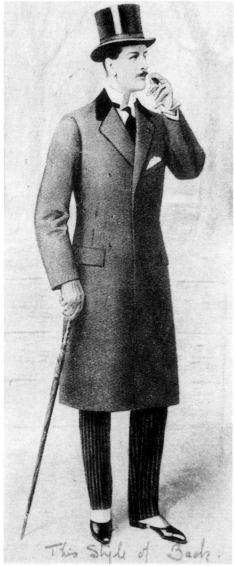

176. **Grafton Fashions for Gentlemen, Autumn and Winter 1924–5**
Anon. lithograph

Note Correct but rather conservative, formal clothes for daytime wear.

Head The models are wearing the correct hats to accompany their suits: a black bowler with the lounge suit (left) and top hat with the more formal Chesterfield overcoat (right). Their hair is short and both men wear small moustaches.

Body The three-piece lounge suit in herringbone tweed (left) is worn with a striped shirt and turned-down collars. The jacket is narrow-fitting and the trousers are also narrow and slightly tapered with turn-ups at the hem. He carries a raincoat or overcoat in the raglan-sleeve style, easier-fitting and less formal than the Chesterfield overcoat on the right with its velvet collar and set-in sleeve. This is probably worn over a frock coat or morning coat which was teamed with striped trousers, and stiff, wing collar; this style of dress was by now very formal.

Accessories Both men wear white handkerchiefs in the breast pocket, gloves and white spats, and carry a walking stick or tightly rolled umbrella. Spats were old-fashioned by this date.

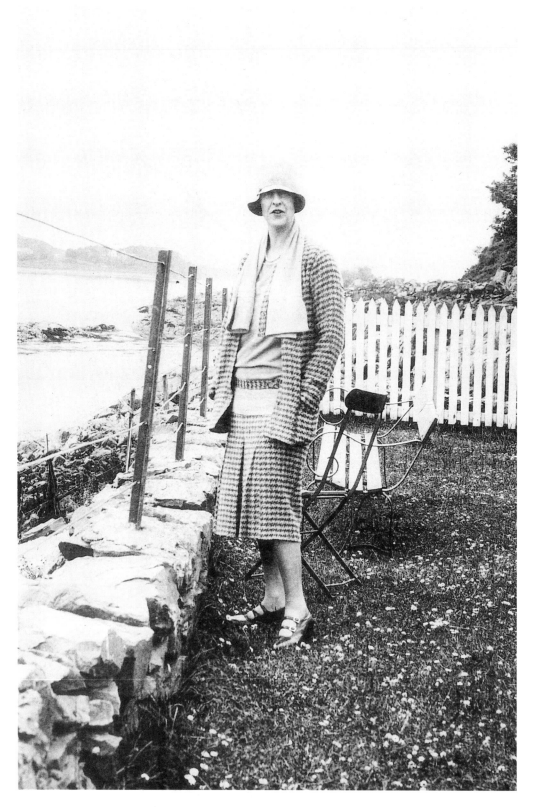

177. The Ranee of Pudukota in a Chanel suit, 1926
Photograph

Note The caption describes the Ranee as wearing 'a famous Chanel suit' and it is typical of the work of the French designer Gabrielle (Coco) Chanel (1883–1971) in the 1920s. Chanel was one of the first to introduce casual, comfortable but very elegant clothes for women in the post-war period. Her jumper suits were often made in soft, pliable, jersey-weave materials in neutral colours.

Head The Ranee's felt cloche hat is pulled well down and fits her head snugly.

Body Her three-piece jumper suit has a checked cardigan jacket and pleated skirt with a long jumper, scarf and belt to match. The hemline is noticeably shorter (having risen in 1925 to just below the knee).

Accessories Her leather shoes have two buckled straps over the instep.

178. Alfred Duff Cooper, 1st Viscount Norwich with his wife, Diana, 1927

David Low

Note Duff Cooper and his wife were well-known figures in London Society during the 1920s, '30s and '40s. Lady Diana Cooper (1892–1986) is generally considered to have been one of the most beautiful Englishwomen of the twentieth century.

Head Duff Cooper's hair is short and neatly trimmed and he wears a small moustache. Lady Diana's short hair curls out at the sides beneath her close-fitting cloche hat with a narrow brim.

Body Lady Diana Cooper wears a knee-length coat over a dress with dropped waistline and pleated skirt. Her husband is in a dark lounge suit with soft-collared shirt and knotted tie.

Accessories She carries a clutch handbag and wears high-heeled shoes.

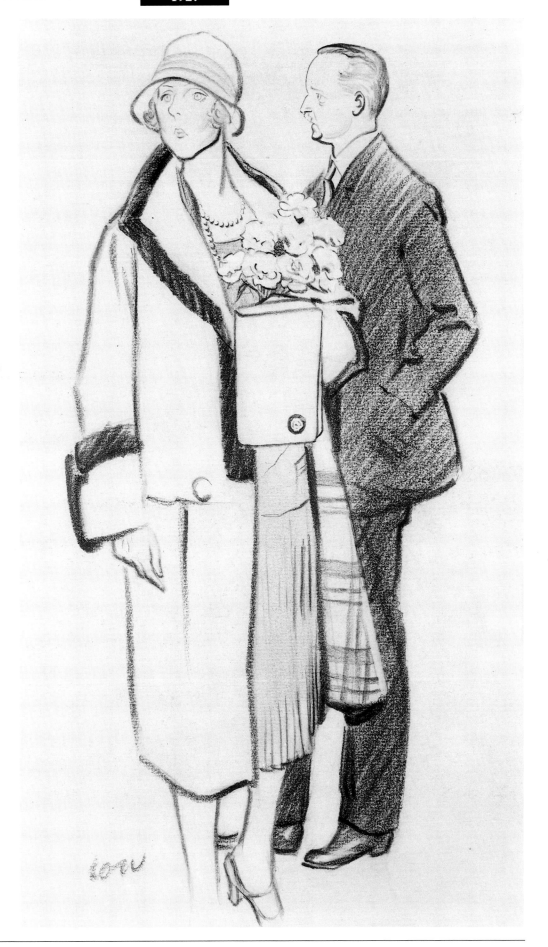

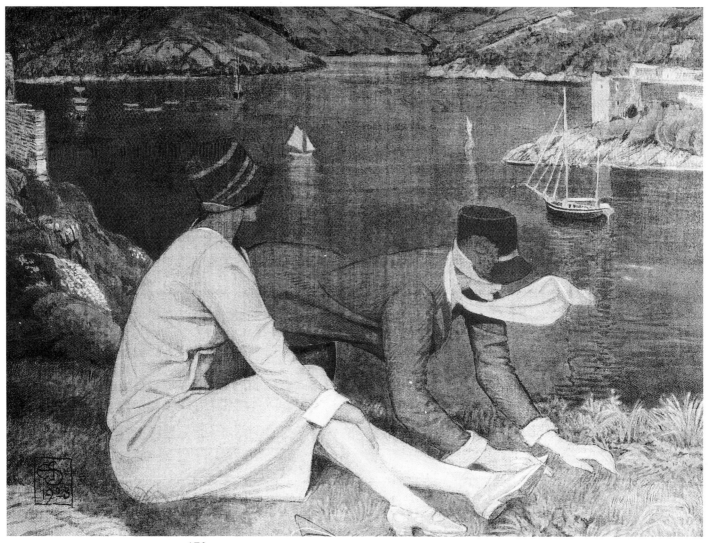

179. **'The Botanists', 1928**
Joseph Southall

Head The late-1920s cloche hat becomes severer in shape and more helmet-like as the brim disappears.

Body The complete lack of shaping in fashionable dress is indicated by the loose folds round both women's waists as they sit and kneel. The skirt just covers the knees.

Accessories The woman on the left wears low-heeled bar shoes suitable for the country walking suggested by the artist.

180. Evening dress by Paquin, *c.* 1928
Anon. illustration

Note In the last two years of the decade dress designers anticipated a reaction against the stark and functional line and tentatively introduced both a longer hemline and gentler shaping over the bust and hips. Eyes were gradually accustomed to a new length by an uneven hemline – in this instance with a skirt longer at the back than the front. The sketch of the rear view of the dress clearly indicates a closer-fitting skirt round the hips.

Head The hair is cut short and shaped to the head in flat, neat waves.

Body The evening dress has a loose, chemise-shaped bodice with the waistline at hip level and a knee-length skirt overlaid with a longer, filmy overskirt which dips to the ankle at the centre back.

Accessories Her only jewellery is a pair of drop earrings; she holds a small evening bag and wears court shoes with Louis heels.

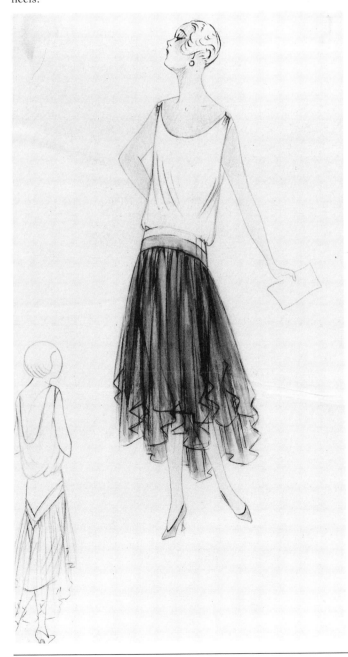

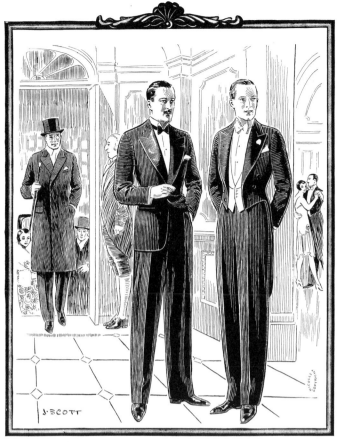

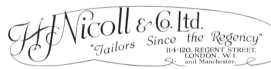

181. Evening wear by H.J. Nicoll & Co. Ltd, *c.* 1929
J. Scott; engraving from H.J. Nicoll & Co. catalogue

Note In 1925 much wider trousers became fashionable for men and were counterbalanced by broader-shouldered jackets; these and a neat fit round the waist made the hips appear slim.

Head Hair is still worn short but can be swept back and kept in place with brilliantine. Small 'toothbrush' moustaches are the only form of facial hair favoured by young men.

Body The usual forms of evening dress are illustrated here; on the left, the less formal dinner jacket worn with a black bow tie. The single-breasted jacket is cut with wide, silk-faced lapels; the shirt has a starched front and stiff, wing collar. On the right is the formal dress suit with tail coat, white waistcoat and white bow tie. Both pairs of evening trousers have silk braid along the outer leg seams.

Accessories On the far left are the outdoor accessories to evening dress: Chesterfield overcoat, top hat, white silk scarf, gloves and cane.

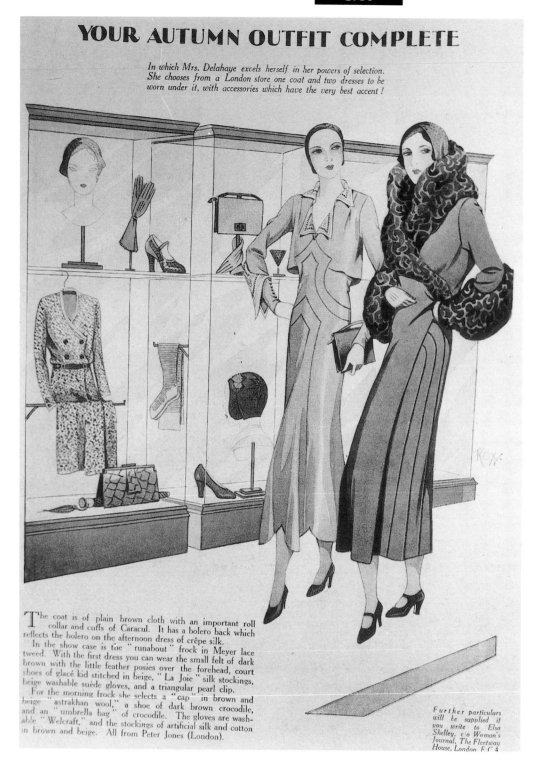

YOUR AUTUMN OUTFIT COMPLETE

In which Mrs. Delahaye excels herself in her powers of selection. She chooses from a London store one coat and two dresses to be worn under it, with accessories which have the very best accent !

The coat is of plain brown cloth with an important roll collar and cuffs of Caracul. It has a bolero back which reflects the bolero on the afternoon dress of crêpe silk.

In the show case is the "runabout" frock in Meyer lace tweed. With the first dress you can wear the small felt of dark brown with the little feather posies over the forehead, court shoes of glacé kid stitched in beige, "La Joie" silk stockings, beige washable suède gloves, and a triangular pearl clip.

For the morning frock she selects a "cap" in brown and beige "astrakhan wool," a shoe of dark brown crocodile, and an "umbrella bag" of crocodile. The gloves are washable "Welcraft," and the stockings of artificial silk and cotton in brown and beige. All from Peter Jones (London).

Further particulars will be supplied if you write to Elsa Shelley, c/o Woman's Journal, The Fleetway House, London E C 4

182. **'Your Autumn Outfit Complete'**
Illustration from *Woman's Journal*, 1930

Note Day clothes and accessories selected by the Fashion Editor, Mrs Delahaye, for *Woman's Journal*.

Head The woman's heads look neat and streamlined with their small and very close-fitting hats. The fashionable 'Dutch cap' shape of the hats can also be seen on the stands.

Body By 1930 the daytime length for dresses is mid-calf and the fashionable silhouette is long and narrow. A diagonal emphasis is indicated by the use of top stitching and the wrap-over style of coat with deep shawl collar. Clothes fit closer to the figure, accentuating the slimness of the hips.

Accessories A range of accessories can be seen in the cases behind and include gloves, bags, shoes, stockings and umbrella.

183. Miss Shelagh Morrison Bell, 1933

Sir John Lavery

Note Lavery's portrait reflects the poised, neat and elegant character of women's fashion in the early 1930s.

Head Her hair is short, parted on one side and waved close to her head.

Body She wears a full-length evening dress with low-cut neckline and narrow shoulder straps. The skirt is cut with fullness fanning out from the hips. A thin silk or chiffon shoulder cape trimmed with dark fur is loosely knotted round her neck and slips over one shoulder.

Accessories Her jewellery consists of large pendant earrings and a bracelet of dark stones.

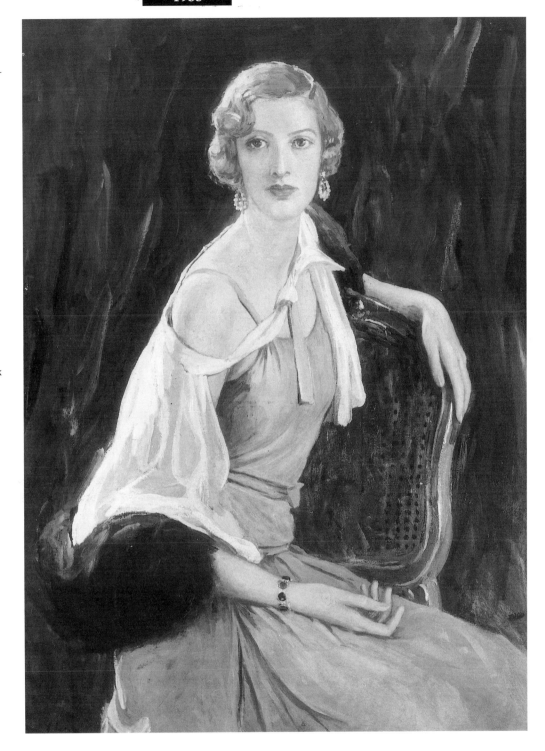

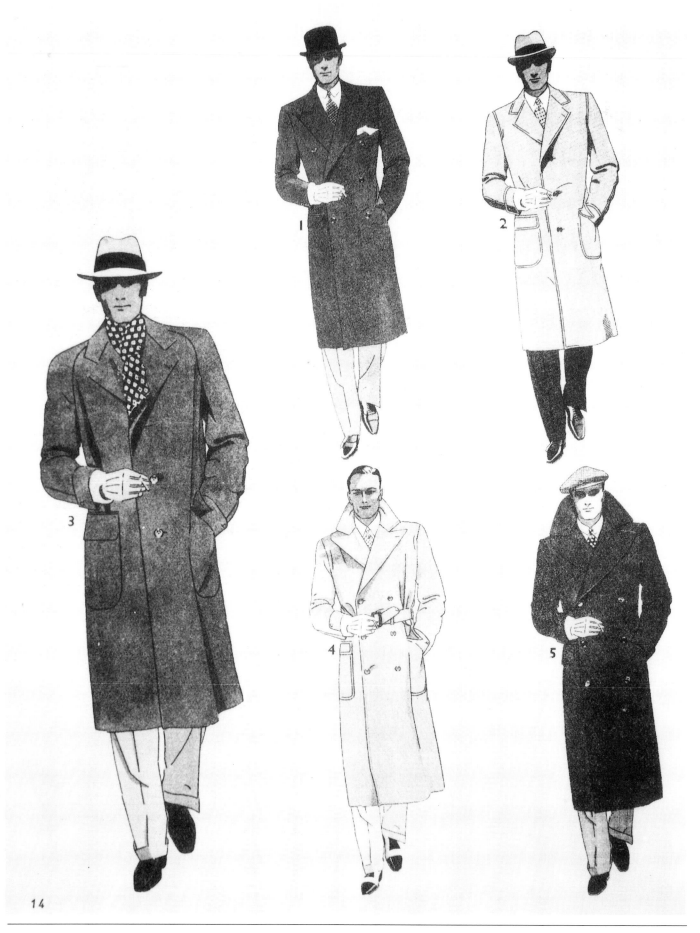

14

184. Men's overcoats by Jaeger, c.1934
Illustration, Jaeger catalogue

Note The fashion artist has caught the stylish manner in which clothes were worn in the 1930s (by both men and women). Hats were often tipped at a slight angle and coat collars turned up.

Head It is still usual for men to wear hats out of doors on almost all occasions although the top hat is rarely seen now. The style of hat depended on the formality of the suit or coat and three types are illustrated here: the formal bowler, less formal snap-brim hat (or trilby) and the casual flat tweed cap.

Body The two most conventional styles of men's overcoats were the fitted coat with set-in sleeves (top left) or the looser-cut coat with raglan sleeves (bottom left). In the 1930s a fashionable variation was the double-breasted overcoat with buckled belt (bottom centre). All the coats here are fashionably cut with wide shoulders; the long lean line emphasizing narrow hips is similar to the ideal silhouette for women at this date.

Accessories The man on the left has a patterned scarf tucked into the neck of his coat. All wear gauntlet gloves.

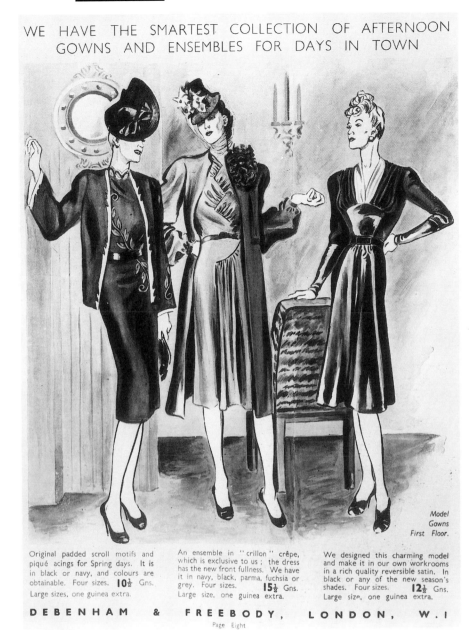

WE HAVE THE SMARTEST COLLECTION OF AFTERNOON GOWNS AND ENSEMBLES FOR DAYS IN TOWN

Original padded scroll motifs and piqué acings for Spring days. It is in black or navy, and colours are obtainable. Four sizes. **10½** Gns. Large sizes, one guinea extra.

An ensemble in "crillon" crêpe, which is exclusive to us; the dress has the new front fullness. We have it in navy, black, parma, fuchsia or grey. Four sizes. **15½** Gns. Large size, one guinea extra.

We designed this charming model and make it in our own workrooms in a rich quality reversible satin. In black or any of the new season's shades. Four sizes. **12½** Gns. Large size, one guinea extra.

Model Gowns First Floor.

D E B E N H A M   &   F R E E B O D Y ,   L O N D O N ,   W . 1
Page Eight

185. Afternoon gowns by Debenham and Freebody, 1939
Illustration from store catalogue

Head The women on the left and right wear their hair swept up and curled at the front. The hats are tall and narrow in shape, tilted to one side and gaily trimmed with ribbon bow, artificial flowers and a veil.

Body The dresses, intended for smart day wear in town, are knee-length and fitted over the bust, waist and hips; the shoulders are padded and the waist tightly belted. The dress and jacket on the left are ornamented with padded scroll motifs; the two on the right are both decoratively ruched across the bust.

Accessories High-heeled court shoes are worn; two of the pairs have open toes, a fashion which appeared in 1936.

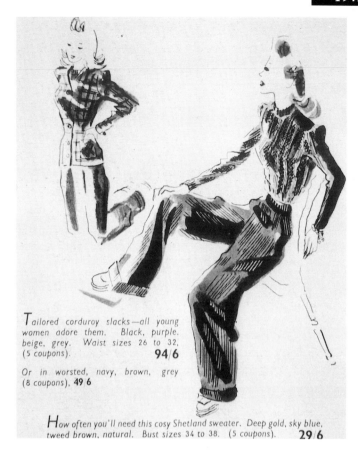

Tailored corduroy slacks—all young women adore them. Black, purple, beige, grey. Waist sizes 26 to 32, (5 coupons). **94/6**

Or in worsted, navy, brown, grey (8 coupons), **49/6**

How often you'll need this cosy Shetland sweater. Deep gold, sky blue, tweed brown, natural. Bust sizes 34 to 38. (5 coupons). **29/6**

186. Tailored corduroy slacks, 1941

Illustration, Harvey Nichols catalogue

Note Trousers had been worn by some women for informal, daytime occasions (especially on the beach) since the 1920s but it was not until the late 1930s that the fashion became very widespread. Slacks proved to be particularly practical and warm during the war – the Harvey Nichols catalogue said, 'all young women adore them'.

Head The hair is shoulder-length with the front rolled back to give it height.

Body The young woman on the right wears a short, knitted Shetland wool sweater and corduroy trousers with wide legs and turned-up hems. The girl on the left has a tailored jacket with her trousers.

Accessories The right-hand model wears a lucky charm bracelet on her left wrist.

187. 'Every Coupon Counts'

Illustration from *Weldon's Ladies' Journal*, 1942

Note The dress patterns featured in this issue of *Weldon's Ladies' Journal* are recommended for their economical use of clothing coupons. Clothes rationing was introduced in June 1941 limiting, with the use of coupons, the acquisition of clothing by civilians. This was followed in 1942 by a series of Making of Clothes (Restrictions) Orders by the Government.

Head The hair is shoulder-length and in some cases worn with a curled fringe or rolled back from the temples. Hats (which were exempt from rationing) have tall crowns.

Body Clothes rationing and Utility regulations limited the design of women's dresses. The early 1940s saw little development apart from an intensification of the features fashionable on the outbreak of war: wide shoulders, narrow waists and short skirts. The dresses illustrated here have attempted some variety in the basic style with yokes, insets and contrasting panels. A classic 'Box Coat for all occasions, all weathers, all seasons of the year' appears on the far left.

Accessories Most of the footwear is heavy and practical. A touch of femininity is given by the bracelets worn by the seated model who also carries a large handbag.

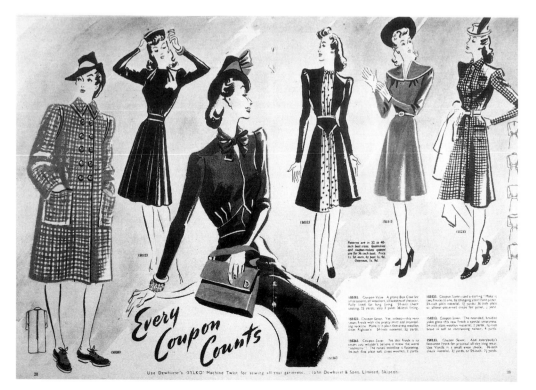

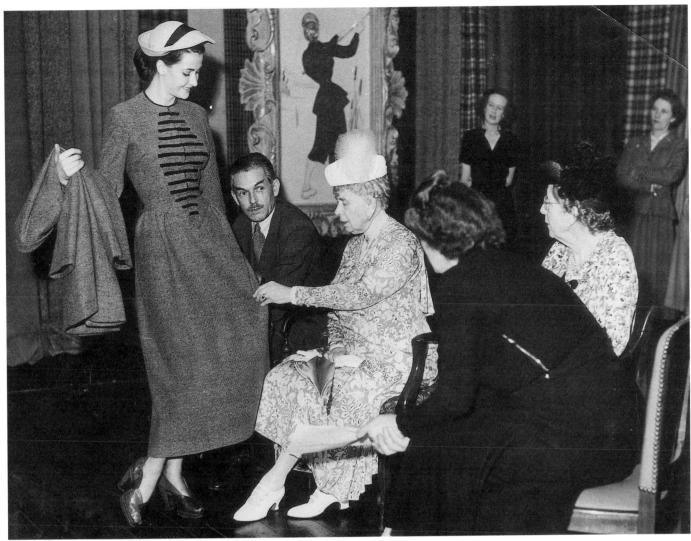

188. Queen Mary inspecting the latest 'New Look' tweeds at the International Wool Secretariat showrooms, London, 1948
Photograph

Note The New Look was greeted with enthusiasm by most women in Britain although many officials disapproved. Clothes rationing was still in force and made the new styles seem extravagant and expensive. However, manufacturers were able to produce an approximation of the line within reasonable prices. This model by the London couturier, Mattli, has far less material in the skirt than Dior would have used. Ironically, Queen Mary's skirt is fashionably long although she had not significantly altered the length of her dresses since the hemline began to rise in 1939.

Head The model's hair is longer than that of the other women in the room but is tightly drawn back.

Body The tweed dress reflects the main features of the New Look – less padding in the shoulders, a fitted waist and longer, fuller skirt. It has a three-quarter-length jacket to match. Queen Mary and her neighbour wear floral print dresses. The light has caught the clumsy metal zip of the black dress in the foreground.

Accessories Queen Mary wears her habitual toque and shoes which are closer in style to the 1920s than the 1940s. The model's open-toed shoes have thick platform soles. Her hat is flat in the crown.

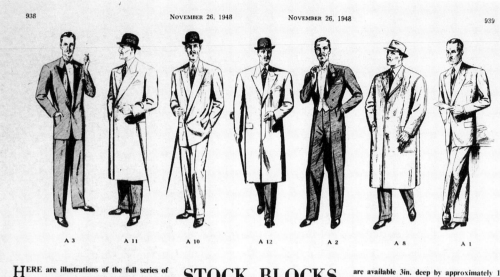

A 3   A 11   A 10   A 12   A 2   A 8   A 1

HERE are illustrations of the full series of our styles in the Stock Block service. Readers will find these stock blocks invaluable for illustrating their local press advertisements, brochures, letterheads, etc. There are at pre-

STOCK BLOCKS

sent thirteen different styles available which we illustrate individually each week. Blocks

are available 3in. deep by approximately 1in. wide (as illustrated), and priced at 19s. 6d. Readers requiring stock blocks should apply to "Stock Blocks," Tailor and Cutter House, Gerrard Street, London, W.1.

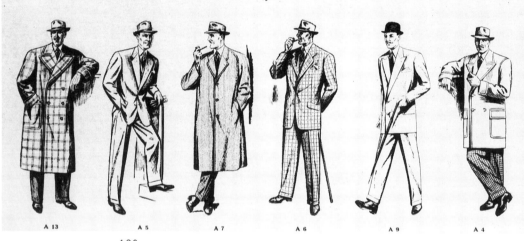

A 13   A 5   A 7   A 6   A 9   A 4

189. 'Stock Blocks'
Illustration from *The Tailor and Cutter*, 1948

Note The 13 figures illustrate the main styles of dress in the post-war male wardrobe: dinner jacket and dress suit for evening wear, double or single-breasted lounge suits for the daytime and several different types of overcoats.

Head Hats are still considered essential but only two styles appear here: the formal bowler and the less formal, soft felt trilby. The hair is cut short. The men are either clean shaven or have small moustaches.

Body The fashionable line is an exaggerated version of the later 1930s style of dress – the shoulders are very broad but jackets taper to fit neatly round the hips. Lapels are wide and long, dropping to a low-set, double-breasted fastening. Trousers are wide with turn-ups. All shirt collars are soft for day wear but the stiff, wing collar still appears with evening clothes.

Accessories Gloves, sticks or tightly furled umbrellas are usual. Half the men are pictured smoking cigarettes or pipes.

190. 'From Narrow to Wide'
Illustration from *Woman's Journal*, 1955

Note Christian Dior was the first couturier to christen each collection with a theme name or line. Probably his most famous, after the New Look, was his 'A' line in 1955, described here as 'the uninterrupted length of bodice from narrow shoulder to banded hip, with the lightly fitted waistline. Avoidance of nearly all trimming gives that completely plain look which is this season's chic.'

Body On the left is a linen dress with full skirt, just below knee-length; next to it is a tailor-made suit in shantung silk with hip-length, fitted jacket and wide, pleated skirt. The strapless ball gown, though its skirt is full, recalls the 'Empire' line with its waistband just below the bust.

Accessories Formal hats and long gloves are worn with the day clothes. Shoes are lighter in appearance, with slimmer, high heels and pointed toes.

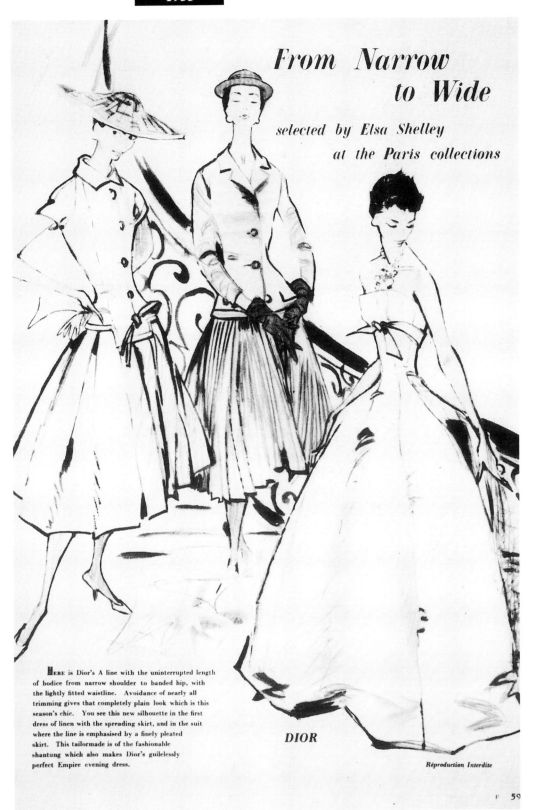

From Narrow to Wide

selected by Elsa Shelley at the Paris collections

HERE is Dior's A line with the uninterrupted length of bodice from narrow shoulder to banded hip, with the lightly fitted waistline. Avoidance of nearly all trimming gives that completely plain look which is this season's chic. You see this new silhouette in the first dress of linen with the spreading skirt, and in the suit where the line is emphasised by a finely pleated skirt. This tailormade is of the fashionable shantung which also makes Dior's guilelessly perfect Empire evening dress.

DIOR

Réproduction Interdite

F 59

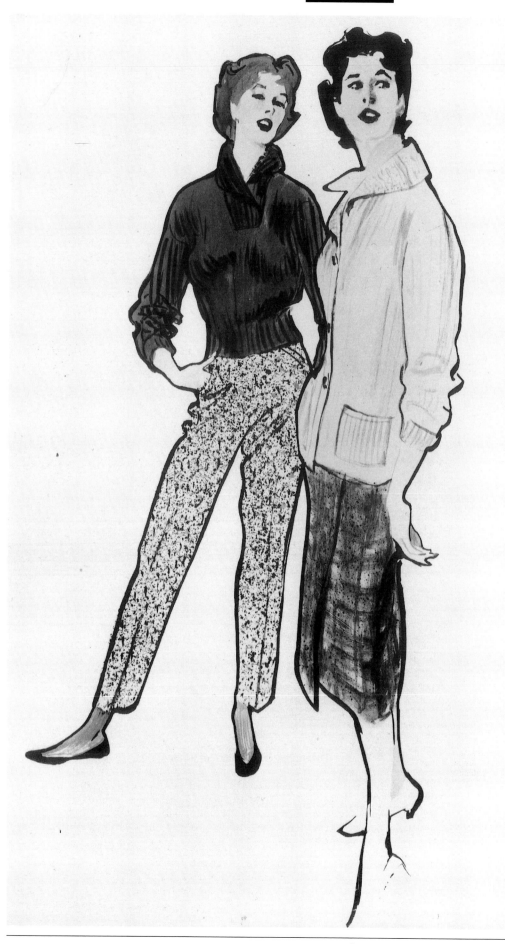

191. Casual clothes by Jaeger, 1956
Anon. illustration

Head In the later 1950s the hair is grown longer and styles become softer and fuller.

Body The model on the left wears a chunky, knitted pullover with a shawl collar, and ankle-length, tweed slacks; the girl on the right has a thick, knitted cardigan with her wrap-over, checked tweed skirt.

Accessories The trousers are worn with flat pumps, the tweed skirt with low-heeled court shoes.

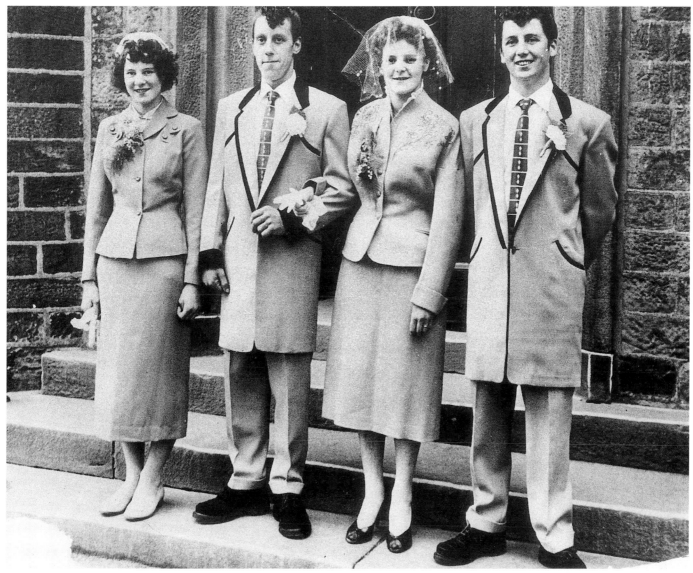

192. **Teddy Boy wedding, Lancaster, 1957**
Photograph

Note A photograph of David Hamm and his bride, Mary Crawshaw with their best man, Bobby Donaghy, and bridesmaid, David's sister Gwen, at St Luke's Church, Skerton, Lancaster on 22 Mary 1957. The two men wear matching powder blue suits edged with black velvet. The Teddy Boy style of dress first emerged around 1952 in the East End and North London and by 1956 could be seen all over Britain before passing out of fashion after 1958. Its characteristic features were a long jacket (retaining the pronounced shoulder-line and 'drape' cut of the 1940s), trousers with straight and very narrow legs (sometimes tapered to the ankle), narrow ties, yellow socks and large, crepe-soled shoes (called 'creepers'). Fancy waistcoats could also be worn and the hair was cut with a long quiff at the front slicked back with grease. Although both men opt for this unconformist style of dress for a church wedding, the bride and bridesmaid in their tailored suits are quite conventionally, if not dowdily dressed for this date. The bridesmaid's skirt is unfashionably long recalling, with her padded shoulders and indented waistline, the fashions of the late 1940s.

Head The girls' hair is short and curled but covers the ears in the longer style favoured towards the end of the decade. Both men have their hair arranged in the classic Teddy Boy 'duck's arse' hair cut. It is noticeable that neither of them wears or carries a hat (an item deliberately discarded by the Teddy Boys).

Body The bridegroom's and best man's matching suits were probably specially tailored for the occasion and are a smart version of the Teddy Boy style. Powder blue was a favourite colour (with black and maroon) and velvet collars, pointing to their Edwardian origins, were often added to jackets. Their shirt collars and ties are moderately conventional (committed Teddy Boys wore much narrower 'bootlace' ties). The bride and bridesmaid wear tailored suits with fitted jackets (over collared blouses) and straight skirts well below knee level. Suits had often been worn for weddings in the 1940s when clothes rationing and post-war austerity made it impossible or uneconomical to purchase wedding gowns or bridesmaids' dresses.

Accessories Both women carry white gloves. The bride's high-heeled and open-toed shoes appear smarter and more fashionable than the bridesmaid's almost flat-heeled courts. All four wear the floral buttonholes usual for weddings since the beginning of the century.

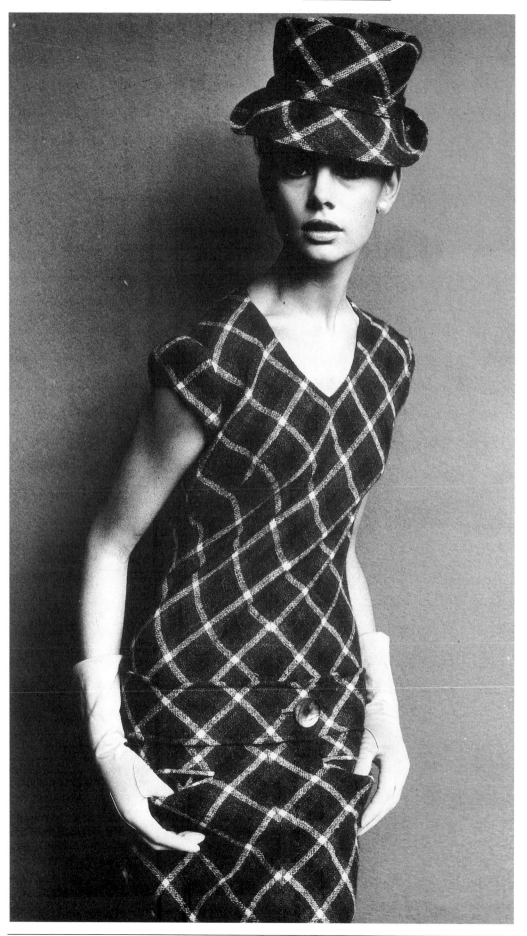

193. Dress and hat by Mary Quant

Photograph from *The Sunday Times*, 1963

Note Mary Quant (born 1934) opened her first shop, Bazaar, in the King's Road, Chelsea in 1955; she began designing and making clothes shortly after and started her wholesale company in 1963. She was a young designer responding to a widely felt need for smart, youthful and inexpensive clothes for other young women in Britain. Her designs were often provocative, aggressive and amusing. The dress is modelled here by Jean Shrimpton who, with Twiggy, was one of the most famous faces of the 1960s.

Head The deliberately masculine trilby style hat is made in checked tweed to match the dress and pulled down to slouch over the eyes.

Body She wears a cap-sleeved, V-necked dress in the sheath shape but with the waistband dropped to the level of the hips. Many of Mary Quant's sleeveless dresses were dual-purpose and could be worn as pinafore dresses over a blouse or sweater by day and on their own (as here) in the evening.

Accessories It is still considered necessary to complete the outfit with bracelet-length, white gloves.

194. Trouser suit by André Courrèges
Illustration from *The Sunday Times*, 1964

Note Trousers were becoming increasingly popular for women and by 1964 were acceptable for both evening and daytime wear although it was not until 1967 that formal trouser suits were generally allowed in expensive restaurants and at Ascot. The French designer André Courrèges (born 1923) launched an influential collection of clothes for the new 'Space Age' in 1964. These were notable for their clean lines and simple shapes, crisply tailored and finished.

Head The model wears one of Courrèges's famous 'baby bonnets' tied under the chin with a bow. The shape of these bonnets was also likened to spacemen's helmets.

Body Courrèges's classic trouser suit is tailored in a firm-textured white cloth with top-stitched seams. The jacket is straight and easy-fitting over slim, straight-legged trousers slit at the front hem.

Accessories The typical Courrèges accessories are short white gloves and white leather boots.

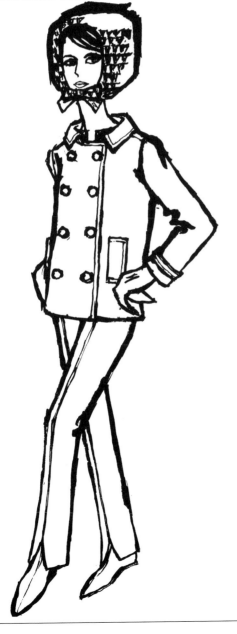

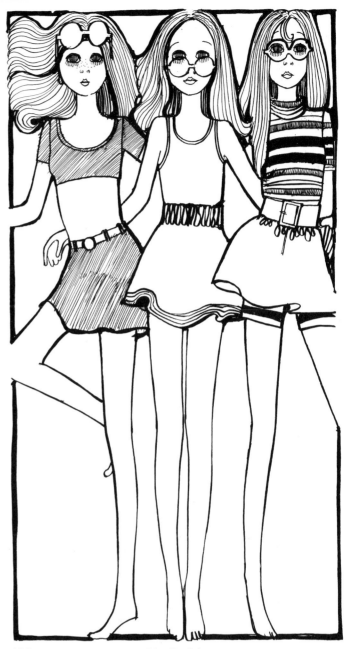

195. Mini-skirts and tops by Gina Fratini
Illustration from *The Sunday Times*, 1968

Note The mini-skirt was at its briefest in 1967–8. This fashion drawing illustrates the ideal image for young women: an adolescent and extremely thin figure with very long legs, a childish face and long, straight hair.

Head The eyes are made-up to look as large as possible. False lashes have been painted under the lower lids and the left-hand model also has freckles painted over her nose.

Body These brief tops, skirts and shorts for summer wear are by the British designer Gina Fratini (born 1934). Their shapes are simple and their only adornment is in the striped patterning and buckled belts.

Accessories Very large, round sunglasses became a fashionable accessory from 1965.

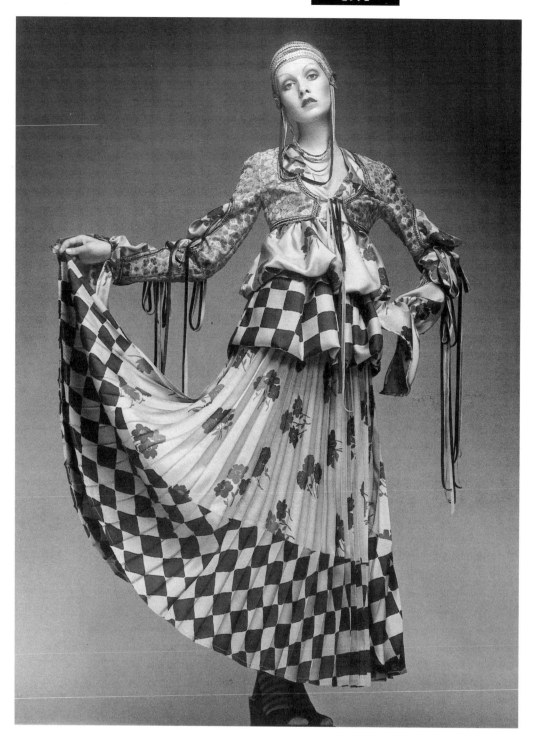

196. Dress by Bill Gibb, modelled by Twiggy
Photograph from *The Sunday Times*, 1971

Note The British designer Bill Gibb (1943–1988) responded to the new taste for romantic and ethnic clothes in the early 1970s. In this example he was clearly inspired by the folk costume of some European or Near Eastern country but there is also a feeling of nostalgia for the dress of an earlier historical period with the full-length skirt and slashed sleeves. Gibb pioneered the use of several different patterned fabrics in one costume – often putting a geometrical with a floral design – an idea which became very popular during the decade.

Head She wears a close-fitting, crocheted wool cap with multiple, uncut strings.

Body Her dress is in several parts; a voluminous, long-sleeved blouse gathered up and billowing out beneath a very short-waisted and tightly-fitting jacket with long, split sleeves fastening with long ribbon ties; the ankle-length skirt is accordion-pleated.

Accessories She has horizontally striped stockings and sandals with high, wedge heels and platform soles (which came into fashion in 1970–1).

XVI Mr and Mrs Clark and Percy, 1970–71
David Hockney
Colour illustration, between pages 128 and 129

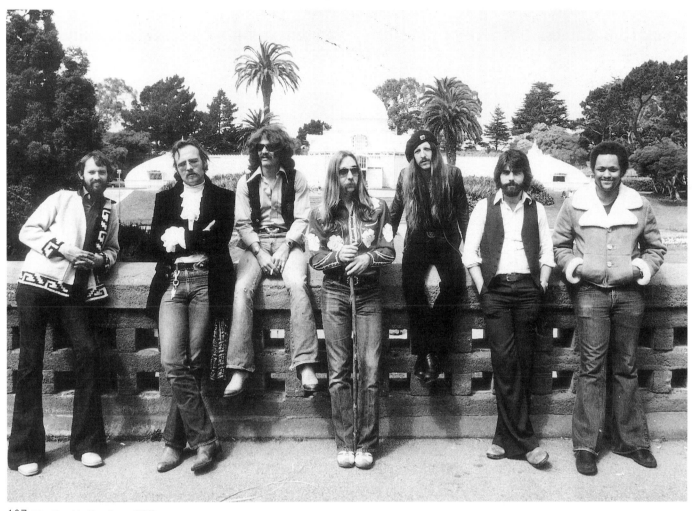

197. **The Doobie Brothers, 1972**
   Warner/Reprise publicity photograph

Note The seven men in this American pop group reflect the influence of the Hippie movement on fashion of the late 1960s and early 1970s although most of them wear the recognized uniform of the young: blue denim jeans and casual shirts. Long hair with a centre parting, beards and moustaches, metal-rimmed spectacles, flower-patterned garments and ethnic clothes were all associated with the Hippies or Flower Children who were 'dropping out' of society at this period. Other elements of fashionable dress can also be found here: long, flared trousers, romantic dress (in the form of historic revivals, for example the frilled jabot and wrist ruffles, second from the left) and the beret (third right) popularly connected with Che Guevara, the South American guerrilla leader and cult figure.

Head There is a wide variety of hair lengths in this picture, ranging from the relatively short to the extremely long (reflecting perhaps a general uncertainty and policy of 'anything goes' in the first years of the decade). But whatever its length and style the hair is evidently well cared-for. Every one of the figures wears a moustache or beard – the moustaches mostly long and drooping in the fashionable 'Mexican' style.

Body The men are all dressed casually in open-necked shirts (having firmly rejected the tie, seen as one of the badges of convention), waistcoats or informal jackets, 'hipster' jeans or trousers and either cowboy boots or training shoes. The trousers of the left illustrate the extreme form of the fashion for a very tight cut over the hips and thighs, flaring widely from the knees to hems which almost sweep the ground. The sharp centre crease of conventional trousers has been abandoned and the hip-level waistband with a deep, buckled belt is usual. The vertical, 'handwarmer' pockets of the jacket on the far right are a new alternative to pockets made useless by the tight fit of the jeans.

Accessories For the same reason, keys are often worn outside the pockets and can be attached by a clip to the belt (second left).

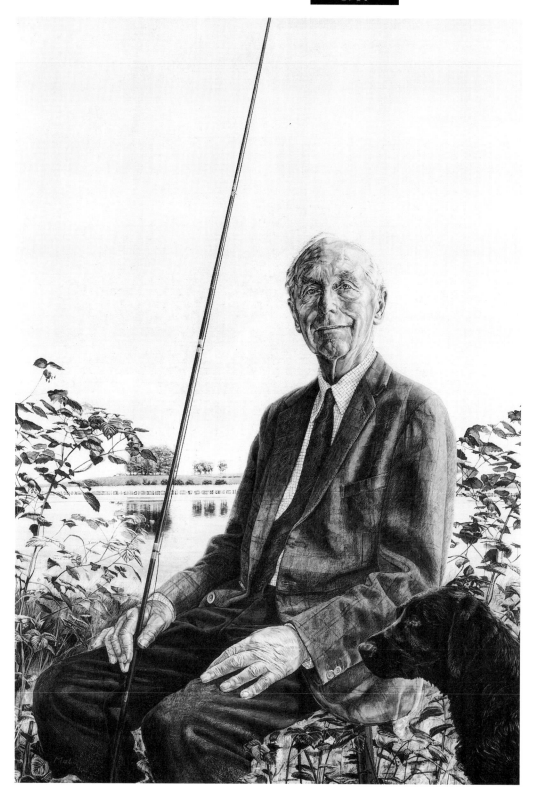

198. Alec Douglas-Home, Lord Home of the Hirsel, 1980
Suzi Malin

Note A relaxed portrait of the Conservative politician and former Prime Minister, Alec Douglas-Home (born 1903). Although he is clearly dressed for fishing in this picture, Lord Home's clothes would hardly look out of place for informal daytime wear in London and are almost dateless, representing a classic style of dress for men which has come to be regarded as particularly English.

Body He wears a checked tweed sports jacket and cloth trousers with a checked shirt and paisley-patterned tie – a form of dress usual for country pursuits.

199. Casual Clothes by Lee Cooper Italia, 1983

Photograph from *Men's Wear*

Note Although denim jeans continued to be popular with both men and women in the early 1980s they were less universally worn than in the 1970s. The shape changed and a straight, very narrow fit was fashionable. A similarity between male and female dress is noticeable with the garments appearing virtually interchangeable.

Head Hair is fairly short and left to look as natural and as casual as possible.

Body Both figures wear loose-fitting, chunky sweaters over slim-fitting jeans. The wide shouldered waistcoat worn by the young man would be equally appropriate wear for the girl.

Accessories Both wear long scarves either left hanging loose or negligently knotted round the neck; both have on wedge-soled, laced sports shoes.

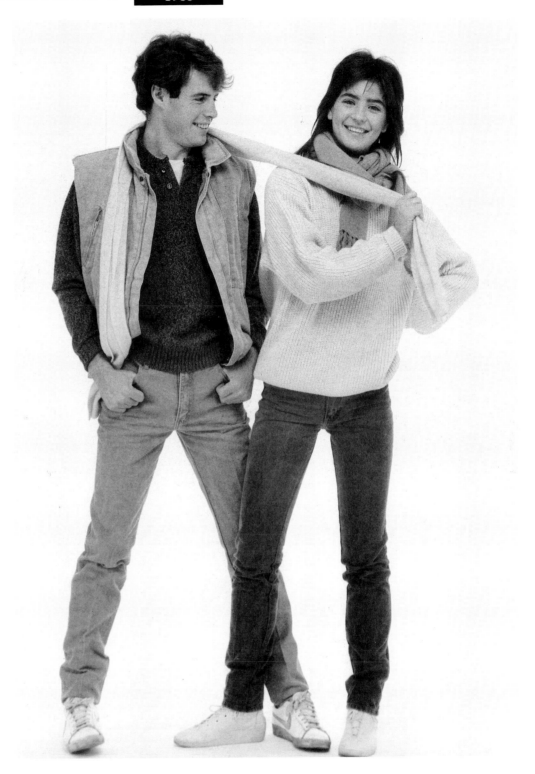

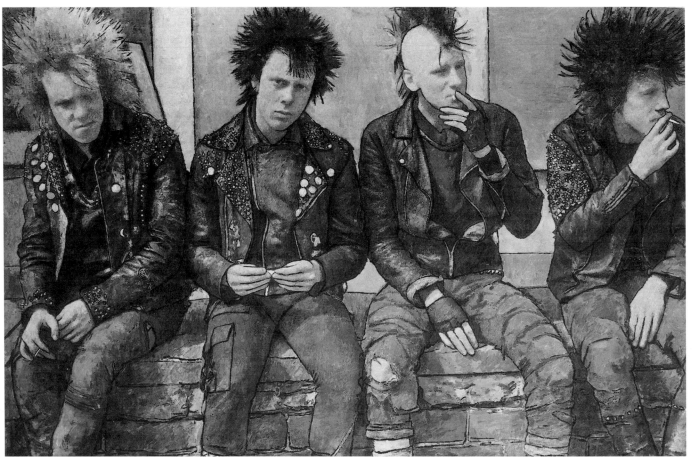

200. **'Smoking – study in Greys', 1984**
Paul Barton R.A.

Note Although the Punk style had made its point and ceased to shock by the early 1980s, it was kept alive by small groups of young people in most provincial British towns.

Head The young men here wear two of the most familiar Punk hair styles – either a halo of stiffened spikes or a 'Mohican' plume (with the sides of the head shaved bare).

Body Their clothes are a modified version of Punk garments: they wear black leather jackets with metal studs on the collar, shoulders and sleeves, with tight, patched and torn jeans.

Accessories Two of the youths have badges pinned to their jackets (almost certainly one of the badges is for the Campaign for Nuclear Disarmament). A third wears fingerless mittens.

SELECT BIBLIOGRAPHY

THIS bibliography is sub-divided into sections listing general books on dress, textiles and accessories, and works relevant to each period covered in the individual volumes in the *Visual History of Costume* series published by B.T. Batsford Ltd in 1983–6. These volumes provide detailed bibliographies for further study. In addition, a number of museums with costume collections publish catalogues from time to time, but they do not always remain in print. Students are advised to consult the *Visual History* series volumes on the eighteenth, nineteenth and twentieth centuries for further details. All the works listed below are published in England unless otherwise stated, and the most recent edition is given.

General

ADBURGHAM, A., *Punch History of Manners and Modes 1841–1940*, Hutchinson, 1961

ALEXANDER, H., *Fans*, Batsford, 1984

ARNOLD, J., *Patterns of Fashion I* c. *1660–1860*, and *Patterns of Fashions II 1860–1940*, Macmillan, 1972

ARNOLD, J., *Perukes and Periwigs*, HMSO, 1970

BALDWIN, F.E., *Sumptuary Legislation and Personal Regulation in England*, Johns Hopkins University Press, Baltimore, 1926

BELL, Q., *On Human Finery*, Hogarth Press, 1976

BOUCHER, F., *A History of Costume in the West*, Thames and Hudson, 1987

BYRDE, P., *The Male Image: Men's Fashions in Britain 1300–1970*, Batsford, 1979

CLARK, F., *Hats*, Batsford, 1982

CUMMING, V., *Exploring Costume History*, Batsford, 1981

CUMMING, V., *Gloves*, Batsford, 1982

CUMMING, V., *Royal Dress: Image and Reality 1580–1986*, Batsford, 1989

CUNNINGTON, P. & LUCAS, C., *Costume for Births, Marriages and Deaths*, A. & C. Black, 1972

CUNNINGTON, C.W. & P., *The History of Underclothes*, Faber, 1981

CUNNINGTON, C.W. & P. and BEARD. C., *A Dictionary of English Costume 900–1900*, A. & C. Black, 1960

DAVENPORT, M., *The Book of Costume*, Crown Publishers, New York, 1972

EWING, E., *Dress and Undress: A History of Women's Underwear*, Batsford, 1978

EVANS, J., *A History of Jewellery 1100–1870*, Faber, 1970

FARRELL, J., *Umbrellas and Parasols*, Batsford, 1986

FOSTER, V., *Bags and Purses*, Batsford, 1982

GINSBURG, M., *An Introduction to Fashion Illustration*, The Compton Press and Pitman Publishing Ltd., 1980

HUGHES, T., *English Domestic Needlework*, Abbey Fine Arts, 1961

MACKRELL, A., *Shawls, Stoles and Scarves*, Batsford, 1986

MANSFIELD, A., *Ceremonial Costume*, A. & C. Black 1980

DE MARLY, D., *Fashion for Men. An Illustrated History*, Batsford 1985

MOORE, D.L., *Fashion through Fashion Plates 1771–1970*, Ward Lock 1971

RIBEIRO, A., *Dress and Morality*, Batsford, 1986

SCARISBRICK, D., *Jewellery*, Batsford, 1984

SQUIRE, G., *Dress, Art and Society 1560–1970*, Studio Vista, 1974

SWANN, J., *Shoes*, Batsford, 1982

THORNTON, P., *Baroque and Rococo Silks*, Faber 1965

VICTORIA AND ALBERT MUSEUM, Department of Textiles and Dress, *Four Hundred Years of Fashion*,

Victoria and Albert Museum and Collins, 1984

WAUGH, N., *Corsets and Crinolines*, Batsford, 1987

WAUGH, N., *The Cut of Men's Clothes 1600–1900*, Faber, 1964

WAUGH, N., *The Cut of Women's Clothes 1600–1930*, Faber, 1968

Fourteenth and fifteenth centuries

EVANS, J., *Dress in Medieval France*, Oxford, 1952

NEWTON, S.M., *Fashion in the Age of the Black Prince: A Study of the Years 1340–1365*, Woodbridge, 1980

SCOTT, M., *A Visual History of Costume, The Fourteenth and Fifteenth Centuries*, Batsford, 1986

Sixteenth century

ASHELFORD, J., *A Visual History of Costume, The Sixteenth Century*, Batsford, 1983

ASHELFORD, J., *Dress in the Age of Elizabeth I*, Batsford, 1988

CUNNINGTON, C.W. & P., *Handbook of English Costume in the Sixteenth Century*, Faber, 1962

DIGBY, G.W., *Elizabethan Embroidery*, Faber, 1963

LINTHICUM, M.C., *Costume in the Drama of Shakespeare and his Contemporaries*, Oxford, 1936

REYNOLDS, G., *Costume of the Western World: Elizabethan and Jacobean 1558–1625*, Harrap, 1951

Seventeenth century

CUMMING, V., *A Visual History of Costume, The Seventeenth Century*, Batsford, 1984

CUNNINGTON, C.W. & P., *Handbook of English Costume in the Seventeenth Century*, Faber, 1972

REYNOLDS, G., See above.

Eighteenth century

BUCK, A., *Dress in Eighteenth-Century England*, Batsford, 1979

CUNNINGTON, C.W. & P., *Handbook of English Costume in the Eighteenth Century*, Faber, 1972

RIBEIRO, A., *A Visual History of Costume, The Eighteenth Century*, Batsford, 1983

RIBEIRO, A., *Dress in Eighteenth Century Europe 1715–1789*, Batsford, 1984

Nineteenth century

ADBURGHAM, A., *Introduction to Victorian Shopping*, David & Charles, 1972

ADBURGHAM, A., *Shops and Shopping 1800–1914*, Allen & Unwin, 1981

BLUM, S. (ed), *Victorian Fashions and Costumes from Harpers Bazaar 1867–1898*, Dover, New York, 1974

BLUM, S. (ed), *Ackermann's Costume Plates; Women's Fashions in England 1818–1828*, Dover, New York, 1978

BUCK, A., *Victorian Costume and Costume Accessories*, Ruth Bean, 1984

CUNNINGTON, C.W. & P., *Handbook of English Costume in the Nineteenth Century*, Faber, 1970

FOSTER, V., *A Visual History of Costume, The Nineteenth Century*, Batsford, 1984

GERNSHEIM, A., *Victorian and Edwardian Fashion: A Photographic Survey*, Dover, New York, 1981

GIBBS-SMITH, C., *The Fashionable Lady in the Nineteenth Century*, HMSO, 1960

GINSBURG, M., *Victorian Dress in Photographs*, Batsford, 1982; paperback, 1988

NEWTON, S.M., *Health, Art and Reason*, John Murray, 1974

Twentieth century

BATTERSBY, M., *The Decorative Twenties*, Studio Vista, 1969

BATTERSBY, M., *The Decorative Thirties*, Studio Vista, 1971

BERNARD, B., *Fashion in the Sixties*, Academy Editions, 1978

BYRDE, P., *A Visual History of Costume, The Twentieth Century*, Batsford, 1986

CARTER, E., *Twentieth Century Fashion, A Scrapbook 1900 to Today*, Eyre Methuen, 1975

CUNNINGTON, C.W. & P., *Englishwomen's Clothing in the Present Century*, Faber, 1952

DEVLIN, P., *Fashion Photography in Vogue*, Thames & Hudson, 1978

DORNER, J., *Fashion in the Twenties and Thirties*, Ian Allan, 1973

DORNER, J., *Fashion in the Forties and Fifties*, Ian Allan, 1975

EWING, E., *A History of Twentieth Century Fashion*, Batsford, 1986

GLYNN, P., and GINSBURG, M., *In Fashion: Dress in the Twentieth Century*, Allen & Unwin, 1978

HOWELL, G., *In Vogue, Six Decades of Fashion*, Allen Lane, 1975

McDOWELL, C., *McDowell's Directory of Twentieth Century Fashion*, Frederick Muller, 1984

DE MARLY, D., *A History of Haute Couture 1850–1950*, Batsford, 1980

PACKER, W., *Fashion Drawing in Vogue*, Thames & Hudson, 1983

VREELAND, D., *Inventive Paris Clothes 1909–1939*, Thames & Hudson, 1978

GLOSSARY/INDEX

After most entries the reader will find numerals indicating illustrations which show examples of the item concerned.

For reasons of space, this *Glossary* cannot be wholly comprehensive: it refers only to costume mentioned in this volume. For example, some fabrics, garments and accessories included here were in existence *before* our starting point of *c.* 1300, but they are only mentioned here in terms of the period covered in this book.

The vocabulary of costume history has always posed semantic problems for historians, and it is difficult – if not impossible at times – to hack a way through the jungle of contemporary nomenclature for fabrics and fashions. One must also be aware of the ways in which words changed their meaning over the centuries, thus requiring constant redefinition. We have tended to describe fabrics in general terms, since it is particularly difficult to disentangle all the contemporary variations. With regard to fashion, however, which is the main theme of this book, we have tried to keep to the words for dress which were in use at the time.

On the whole, unless the foreign name is widely understood, we have used English words. This is not necessarily the case in the late medieval period, for even the English themselves did not always call their garments by English names, preferring French or Latin. Where the French word is used, it is possible that there were minor national differences in the styles of the garments which now seem to share the same name, differences of which we are no longer aware. So we have called the major garments by English names where known, when discussing English dress, and French terms have been used when talking of Franco-Flemish dress.

Some of the limitations of this Glossary must be stated here. Certain aspects of dress and appearance are obvious to the eye and are unequivocal in use or construction; these are mentioned here only at a point when change occurs. On the other hand, words were sometimes coined to describe particular fashions which had only a temporary life span, and these we have tried to eliminate wherever possible, having neither the space nor the inclination to list every minor novelty.

a shirt or smock; 58

Falling band (m & f), 16th and 17th centuries: a turned-down collar held at the centre front by ties; 61, 69

Bandeau (f), 19th and 20th centuries: a narrow band worn round the head crossing the forehead just above the eyes; sometimes called a Grecian-style fillet; 126, 128, 169

Banyan: see *Gown*

Bar shoes: see *Shoes*

Basque (m & f), 16th to 20th centuries: a deep, shaped band or tab-like bands of material attached below the waist of a doublet or bodice; 61, 71

Bavolet (f), 19th century: a curtain of fabric attached to the back of a bonnet to shade the neck; 145

Beaver: an amphibious soft-furred rodent from North America, a principal raw material for hats in the 16th to 18th centuries; the fur fibres were combed out of the skin and made a glossy, waterproof fabric; see *Hats.*

Beret: see *Bonnets/caps*

Bertha: see *Collar*

Bicorne: see *Hats*

Billiment (f), 16th century: a decorative border often made of gold and studded with jewels that was used to edge the upper curve of a French hood and the lower curve; also worn separately as a hair ornament; 38, 39, 42, 47, 54

Blackwork 16th and 17th centuries: a type of embroidery of Spanish origin, using black silk to stitch stylized or naturalistic motifs on linen or silk; 38, 40, 42, 54, 63, 68

Blouse (f), 19th and 20th centuries: a woman's loose, lightweight, sleeved bodice visible to the waist; it first became fashionable in the 1860s worn with a skirt and – in the 1890s – with a tailor-made costume; 150, 164, 167, 192

Boater/Sailor hat: see *Hats*

Bobbin lace: see *Lace*

Bombast 16th to 18th centuries: a type of padding used in doublets, hose, coats etc, originally made from cotton wadding.

Bongrace (f), 16th and early 17th centuries: a flat, stiffened rectangular section of material projecting over the forehead and hanging down to the shoulders, worn over a *coif* (q.v.); 56

Bonnet/cap (m & f), 14th to 20th centuries: these terms are sometimes confused and used interchangeably though there are subtle differences; a *bonnet* is generally a soft, semi-

structured form of headwear with both crown and brim, while a *cap* is usually a closely fitting head-covering of unstructured material with an optional brim or edging.

Beret (m & f), late 19th and 20th centuries: a cap of felted wool; 197

Bonnet (m & f), 16th century: general term for headwear – excluding hats; sometimes categorized, as in the *Milan bonnet* (m), which was popular in the first four decades of the century – this had a pleated crown and upturned brim slit on each side; 34, 36, 41, 44, 52

Coif (m & f), 14th to 17th centuries: a term used for a closely fitting cap sometimes tied under the chin; 3, 46

Cornette (f), 19th century: a bonnet-shaped cap, tied beneath the chin, sometimes pointed at the back; 129

Dormeuse (f), 18th century: similar to a *mob cap* (q.v.), with curving flaps at the sides, but usually more decorated; frilled lappets were added in the 1770s; 118, 122

Jockey cap (m), 18th and early 19th centuries: a cap made of velvet or cloth with a hatband buckled at the front, above the peak – this style was worn for riding and other sports; 100

Marie Stuart (f), mid-18th and 19th centuries: a cap with a distinctive dip in the centre front, imitating the heart-shaped caps worn by Mary, Queen of Scots; 135

Mob cap (f), late 18th century: a cap with a puffed-out crown, deep border and pendant side pieces which could be tied under the chin; the latter were often omitted later in the century as the width of hairstyles increased; 103

Nightcap (m), 16th and 17th centuries: an informal cap constructed from four conical sections of material and an upturned border, usually made from embroidered linen; cf *Turban*

Pinner (f), 18th century: a plain scarf over a lace headdress early in the century; later a circular cap surrounded by a frill of linen and with optional *lappets* (q.v.); 100, 106

Round-eared cap (f), 18th century: a cap shaped to curve round the face to the ears or below, with a frilled or lace-edged border at the front and sides, sometimes worn with lappets; 109

Spoon bonnet (f), 19th century: colour XII

Sun-bonnet (f), 18th to 20th centuries; 124, 164, colour XIV

Turban (m & f), 18th to 20th centuries:

a cap composed of material folded and stitched to simulate this oriental style of headwear; 109

Boothose (m), late 16th to mid-17th centuries: an overstocking, or detachable band with an embroidered or decorated edge turned down over a boot; 72, 77, 80

Boots (m & f), 14th to 20th centuries: 57, 70, 72, 77, 194

Ankle/Half boots (m) 14th to 20th centuries: short boots reaching to just above the ankle; 5, 6, 18, 20, 23, 146, 163

Cowboy boots (f), 20th century: 197

French top-boots (m), 18th century: 129

Hessian boots (m), late 18th and early 19th centuries: knee-length boots with a heart-shaped peak at the front, often decorated with a central tassel; 127

Hussar buskins (m), late 18th and early 19th centuries: calf-length boots with a dip at the front top edge, and a tassel on each side; 123

Bourrelet (m & f), 14th and 15th centuries: a French term for a padded roll, initially found as part of female headdresses and then absorbed into men's headwear as a feature on hoods and chaperons; 20, 22

Bowler hat: see *Hats*

Box coat: see *Coats*

Brassière (f), 14th and 15th centuries: French term for a small bolero-like jacket, usually of black silk or velvet; worn under the *robe* (q.v.) by women from c. 1485 onwards.

Breeches (m), 16th to 20th centuries: an alternative style of lower body and legwear to *trunkhose* (q.v.) from c. 1570 onwards; worn with separate stockings they covered the area from the waist to the knee; 57, 61, 66, 70, 72, 73, 77, 80, 82, 85, 86, 90, 92, 100, 102, 107, 108, 112, 116, 120, 125. See also *Knickerbockers* and *Plus-fours*

Petticoat-breeches, (m), 17th century: primarily a court fashion; immensely wide legs pleated into a waistband but not held at the knee; 79, 83

Venetians (m), 16th and early 17th centuries: full breeches closed at the knee, voluminous, close-fitting or pear-shaped; 58

Brilliantine (m), 20th century: a type of hair oil; 181

Brocade 14th to 20th centuries: a richly patterned silk fabric with a woven-in pattern in gold, silver or contrasting-coloured yarn – the pattern might be floral or geometric and was

sometimes raised above the silk
ground; 29, 36, 81, 101, 136

Broderie anglaise 19th and 20th centuries:
cutwork embroidery, usually in
cotton – a pattern of small round or
oval holes is cut into the fabric and
overcast, and interspersed with
motifs in satin stitch and stem stitch;
150

Brunswick: see *Gown*

Buckram 16th to 20th centuries: a coarse
cloth made from gummed linen or
hemp, used for lining and stiffening
coats and other garments

Buff 16th to 19th centuries: a stout dull-
yellow leather made from ox or
buffalo hide; 72

Buffon (f), 18th century: a large, often
starched handkerchief, bunched up in
front over the bosom; popular in the
1780s.

Busk (f), 16th to 19th centuries: a long,
flat, narrow piece of metal or
whalebone inserted at the centre front
of the *corset* (q.v.) to give it a rigid
line

Bustle (f), 19th century: a pad or frame
worn beneath a petticoat to extend
the back of the upper skirt; 153, 158,
159

  Bustle pad (f), late 18th and 19th
  centuries: diminutive form of the
  bustle

  Rump (f), 18th century: a small,
  crescent-shaped hip pad placed
  beneath the dress at either the back
  or sides; 122

C

Calash: see *Hood*

Calico late 17th to 20th centuries: a cotton
cloth with a printed pattern in one or
more colours

Cambric 18th to 20th centuries: a fine
linen cloth, originally from Cambrai;
term later used to describe fine,
lightweight cotton

Camlet 14th to 19th centuries: a fabric of
mixed yarns, originally silk and
camelhair but, by the 18th century,
usually a mixture of silk and wool

Cane/walking stick (m),
  17th century; 70
  18th century; 98, 99
  19th century; 128, 132, 134, 141
  20th century; 168, 171, 176, 181, 189

Canions (m), 16th and 17th centuries:
short, fitted extension between
trunkhose (q.v.) and the upper leg
above the knee; 49, 61, colour IV

Cape: see *Cloak*

Caped hood: see *Hood*

Carcanet (f), 16th century: a heavy
necklace made of gold and gemstones;
42

Cardigan (m & f), 19th and 20th
centuries: an unstructured jacket of
knitted wool; 191

Caul (f), 14th to 16th centuries: a hairnet
made of gold thread or of silk, and
lined and decorated; 14, 43, 53,
colour III

Chanel, Gabrielle (1883–1971): 177

Chapeau bras: see *Hat*

Chaperon (m & f), 14th and 15th
centuries: generic French term for a
hood, often incorporating long
pendant strips; 18, 23

Chemise (m & f), 14th to 19th centuries:
originally a French term for the linen
undergarment worn by both sexes in
the 14th and 15th centuries; from the
16th century it refers only to the
loose-fitting and unshaped
undergarment of linen or cotton worn
by women until the end of the 19th
century; 17, 35, 38, 39, 42, 46, 78, 81,
87, 103, 129

  Chemise dress (f), late 18th to 20th
  centuries: an outer garment of similar
  loose cut to the undergarment; 125,
  180, colour XV

  Chemisette (f), 19th century: in the first
  half of the century a high-necked,
  sleeveless muslin half-shirt, worn as a
  fill-in for low-necked dresses; by the
  1860s a long-sleeved blouse: 126, 133,
  135, 150

Chenille late 17th to 20th centuries: a
furry-looking silk thread with a long
pile, rather like a caterpillar in
appearance; 147

Chesterfield: see *Coat*

Chiffon 19th and 20th centuries: a semi-
transparent, lightweight silk; 183

Chin-clout (f), 16th century; a large square
of material worn over the chin, seen
in depictions of country women, *cf*
Wimple; 46

Cloak (m & f), 14th to 20th centuries: a
general term used to describe all
loose, sleeveless garments of varying
length which served as the outermost,
protective layer of clothing; 1, 29, 41,
76, 98

  French cloak (m), 16th and 17th
  centuries: a long, full cloak worn
  draped informally over the left
  shoulder

  Spanish cloak (m), 16th and 17th
  centuries: a short, full cloak with a
  hood

Cloche hat: see *Hat*

Clocks (m & f), 16th to 19th centuries: an

embroidered or woven design in
contrasting or matching silk on the
inner and/or outer legs of stockings;
64, 129

Close-bodied gown: see *Gown*

Cloth 14th to 20th centuries: although this
term is used for any woven fabric, it
normally refers to a closely woven
material of fine-quality wool

  Cloth of gold 14th to 20th centuries: a
  material woven with a warp of pure
  gold thread and a weft of silk;
  sometimes both were of gold

Coat (m & f), 16th to 20th centuries: a
general term for a sleeved, front-
fastening outer garment, with knee-
length or longer skirts; *cf Cote*; 57 80,
91, 145

  Dress coat (m), 19th and 20th centuries:
  a man's formal tail-coat, cut square
  across the waist; 159, 181

  Frock coat (m), 18th to 20th centuries: a
  sporting and informal coat which first
  appeared in fashionable circles in the
  1720s; it had a small turn-down collar
  and sleeves with shallow cuffs or
  decorative slits; it became acceptable
  as formal wear by the last quarter of
  the 18th century. In the 19th and
  20th centuries it was a skirted, knee-
  length coat characterized by its
  straight front edges; 100, 120, 128,
  163, 166, 170

  Morning coat (m), 19th and 20th
  centuries; a tail coat with curved
  front edges; originally a riding coat, it
  evolved into general day wear; 134,
  146, 170

  Persian vest (m), 17th century; a loose
  coat held by a sash or belt,
  introduced into England by Charles
  II in 1666

  Tail coat (m), 19th and 20th centuries:
  see *Dress coat, Morning coat*

Overcoat (m & f), 19th and 20th centuries:
a heavy top-coat, usually loose rather
than fitted; 156, 184, 189

  Box coat (f), 20th century: a fashionable
  style of the 1930s and 1940s, with
  padded, square shoulders and loosely
  fitted around the waist; 187

  Chesterfield (m), 19th and 20th
  centuries: a variant of the frock coat,
  first named after the 6th Earl of
  Chesterfield in the 1840s, and worn
  as a formal overcoat; it was fitted and
  slightly waisted, and often with a
  velvet collar; 161, 168, 181

  Greatcoat (m), 17th and 18th centuries:
  earlier term for an overcoat; 108, 131

  Paletot (m), 19th century: French term
  for overcoat; applied in the mid-

century to short, loose coats, usually
without a waist seam and popularly
known as Pilot coats; 141

Pelisse (f), 19th century: a fitted coat
worn early in the century; 132

Raincoat (m & f), 19th and 20th centuries:
an overcoat treated to resist rain; 176

Wrapover (f), 20th century; 182

Codpiece (m), late 15th and 16th centuries:
a padded ornamental pouch attached
by *points* (q.v.) to the hose and
concealing the opening at the front of
the hose; 36, 40, 41

Coif: see *Bonnet/Cap*

Collar (m & f), 14th to 20th centuries: a
band of material attached to the
neckline of any under or upper
garment

Bertha (f), 19th century; a deep collar
falling as a continuous band from a
low neckline; 139, 143

Cape collar (m), 18th to 20th centuries:
a deep collar similar to a shallow
cape, attached to garments such as
greatcoats (q.v.); 108, 115, 123, 140

Roll collar (m), 19th century: a
shallower version of a *shawl collar*
(q.v.), often, early in the century,
with M-notch lapels; 134, 137, 140

Shawl collar (m & f), 19th century: a
collar continuous with the lapels; (m)
131, 137, 145, 150, 157; (f) 182, 191

Wing collar (m), 19th and 20th
centuries: a standing collar with the
two front points turned down;
sometimes called a butterfly collar;
160, 163, 167, 176, 181

Commode (f), late 17th and early 18th
centuries: originally the wire frame
which held-up the female headdress
of the 1690s, but by the beginning of
the 18th century the headdress itself.
It was composed of a linen cap with
lace edging and layers of pleats raised
above the head and supported by a
wire frame; it also had two lappets
either pendant or pinned up; 91,
colour VII

Copotain: see *Hat*

Cornette: see *Bonnet/Cap* and *Tippet*

Cossacks: see *Trousers*

Courrèges, André (1923–   ), 194

Corset (f), 16th to 20th centuries: until the
18th century a boned, sleeveless
bodice which in England usually
laced behind; the front was either
plain or embroidered, the more
decorative versions acting as a
stomacher (q.v.). From the 18th
century a tight-fitting, rigid
undergarment which moulded the
bosom and compressed the waist into

the fashionable silhouette (*cf Stays*);
129

Cote (m & f), 14th and 15th centuries:
French term, sometimes used in
English, for a garment worn over the
chemise (q.v.), and under the *robe*
(q.v.) of both sexes. Women's cotes
laced up the centre front of the
bodice, and had short sleeves to
which false sleeves of more elaborate
materials could be attached. The cote
lost its importance in the male
wardrobe by the end of the 14th
century, but reappeared looking like a
tighter, inner robe in the last 20 or so
years of the 15th century; 29

Cote hardie (f), 14th and 15th centuries:
a garment for women which had the
social acceptability of the robe, but
the tight bodice of the cote, but
without the latter's visible front
lacing; it had full-length sleeves of
matching material; 10

Court shoe, see *Shoe*

Couture/Haute couture/Couturier 19th and
20th centuries: *couture* is taken from
the French for 'sewing', but its usual
meaning is 'dressmaking'. *Haute
couture* is the term applied to the
design and making of fashionable
clothing. *Couturier/ière* is the term for
the dressmaker or dress designer

Crape (*Crêpe*) 18th to 20th centuries: thin
silk gauze, or a silk and worsted
fabric used for mourning

Crinoline (f), 19th and 20th centuries: a
petticoat (q.v.), distended by hoops of
cane, steel or whalebone; introduced
in 1856; 147, 148, 150

Cravat (m), 17th to 20th centuries: a long
strip of fabric wound around the
neck, tying in front with a knot or
bow; 83, 92, 127, 144, colour VI

Steinkirk (m), 17th and 18th centuries:
a method of wearing the cravat,
loosely twisted in front with one or
both ends pushed through a
buttonhole. Supposedly derived from
the battle of Steinkirk (1692) when
French soldiers, taken by surprise,
had to dress quickly; 97

Cuff (m & f), 17th to 20th centuries: the
turned-back bottom edge of a sleeve

Boot cuff (m), 18th century; a deep,
round cuff reaching to the elbow, 99,
102

à la marinière (m), 18th century: a
small, round cuff with a vertical flap,
often scalloped and edged with three
or four buttons; 112

Cutwork: see *Lace*

D

Dagging/jaggs (m & f), 14th and 15th
centuries: serrated edges of clothing,
at the hem and cuffs of men's clothes
but usually only the cuffs of women's;
created by the use of specially shaped
metal cutters. Introduced in the early
1340s, at its most lavish c. 1380–1420,
but continued in modified form until
c. 1440; 6, 17, 18

Damask 14th to 20th centuries: a heavy
woven cloth with a reversible pattern
produced by alternating plain and
satin weaves using silk or linen or
wool or mixtures of these yarns; 103,
130

Debenham & Freebody: 185

Décolletage (f), 14th to 20th centuries: the
low neckline of women's dress

Denim 19th and 20th centuries: a twilled
cotton fabric from Nîmes in France
(*serge de Nîmes*), used for working
clothes such as *Jeans* (q.v.)

Dinner suit: see *Suit*

Dinner jacket: see *Jacket*

Dior, Christian (1905–1957): 190

Directoire: the period of government in
France from 1795 to 1799. The term
was used to describe the revival, in
the first decade of the 20th century,
of the style of dress of that era; 169

Doeuillet (1900–1928): colour XV

Doublet (m), 14th to 17th centuries: a term
used from the late 14th century for a
hip-length or waist-length garment
with padded body and worn,
primarily by men, over the shirt. The
hose (q.v.) were laced to it, sometimes
under the 'skirt', and armour could
be anchored to it by suitably placed
laces. It continued as a fashionable
garment for men until c. 1670 and
was laced or buttoned at the front;
21, 44, 64, 77

Dormeuse: see *Bonnet/Cap*

Drawers (m & f), 14th to 20th centuries:
the equivalent of modern underpants;
first worn by English women in the
early 19th century; usually knee-
length or ankle-length; 129

Dress coat: see *Coat*

Dress suit: see *Suit*

E

Echelles (f), 17th and 18th centuries: a
decorative arrangement of ribbon
bows placed in diminishing size down
the front of a *stomacher* (q.v.); 88, 107

English hood: see *Hood*

Epaulette (f), 19th and 20th centuries: an
ornamental shoulder-piece in the

form of a short cap or wing at the top of the sleeve; 152

Ermine 14th to 20th centuries: the winter coat of the ermine, a member of the weasel family, which turns completely white in winter except for the tip of its tail; each black spot on white fur is supposed to be an ermine's tail, but the effect was often obtained by using scraps of black lambskin. The use of ermine was limited to royalty, according to sumptuary legislation, but the aristocracy wore it, or imitations of it, in the medieval and early modern period. Its use diminished from the 17th century onwards, except for official and ceremonial dress; 12, 31, 59, 133

F

Falbala/furbelow (f), 17th and 18th centuries: a horizontal flounce of material or lace on the *petticoat* (*q.v.*); 88, 91, 92, 95, 102

Falling band: see *Band*

Falls (m) early 18th to mid-19th centuries: a form of closure for breeches, trousers and pantaloons, by means of a falling flap at the front which buttoned to the waist; 108, 140

Fan (f), 16th to 20th centuries: a fashionable female accessory, made from a variety of materials; 47, 62, 106, 156, colour V

Farthingale (f), 16th and 17th centuries: an understructure, formed from hoops of cane, wood, metal or whalebone, which increased in circumference from the waist to the ankle – a French farthingale was wheel-shaped; a Spanish farthingale was bell-shaped; 39, 60, 62

Figured fabric 19th and 20th centuries: a fabric woven with a pattern but without additional threads of a different yarn or colour; cf *Brocade* and *Damask*; 142

Fillet: see *Bandeau*

Fontange (f), late 17th century: a high, tiered headdress of wired lace or linen frills attached to a small linen cap worn at the back of the head; cf *Commode*; 88

Forepart (f), 16th century: a decorative, triangular front part of an otherwise plain underskirt; 38, 39, 42

Fourreau, corsage en (f), 18th century: a style of cutting the bodice in one with the skirt by means of a central panel at the back; used infrequently throughout the first half of the 18th

century, but most popular from the 1750s; 122

Fratini, Gina (1934–): 195

French cloak: see *Cloak*

French farthingale: see *Farthingale*

French hood: see *Hood*

Frock (f), 19th and 20th centuries: originally a term applied to the dress worn by children, it referred, in the 19th century, to a dress with bodice and skirt in one piece, usually fastened behind; in the 20th century it became synonymous with a woman's dress

Frock coat: see *Coat*

Frogging (m & f), 16th to 20th centuries: decorative rows of looped braid fastenings arranged down the front of a garment; 47, 131

Frontlet (f), 15th & 16th centuries: the front section of a headdress introduced at the end of the 15th century; usually a band of black velvet worn across the front of the head; 30, colour II

G

Gable: see *English hood*

Gaiters (m), 19th and 20th centuries: protective leggings fastened with buttons or straps and extending over the foot

Gaiter bottoms (m), 19th century: a term applied to trouser bottoms when the side seams curve forward to produce a flared front to accommodate the foot; 141

Garters (m & f), 14th to 20th centuries: ornamented bands of silk or ribbon that secured stockings; from the 19th century these were often elasticated; 12, 36, 49, 61

Gauging 19th and 20th centuries: a technique of gathering skirts, by which the fabric is finely pleated, together with its lining, and sewn to the bodice at alternate pleats

Gauze 15th to 20th centuries: a very thin, open-weave transparent silk or cotton material; 29, 54, 59, 60, 68, 107, 118, 122, 135

Gibb, Bill (1943–1988): 196

Gingham 18th to 20th centuries: originally Indian, this term was applied to cotton fabric made from dyed yarn; 124

Gloves (m & f), 14th to 20th centuries: covering for the hands and individual fingers and thumbs, made from a variety of materials, including leather, wool silk etc; cf *Mittens*; 36, 58, 62, 86, 94, 123, 141, 161, 167, 194

Gore 19th and 20th centuries; a triangular-shaped panel in a skirt, adding width at the hem without increasing fullness at the waist; 130, 162

Gorget (m), 16th to 18th centuries: steel collar to protect the throat, worn by the military and some civilians as a mark of distinction; 50, 72

Gown (m & f), 14th to 17th centuries: a garment worn by both sexes, and apparently introduced *c.* 1360. The term, although not the shape of the garment, was used thereafter to denote any formal outer, sleeved garment, regardless of length and shape. From the 16th century the term usually meant a formal, conservative, official garment; 12, 13, 15, 16, 19, 20, 21, 26, 30, 36, 53

Gown (m), 17th to 20th centuries: a loose garment worn before a person is formally dressed; synonymous with dressing gown, morning gown or nightgown; 81, 89, 130

Gown (f), 17th and 18th centuries: a loose garment, worn informally, which developed into the semi-formal fitted gown of the 1680s which was held at the waist with a sash or belt

Banyan (m), 18th century: a slightly fitted man's dressing gown, often double-breasted and usually calf-length; the name derives from the name for a Hindu trader in the province of Gujerat – it was, erroneously, thought that they wore this type of garment; 109

Brunswick (f), 18th century: a *sack* (*q.v.*), of varying length, with a buttoned-up false bodice front, and long, tight sleeves; 113

Greatcoat dress (f), 18th century: a fashionable style of the 1780s, worn as either a closed robe, buttoned to the hem, or more usually worn just closed to the waist, the overskirt falling away on either side to show the petticoat; sleeves were tight to the wrist; the caped collar and contrasting revers of the male coat were often adopted

Houppelande (m & f), 14th and 15th centuries: a term introduced in France at about the same time as 'goun'/'gown' in England, presumably to describe a similar garment. Its most characteristic form is that seen *c.* 1380–*c.* 1420, when it had very wide, hanging sleeves. The term gradually fell into disuse to be replaced by gown; 12, 18

Loose gown (f), 17th century: an overgarment falling in loose folds from the shoulders; 63, 81

Mantua (f), 17th and 18th centuries: an open robe worn with a petticoat and stomacher; the distinctive feature comprised the elaborate arrangement of the back drapery of the overskirt, which, in its final form, in the 1730s, consisted of a narrow train; 88, 91, 92, 93 101, 102

Nightgown (f), 16th to 18th centuries: a loose, lined or unlined informal open gown, or a loosely fitted closed robe; from the mid-18th century it was a more formal, fitted open gown worn with a contrasting petticoat

Polonaise (f), 18th and 19th centuries: an open gown consisting of a bodice with a draped overskirt ruched up into swags. This style was revived from the mid-1860s onwards; those of the late 1870s were so long as to be almost indistinguishable from a dress; 155, 156

Robe à l'anglaise (f), 18th century: a fitted gown worn throughout the 18th century in England. It had a variety of bodices including the stomacher front, the compère (buttoned front), a false waistcoat sewn to the lining of the inner sides of the bodice, and a plain closed front. In the 1770s it assumed a hybrid form, combining the fitted back of the mantua (q.v.) bodice with the back pleats of the sack (q.v.), but so reduced in size that they eventually became seams; the fourreau (q.v.) back was usual in the 1770s, but in the 1780s there was a complete division at the waist; 122

Sack (sacque) (f), late 17th and 18th centuries: originally an informal gown or negligée. In its early form it hung loose at the back and front, falling from neck to hem in a pyramid shape; in this form it continued to be popular in the first half of the 18th century for pregnant women. In the early years of the 18th century it had loose pleats unstitched at the front and the back and was worn either with the front seamed from just below the waist, or it was completely open, revealing the petticoat. In the 1730s the pleats became more structured, set in two double box-pleats, and the bodice became closer fitted to the body. In the 1750s the sack, worn as an open robe, had virtually replaced the mantua (q.v.) as formal dress. During the 1770s it

went out of fashion but was retained for certain court occasions; 103, 106, 111

Greatcoat dress: see Gown

Guards (m & f), 16th and early 17th centuries: bands of material used either as a decorative border or to cover a seam; made of a material and colour contrasting with the garment; 46

H

Hair – facial and styles

Dundreary (m), 19th century: long side whiskers extending to the collar; named after the fictional 'Lord Dundreary'; 149

Lovelock (m & f), late 16th and early 17th centuries: a long, curled lock of hair arranged to fall over one shoulder; 71

Mutton-chop (m), late 19th and 20th centuries: similar to the Dundreary whiskers, but more closely trimmed

Pickdevant (m), late 16th century: a short, pointed beard worn usually with a brushed-up moustache; 57, 58

Queue (m), 18th century: a lock of hair tied or knotted at the nape of the neck; 102

Quiff (m), 20th century: a lock of hair either pressed down over the forehead or brushed-up from the brow; 192

Tête de mouton (f), 18th century: a tightly curled hairstyle resembling a sheep's fleece; 105

Titus, à la (m & f), late 18th and early 19th centuries: a term applied to hair worn short and tousled in the manner of the Roman emperor of that name; 126, 127

Handbag (f) 18th to 20th centuries: during the 20th century handbags became an essential female accessory; they developed from small fabric drawstring 'Dorothy' bags into versions made from leather for day wear and rich silk and beaded materials for evening wear; 182, 187

Clutch: 178
Dorothy: 170
Evening: 180
Reticule 18th and 19th centuries: the word may derive from the Latin reticulum (net); small netted purses were sometimes carried by women in the 18th century. By the late 18th century they carried small fabric bags fastened with a drawstring; throughout the 19th century small bags of fabric and leather were used;

118, 132, 161

Hanger (m), 16th and 17th centuries; a belt worn diagonally across the body from which a sword was suspended; occasionally called a baldrick; 41, 50, 61, 72

Harrods: 170

Hat (m & f), 16th to 20th centuries: a term used for a head covering of a formal, structured variety with both crown and brim; hats were not much worn by women before the late 16th century, and were sometimes confusingly described as a bonnet (q.v.) or hood (q.v.)

Beaver (m & f), 16th to 18th centuries: a shorthand term used to describe a hat made from expensive beaver fur; 53, 57, 71, 73, 80, 86, 94, 97, 108, 112, 123

Bicorne (m & f), late 18th and 19th centuries: a modern term for a hat with a brim turned up at the front and back, the front blocked into a slight peak, often trimmed with a rosette or cockade; 117, 128

Boater (m & f), late 19th and 20th centuries: a stiff straw hat with a shallow crown and straight brim; 151, 164, 167

Bowler (m), mid-19th to 20th centuries: a felt hat with a stiffened domed crown and narrow curled brim; 150, 156, 170, 172, 176, 189

Chapeau bras (m), 18th to 20th centuries: a crescent-shaped opera hat which could be folded flat; 128

Cloche (f), 20th century: a bell-shaped hat with a deep crown and small brim, or without a brim; 175, 177, 179

Copotain (m), late 16th century: a hat with a high conical crown, also called a 'sugar-loaf' because of its shape; 58

Mousquetaire (f), 19th century; a low-crowned, wide-brimmed hat with a feather plume, inspired by those worn by 17th-century musketeers; 145

Panama (m), 20th century; a summer hat of fine, flexible straw similar in shape to a trilby (q.v.); 171

Picture (f), 19th and 20th centuries; low-crowned, wide-brimmed hat derived from those worn in 18th-century portraits; 163

Pork-pie (m & f), 19th and 20th centuries: a small, round hat with an upturned brim almost flush with the crown; 148

Round (m & f), late 18th century: a style which became fashionable in the

1770s, especially for riding, it had a round, flat-topped crown, was usually made of *beaver* (*q.v.*), and had a flat brim; 121, 123, colour X

Sailor (m & f), 19th and 20th centuries; a low-crowned, narrow brimmed straw hat, similar to a boater (*q.v.*); 156, 164

Top (m), late 18th to 20th centuries; a style of hat with a tall, blocked crown and stiffened, curled brim, varying in width and height according to period; 123, 132, 163, 168

Toque (f), 19th and 20th centuries: a small, round hat, usually raised above the head and with little or no brim; 156, 161, 188

Tricorne (m & f), 18th to 20th centuries: a modern term for a hat cocked into an equilateral triangle with the point worn at the front; 90, 94, 95, 112, 128

Trilby (m & f), late 19th and 20th centuries: a soft felt hat with a crease in the crown from back to front, and a curled brim; 184, 189, 193

Tyrolean (m & f), late 19th and 20th centuries: a small felt hat with a shallow brim and feather decoration, inspired by the headwear worn in the Austrian Tyrol; 155

Hobble skirt (f), early 20th century: a style of skirt which fitted tightly around the lower leg, restricting movement; front jacket illustration; colour XIV

Hood (m & f), 14th to 20th centuries: a soft, loose head-covering extending to and often covering the shoulders; 5

Calash (f), 18th and 19th centuries: a folding hood made of silk and built up over arches of cane; 117, 124

Caped hood (f), 18th century: a soft hood extending into a shoulder cape; 99

English hood (f), late 15th to mid-16th centuries: also known as a 'gable' or 'pediment headdress', this consisted of a stiffened, pointed arch which framed the face; it existed in various forms from the late 15th century until its disappearance; 33, 34, 35

French hood (f), 16th century: a small hood worn on the back of the head with a curved front border and horse-shoe-shaped curve on the top of the crown; 39

Scarf (f), 18th century: a length of fine material worn over the head and tied under the chin; 104

Hose (m), 14th to 17th centuries: the covering for a man's body from waist to feet. The term hose was usually applied to the upper portion, but did not denote stockings until the mid-17th century; 11, 28, 40

Trunkhose (m), 16th and early 17th centuries: short, substantially padded round hose, often worn with *canions* (*q.v.*); 55, 61, colour IV

Houppelande: see *Gown*

J

Jabot (m & f), 19th and 20th centuries: a frill or ruffle, usually of lace and worn at the neck and decorating the front of a shirt or blouse; 197

Jacket (m), 14th to 20th centuries: in the early periods a sleeved or sleeveless short body-garment, related in some way to the doublet and also to the jack – a cheap form of body armour with metal plates sewn into cloth. By the 16th and 17th centuries it was worn over the doublet. In the 18th century it was a working-class garment, but by the mid-19th century it was an acceptable part of a man's suit, replacing the coat for informal occasions.

Blazer (m), 19th and 20th centuries: a single- or double-breasted jacket, sometimes of striped cloth, associated with outdoor or sporting events

Dinner jacket (m), late 19th and 20th centuries; 181

Lounge jacket (m), 19th and 20th centuries: a short jacket, worn informally; when accompanied by matching waistcoat and trousers, it became a lounge suit; 149, 150, 151, 157, 162, 164, 167, 170, 171, 172, 176, 178

Monkey jacket (m), 19th century; 141

Norfolk jacket (m), 19th and 20th centuries: a loose fitting jacket with vertical pleats, belted at the waist; usually worn with knee-breeches in the country

Pea jacket (m), 19th century; 141

Reefer (m), 19th and 20th centuries: a double-breasted jacket with a low collar and small lapels; worn for sailing and yachting, and taken up in the 1880s popular informal wear

Sports jacket (m), 20th century: 198

Jacket (f), 16th to 20th centuries: an informal, fitted or unfitted alternative to the bodice, worn with a skirt and/or an overgown in the 16th and 17th centuries; 59, 63, 68

In the 18th and 19th centuries it was worn as an upper garment for outdoor wear and for sports, and later as part of the tailor-made costume of the late 19th century; 95, 117, 121, 161, 162, 164

Its use continued, as part of a suit, or worn with a skirt or trousers into the 20th century; 173, 177, 185, 186, 192, 194

Leather jacket (m & f), 20th century; 200

Spencer (f), late 18th and early 19th centuries: a short-waisted, long-sleeved jacket; 131

Jaeger: 184, 191

Jeans (m & f), 19th and 20th centuries: American working trousers of thick cotton, usually blue, worn from the mid-19th century onwards; in the mid-20th century adopted by young men, women and children as informal wear; 197, 199, 200

Jerkin (m), 16th and 17th centuries: a garment usually worn over the doublet, mostly sleeveless or with attached hanging sleeves; 36, 40, 45, 61

Jersey (m & f), 19th and 20th centuries: a knitted top, originally worn by sailors, but adopted for informal wear by both sexes from the 1880s onwards, *cf Sweater*; 164

Jersey weave 20th century: a plain-knit, ribbed fabric of wool, silk, cotton or synthetics, with a degree of elasticity, used principally for informal wear; 177

Jockey cap: see *Bonnet/Cap*

Jumper suit: see *Suit*

K

Kerchief/handkerchief/neckerchief (f), 16th to early 19th centuries: a large square of material folded and worn round the neck and shoulders; 46, 73, 74, 75, 103, 105, 111, 136, colour X

Kersey 14th to early 19th centuries: coarse, lightweight narrow wool cloth

Kirtle (f), 14th to 16th centuries: an inner garment, worn over the smock. The term replaced *tunic* (*q.v.*) at about the turn of the 14th and 15th centuries, although the function of the garment – to provide an early form of corseting – does not seem to have altered. From the late 15th century this term denoted both bodice and skirt, sewn or tied at the waist, but after *c.* 1545 it referred to the skirt only; 22, 34, 37, 46

Knickerbockers (m & f), late 19th and 20th centuries: a variety of breeches, but cut several inches fuller and wider than ordinary knee breeches. They were popular for country and sporting wear in the late 19th century. A longer, looser version was fashionable in the 1920s, known as plus-fours; 174

Knotting 17th and 18th centuries: a popular pastime from the late 17th century, this consisted of knotting silk or linen thread into a decorative braid for furnishings or small items of clothing such as tassels and fringes; 118

L

Lace 16th to 20th centuries: decorative bands with open-work designs, originally made by hand from linen thread, later made on machines from cotton and synthetic yarns

Blonde lace 18th and 19th centuries: lace of an almost transparent fineness made from undyed silk; 107, 111, 136

Bobbin lace 16th to 20th centuries: a fine, patterned lace made by interweaving threads attached to bobbins; 103, 143

Cutwork 16th and 17th centuries: lace of Italian origin, sometimes called *reticella*, made by cutting and over-stitching squared designs; 54, 63, 65

Needlepoint lace late 16th to 20th centuries: lace made with a needle and thread on a parchment pattern

Lappet (f), 16th to 19th centuries: during the 16th century this was the decorated border of an *English hood* (*q.v.*) that was extended so that it hung down on each side of the face; 32, 33

After *c.* 1525 these lappets were turned-up at ear level and pinned to the crown; 34, 35

From the late 17th century onwards, lappets were long linen or lace streamers appended to a cap or headdress and worn either pendant or pinned up; 88, 97, 100, 101, 118, 144

Lawn 15th to 20th centuries: a material woven from processed flax, this was the finest and most expensive variety of linen; it was used for a wide range of dress accessories; later the term was also applied to fine, lightweight cotton; 37, 63, colour IX

Leading strings (m & f), 16th to 19th centuries: long ties attached to the back of the dress of young children of both sexes, allowing them to walk without straying or falling; 93

Liberty: 157, 173

Liripipe (m), 14th and 15th centuries: long, narrow strips of cloth which hung from men's hoods

Loose gown: see *Gown*

Louis heel (m & f), 19th and 20th centuries: a high heel, waisted or curved inwards, inspired by 18th-century French footwear for both sexes, but fashionable in the late 19th and 20th centuries, primarily for women; 180

Love lock: see *Hair*

M

Mannequin (m & f), 19th and 20th centuries: a person, usually a woman (the term *fashion model* which is used mainly today, can refer to either sex) who displays clothes by wearing them; a clay figure or dummy used for the display of clothes in a shop or museum; 118, 193, 196, 199

Mantle (m & f) 14th to 19th centuries: a popular outer garment similar to a full ankle-length cloak until the end of the 14th century, fastened usually on the shoulder for men, and tied in front for women. After that time the mantle was mainly restricted to religious, official and ceremonial use; 20, 33, 34

The mantle re-emerged in the fashionable female wardrobe in the 19th century; it could take the form of a cloak (in varying lengths), or a loose-fitting wrap half-way between a coat and a cloak, with wide sleeves or armhole slits; sometimes it could have a hood and/or a collar; there were many individually named variations, some (though rarely) worn by men; 126

Pelerine (f), 18th and 19th centuries: small shoulder mantle sometimes with long front pendants; also known in the 19th century as a *fichu-pelerine*; 99, 119, 122, 136, 138, 156

Mantua: see *Gown*

Marie Stuart cap: see *Bonnets/Caps*

Marocain 20th century: a silk or wool fabric with a crêpe weave; 175

Mattli, Giuseppe Gustavo (1907–1982); 188

Milliner: a seller of fancy goods and fashionable accessories, the term deriving from the fact that many of these items came originally from Milan. By the late 17th century, some informal items of dress were sold alongside accessories such as fans, gloves etc, and trimmings such as lace. The term is not associated solely with headwear until the early 20th century

Miniver 14th and 15th centuries: the fur of the grey squirrel, arranged in shield-like rows, with the white belly forming the 'shield' within a narrow frame of grey; reserved for royalty and nobility partly because of the sheer numbers of skins required to line a garment

Mi-parti (also *motley*) 14th and 15th centuries: the practice of splitting a garment visually in two, having the right half in one colour or pattern, and the left half in another. This was particularly fashionable for entire wardrobes from *c.* 1320 to *c.* 1370, but remained in use for men's hose until at least the end of the century, and for liveries well into the next century; 12

Mittens (m & f), 16th to 20th centuries: type of hand-covering (of varying length) which (i) contained the fingers and thumb within one enclosed section of material; (ii) retained the fingers in one section with the thumb separately enclosed; or (iii) allowed the fingers to remain uncovered beyond the line of the knuckles; 119, 138, 200

Mob cap: see *Bonnets/Caps*

Modesty piece (f), 18th century: a small piece of lace or linen fixed to the top of the *stomacher* (*q.v.*) and covering the décolletage; 96

Morning coat: see *Coat*

Morning suit: see *Suit*

Mousquetaire hat: see *Hats*

Muff (m & f), 16th to 20th centuries: a flat or tubular, often padded, covering for the hands, often made of fur or a rich decorative material; 34, 133, 165

Mules: see *Shoes*

Muslin 18th to 20th centuries: very fine semi-transparent cotton, initially imported from India from *c.* 1670, then produced in England from the late 18th century; 93, 125, 135, 154

N

Nankeen 18th and 19th centuries: plain, closely woven cotton, usually buff in colour, for men's informal summer breeches, from the 1780s into the early 19th century; 125

New Look (f), 20th century: the style of dress introduced by Christian *Dior* (*q.v.*) in 1947; it had a fitted bodice and a long, full skirt; 188

Harvey Nichols: 186

H.J. Nicoll & Co: 181

Nightcap: see *Bonnets/Caps*

Nightgown: see *Gown*

Nylon: the first synthetic fibre of the 20th century, discovered through research by the American chemical firm du Pont. Commercial production in the USA began in 1939 and nylon stockings were available by 1940. It has been made in Britain since 1941 under the trade name Bri-nylon.

O

Overcoat: see *Coat*

P

Panama hat: see *Hats*

Panes (m & f), 16th and 17th centuries: strips of material, similar to broad ribbons, caught at each end into the main construction of a sleeve, doublet, bodice or hose; 48, 50, 61, 70

Panier (f), 18th and 19th centuries: the 18th-century French word for a hooped petticoat, from which the 19th-century revival term *pannier* arose to describe part of a skirt or overskirt which is looped up in a puff on the hips; 153

Pantaloons: see *Trousers*

Paquin, house of, founded 1891, closed 1956; 180

Parasol (f), 17th to 20th centuries: light ornamental umbrella to shield ladies from the sun; 145, 150, 151, 154, 163, 164, 167

Partlet (m & f), 16th and 17th centuries: decorative accessory that covered the upper part of the chest and fastened at the front; 33, 37, 51, colour III

Paste 18th to 20th centuries: glass cut and polished into gem-like forms, and in imitation of precious stones; 111

Patent leather late 18th to 20th centuries: a very glossy leather made from hide coated with layers of varnish or lacquer; 127, 181

Pattens: see *Shoes*

Peascod belly (m), 16th and 17th centuries: the distortion of the main body of a man's doublet by the addition of extra padding above the waistline; fashionable from *c*. 1575 to *c*. 1605; 48, 56

Pelerine: see *Mantle*

Pelisse see *Coat*

Persian vest: see *Coat*

Petticoat (f), 16th century to 20th century: an underskirt, sometimes called an *under-petticoat*. From the 19th century the term always means an undergarment

Petticoat breeches: see *Breeches*

Pickadil (m & f), 16th and early 17th centuries: a tabbed or scalloped border as a form of decoration on the sleeve or skirt of the bodice/doublet; 48, 49. See also *Tabs*

Also a standing frame with horizontal tabs attached to the back of the doublet and used to support a ruff or standing collar.

Pickdevant: see *Hair*

Picture hat: see *Hats*

Pièce (m & f), 15th century: French term for a small piece of cloth, often of velvet or satin, worn across the chest for warmth or modesty; not much required before *c*. 1450 when the robes of both sexes began to be worn rather open at the centre front chest; 29

Pinking

(i) a decorative pattern of small holes or slits on material and leather; 16th to mid 17th centuries; 45, 48, 61

(ii) raw edge of fabric cut in zig-zags or scallops; mid 17th to 20th centuries

Pinner: see *Bonnets/Caps*

Plastron (f), 19th century: a loose panel of fabric inserted down the centre front of a bodice, creating the effect of a waistcoat; 158

Plus fours (m), 20th century: a style of *knickerbockers* (*q.v.*) popular for golfing wear in the 1920s and 1930s: the term may derive from the extra four inches in length which gave the breeches the requisite fullness over the knee, but it is also said to come from a golfing expression; 174

Points (m & f), 15th to 17th centuries: metal-tagged ribbon or lace ties used to attach doublet to hose (70), or as a decorative conceit on bodice/doublet/coat; 83

Poiret, Paul (1879–1944); 169

Polonaise: see *Gown*

Pomatum (m & f), 18th and 19th centuries: scented ointment used to dress the hair

Pompon (f), 18th century: small ornament for the hair, of feathers, ribbons, flowers or jewels, which could be worn on its own or with a cap. Named after Madame de Pompadour, it was introduced in the 1740s, but was most popular in England in the 1750s and 1760s; 111, 113

Pork-pie hat: see *Hats*

Poulaines: see *Shoes*

Pourpoint (m), 14th and 15th centuries: French term for garment similar to doublet; the word may have a

military origin from the 'points' used to tie on pieces of armour; 23

Princess dress (also known as *en princesse*) (f), 19th century: a style of dress without a waist seam, perhaps called after Princess Alexandra; 155

Puffs (m & f) 16th to mid-17th centuries: decorative effect produced when material was drawn out through slashes and *panes* (*q.v.*); 35, 36, 38, 70

Pullover: see *Sweater*

Pumps: see *Shoes*

Punk (m & f), a street fashion of the mid-to-late 1970s characterized by the use of leather, chains, torn clothes, and brightly coloured, exotic hairstyles; 200

Q

Quant, Mary (1934–   ); 193

R

Raincoat: see *Coat*

Reticella: see *Lace*

Reticule: see *Handbag*

Robe (m & f), 14th and 15th centuries: from the Latin *roba*, a robe in the 14th century means a suit of clothes for men or women; 1

This definition is retained into the 15th century when a ceremonial outfit is concerned. In everyday terms, however, from *c*. 1430, *robe* comes to be the word used in France for the outer, sleeved garment of men and women; 23, 28, 29

Robe à l'anglaise: see *Gown*

Robe à la française: see *Gown*

Robings (f), 18th century: the edges of the bodice and open skirt, bordered with flat sewn-down revers generally double; until the middle of the century the robings reached to the waist, but later they were usually carried to the hem; 101, 104, 111

Round-eared cap: see *Bonnets/Caps*

Round hat: see *Hats*

Ruching 16th to 20th centuries: decorative manner of gathering, pleating and folding material to enhance its three-dimensional qualities, when used as a trimming

Ruff (m & f), 16th to mid-17th centuries: originally the frill that edged the standing collar of a shirt, by the 1570s it had become a separate article, consisting of radiating stiffened pleats of linen or lace attached to a neckband, and often constructed in multiple layers; 44, 47, 50, 55, 63, 64, 65

Ruffs could also be attached to the sleeves at the wrist; 45, 50

Neck ruffs occasionally appear in women's dress as part of the vogue for revivals of historical costume in the 18th and 19th centuries

Rump: see *Bustle*

Russet 14th to 16th centuries: coarse woollen homespun material largely used by country people

S

Sable luxurious brown fur of the sable marten worn by royalty, nobility and the wealthy, late medieval period onwards

Sack/sacque: see *Gown*

Scarf hood: see *Hood*

Shag 16th and 17th centuries: thick-piled, long-haired cloth with some rough fur in its composition, used to line garments

Shantung silk 20th century: a plain weave cloth of wild or slubbed silk (i.e. with surface irregularities); 190

Shift: see *Chemise*

Shirt (m) 14th to 20th centuries: a term used in England for a man's sleeved linen (usually cotton in the 20th century) undergarment; 3, 21, 40, 72, 97, 137, 166, 174, 197

In the 20th century the word is sometimes used for a tailored woman's *blouse* (*q.v.*).

T-shirt (m & f), 20th century: informal shirt, usually made of jersey-knit cotton, with a round neck and short sleeves; 199

Shoes (m)

Cracows 14th and 15th centuries: shoes with elongated toes, often, by the 1390s, tied to the knee with chains; in French, *poulaines*; 10, 12, 18, 23

Crêpe-soled shoes 20th century; 192

Startups 16th to early 17th centuries: loose, leather shoes worn by countrymen; 57

Shoes (m & f)

Brogues 20th century: strong leather shoes particularly associated with country- and sportswear; 174

Mules 16th to 20th centuries: a type of informal backless shoe or slipper; 59, 89, 109, 130

Pattens 14th to 19th centuries: wooden-soled shoes, with ridges under the heel and ball of the foot, to raise the wearer above the mud and filth of the streets, and to lessen the wear on leather soles

Pumps 18th to 20th centuries: light shoes, usually low-cut, with heels of varying heights; 116, 133, 137, 191

Sports/training shoes 20th century: shoes designed for sportswear with light leather or cloth uppers and rubber soles; worn as informal footwear from the late 1970s; 197, 199

Shoes (f)

Bar shoes 20th century: shoes fastened with one or more straps across the instep; 178, 179

Court shoes 20th century: heeled shoes with a low-cut front and usually no fastening; 174

Open-toed shoes 20th century; 185

Platform shoes 20th century: shoes with a very deep sole and corresponding heel; first appeared in the late 1930s and the 1940s; revived in the 1970s; 188, 196

Wedges 20th century: shoes with the sole and heel formed in one wedge; 186, 196

Skeleton suit (m), late 18th/early 19th centuries: a boy's suit consisting of a pair of ankle-length trousers buttoning onto a sleeved jacket, usually of matching material; 125

Slashing (m & f), late 15th to mid-17th centuries: slits of varying lengths cut in a garment and arranged in a pattern; 36, 48, 50, 65

Sleeves (m & f)

Hanging sleeve 15th to mid-17th centuries: a pendant sleeve, slit to allow the arms through (28, 36) or a false decorative sleeve matching the gown, jerkin, doublet or bodice; 53, 58, 60, 64, 65, 68

Raglan sleeve mid-19th and 20th centuries: a wide sleeve, not set into a round armhole but tapering to a point at the neckband; 184

Trunk sleeve late 16th and early 17th centuries: sleeve with a very wide top part, the swollen shape achieved by padding, and narrowing to a closed wrist; 60

Sleeves (f),

Bishop sleeve 19th century: long, full sleeve, gathered to the wrist; first mentioned 1855; 147, 149

Gigot sleeve (also known as 'leg-of-mutton') 19th century: sleeve with very full puffed shoulder but tapering to a narrow wrist; fashionable in the late 1820s and 1830s, and revived in the 1890s; 136, 138, 162, 164

Mancheron 19th century: a short flat oversleeve; 132

Pagoda sleeve late 17th to 19th centuries: a sleeve tight to the upper arm and flaring below the elbow; 144, 153

Smock (f), 14th to 19th centuries: the female equivalent to the male shirt; see also *Chemise*

Solitaire (m), 18th century: black ribbon from the bag of a wig, which was brought round from the back and tied in front over the stock; 112, 116

Spangles small thin pieces of metal used to decorate dress from the late 15th century to the late 19th century, when the term *sequins* began to be used; 43, 54, 59, 64, 69

Spanish cloak: see *Cloak*

Spanish farthingale: see *Farthingale*

Spats (m), 19th and 20th centuries: short gaiters reaching just above the ankle and buttoned on the outer side; 163, 176

Spencer: see *Jacket*

Sports jacket: see *Jacket*

Stays (m & f), 16th to 20th centuries: more usually a pair of stays. An undergarment (laced usually at the back) and reinforced with whalebone, cane or steel bands; it contained or re-shaped the human figure from chest to waist; from the late 18th century onwards the French term *corset* (*q.v.*) was often preferred; 129

Steinkirk: see *Cravats*

Stock (m), 18th and 19th centuries: a made-up, stiffened neckband fastening behind; 112, 134

Stockings (m & f), 16th to 20th centuries: tailored from cloth or knitted by hand or machine, they were made from a wide range of materials, silk being the most expensive; 49, 58, 61, 70, 98, 120, 129, 130, 174

Stomacher

(i) (m & f): a decorative section of material which covered the low cut V- or U-shaped doublet or gown opening, in the late 15th and early 16th centuries; 22

(ii) (f): an inverted triangle of stiffened and decorated material placed between the edges of an unclosed bodice, and held by ties, pins, or lacing; it was worn from the late 16th century to the late 18th century, and the style was occasionally imitated in the 19th century; 56, 60, 71, 88, 92, 109

Streamer: see *Tippet*

Suit (m & f), Term used, from the late 17th century onwards, for a complete set of clothing, although not necessarily in matching material:

Dinner suit (m), coat, waistcoat and

V

Vandyking late 18th and 19th century: zig-zag edgings supposedly imitating the pointed lace collars and cuffs of the 17th century as depicted in portraits by van Dyck; 132

Velvet A material woven originally from silk with a short dense pile; it could be either plain or figured, the latter being woven in two colours with two and sometimes three piles; from the late 18th century velvet was also made from cotton, and in the 20th century from nylon; 28, 38, 87, 147, 172

Venetians: see *Breeches*

W

Waistcoat (m), 17th to 20th centuries: a close-fitting jacket which in the 17th and 18th centuries had sleeves, but from the mid-18th century onwards was usually sleeveless; it could be single- or double-breasted, with or without a collar; 86, 91, 94, 112, 123, 137, 144, 153, 171, 181, 197

Waistcoat (f), late 16th to 20th centuries: informal sleeved or sleeveless jacket/bodice worn with a skirt; late 16th to 18th centuries. See also *Jacket*. A sleeved/sleeveless waistcoat cut on masculine lines was sometimes worn with the riding habit in the 17th and 18th centuries. In the 19th century, sleeveless waistcoats were sometimes worn with carriage dresses, and with tailor-made costumes. In the 1960s and 1970s a waistcoat was sometimes worn with a formal trouser suit; in the late 20th century an informal waistcoat (usually knitted) can be worn with a range of casual clothes

Warp-printing 18th and 19th centuries: textile designs with slightly blurred patterns produced by dyeing the warp threads before weaving; 144

Watch chain 19th and 20th centuries: a long chain attached at one end to the watch, worn in the waistcoat pocket and fixed through a chain hole in the front edge of the opposite side of the waistcoat; 144, 150, 171

Watered silk 18th to 20th centuries: a corded silk pressed between heated rollers so that the crushed cords reflect the light in wave-like patterns; 139

Wide-brimmed hat: see *Hats*

Wig (m & f), a shortened version of the word periwig which, in turn, derives from the French *perruque*. Hair (human or animal – very rarely it might be vegetable fibre) was woven on to a base and then styled in the current fashionable manner. Such wigs became fashionable in the mid-17th century (80, 84, 90) and remained so throughout much of the 18th century. Occasionally wigs were worn by women, most notably with riding habits in the late 17th and early 18th centuries; 95

Bob wig 18th century: a wig made undivided into sections, with all-over curl or frizz; the short bob came to just below the ears, the long bob to the shoulders. They were informal or undress wigs, worn mainly by the professional and middle classes from the 1720s onwards; 100, 102

Campaign wig early 18th century: deriving from Marlborough's military campaigns, it had two knotted locks hanging over each shoulder, and a long curl at the nape of the neck. The name was sometimes applied to any wig where part of the hair was knotted; 94, 96

Toupet 18th century: the often elevated front section of the wig, or the natural hair combed over a padded roll

Tie/tye wig 18th century: a wig with the hair drawn back and tied with a ribbon at the nape of the neck; 108

Wimple (f), 14th and 15th centuries: a term used here to describe the cloth which covered the chin of all women at the start of the 14th century, and then was gradually relegated to widows: see *Chin clout*; 2, 26

Wing (m & f), mid-16th to mid-17th centuries: band of stiffened material hiding the join between sleeve and armhole; it could be decorated in a variety of ways; 44, 49, 51, 61, 70

Z

Zip: an edge-to-edge slide fastener with interlocking teeth made of metal and later nylon; introduced in the early 20th century; 188